VOLUME 1

DISEASE CONTROL PRIORITIES • FOURTH EDITION

Country-Led Priority Setting for Health

Scan to see all titles in this series.

DISEASE CONTROL PRIORITIES • FOURTH EDITION

SERIES EDITORS

Ole F. Norheim
David A. Watkins
Kalipso Chalkidou
Victoria Y. Fan
Muhammad Ali Pate
Dean T. Jamison

VOLUMES IN THE SERIES

Country-Led Priority Setting for Health
Pandemic Prevention, Preparedness, and Response
Interventions Outside the Health Care System
Universal Health Coverage: Priorities and Value for Money

VOLUME EDITORS

Ala Alwan
Mizan Kiros Mirutse
Pakwanja Desiree Twea
Ole F. Norheim

Disease Control Priorities

This fourth edition of *Disease Control Priorities (DCP4)* builds on the first three editions, all published by the World Bank. Using experiences from collaboration and capacity strengthening in a select number of low- and middle-income countries, *DCP4* summarizes, produces, and helps translate economic evidence into better priority setting for universal health coverage, public health functions, pandemic preparedness and response, and intersectoral and international action for health. *DCP4* aims to be relevant for countries committed to increasing public financing of universal health coverage and other health-improving policies, recognizing the need to set priorities on their path toward achieving the Sustainable Development Goals and beyond. The project is a collaboration between the World Bank and the University of Bergen, Norway, to develop and co-publish *DCP4* in four volumes with broad inputs from individuals and institutions around the world. These plans will likely evolve in the course of the work.

More people live longer and have better lives today compared to any other time in history. The world's population is aging at dramatic speed. Improved living standards and new technologies are driving this change. However, we live in times of increased risks. No country can afford all technologies that are effective at improving health and well-being—and progress is unequal. The COVID-19 (coronavirus) pandemic has emphasized the vulnerability of countries when a threatening new infection affects life, the health system, work, and the economy. Climate change is another major challenge. Those already worse off are especially affected, both by direct and indirect effects on the health system, the economy, and the environment. During times of crisis, health care providers and policy makers must decide whom to prioritize and which programs to protect, expand, contract, or terminate.

These challenges are not unique to pandemics and climate change. Resource allocation decisions under scarcity are always being made, creating winners and losers when compared to the status quo. Such decisions may exacerbate or ameliorate existing inequities, which are often substantial. These risks are not the only reminders of the importance and urgency of priority setting in global health;

in many low-income countries, the unfinished agenda with respect to infections and maternal and child mortality competes with increasing needs to prevent and treat chronic conditions such as cardiovascular diseases, cancer, and mental health. How should countries prioritize among infectious diseases, maternal and child health programs, and prevention of noncommunicable diseases? How should a health ministry define essential health benefit packages to be financed under universal health coverage reforms? Priority setting is key, and we now have the experience and the tools needed to improve and implement decision-making support for more efficient and fair resource allocation on the path toward better health and well-being for all.

Disease Control Priorities provides a periodic review of the most up-to-date evidence on cost-effective and equitable interventions to address the burden of disease in low-resource settings. *DCP3* included nine volumes laying out a total of 21 essential intervention packages that contained 218 unique health sector interventions and 71 intersectoral policies. Each essential package addressed the concerns of a major professional community and contained a mix of intersectoral policies and health sector interventions. Since then, several countries have used this evidence and translated it into revised health system priorities. In many countries, experts from the World Health Organization and the World Bank have been substantially involved. Key results have been published in a series of high-impact journal articles. *DCP3* relied primarily on cost-effectiveness analysis to evaluate interventions, using benefit-cost analysis in some cases to address the overall impacts on social welfare. It also introduced a new and extended cost-effectiveness analysis method to account for the equity and financial protection impacts of extending coverage of proven effective interventions. *DCP4* builds on these methods but differs substantially from its predecessors by adopting a country-led approach to priority setting.

Ole F. Norheim
David A. Watkins
Kalipso Chalkidou
Victoria Y. Fan
Mohammed Ali Pate
Dean T. Jamison

VOLUME **1**

DISEASE CONTROL PRIORITIES • FOURTH EDITION

Country-Led Priority Setting for Health

Editors

Ala Alwan

Mizan Kiros Mirutse

Pakwanja Desiree Twea

Ole F. Norheim

WORLD BANK GROUP

Contents

Foreword by Justice Nonvignon

Growing up in a rural area near Accra, I often heard stories of neighbors dying of malaria, leading me to believe that there was little we could do to lessen the impact of poverty-related diseases like malaria, except for praying. During that period, many families strived to secure basic health services, which were not readily accessible, so that their children could thrive, live longer, and be happy. They did everything to save their children, often sacrificing their meager household resources and other basic needs. Even at such a young age, I understood that resources were limited or not available in the quantities we would expect. The daily reminder came when we would make many demands of our parents, and they would often remind us that they did not have the resources to meet all our demands, despite their best efforts to address our most pressing needs. They tried to inform us and, if possible, convince us of the challenges.

Just as children rely on their parents to allocate limited resources among their limitless wants and needs, the public expects decision-makers to distribute resources in an equitable, fair, and transparent manner. But, in practice, how do decision-makers—at national and subnational levels—decide for which needs to channel the limited resources first, and how, at any given time? Most of the time, the decision is based on individuals' or small groups' opinions and recommendations and happens implicitly for various understandable reasons, such as a large disparity between needs and available resources; a fear of accountability; limited system capacity; and a lack of contextualized framework, evidence, and tools to guide priority-setting decisions.

Low- and middle-income countries face ever-increasing health needs without much increment in the pot of funding. For instance, the growing burden of noncommunicable diseases further strains the already stretched health system. The priority-setting challenges also affect existing prioritized programs. For example, the growing number of vaccines available to countries (with malaria and HPV vaccines lately joining the introduction train in many African countries) raises the hope of delivering better health to the population, but it also means decision-makers face the dilemma of deciding where to cut off to introduce these newer and more expensive vaccines. Such vaccine introductions have a high risk of crowding out other equally important health services or investments. These considerations are a day-to-day dilemma for decision-makers, especially in low- and middle-income country settings.

There is growing interest and effort in many countries to introduce and strengthen priority-setting systems to systematically address such dilemmas and improve efficiency, fairness, and transparency. One of the cross-cutting challenges reported by the majority of African Union Member States is capacity issues, such as a lack of contextualized frameworks, data and evidence, analytic tools, and trained human resources—and many countries frequently request technical support.

Recognizing this issue as a major challenge to the scale-up of priority setting in Africa, the Africa Centres for Disease Control and Prevention began an effort in 2022 to develop a harmonized continental framework for evidence-informed priority setting, as well as options to support African Union Member States in its implementation. In addition, a guidance document on how to contextualize priority setting for public health emergency preparedness and response was developed. These two efforts led to interactions with experts and policy makers from ministries of health and finance and quasi-health sectors in 44 of 55 countries over a period of 18 months. The interactions (in the form of interviews, in-person workshops, and consultative sessions) led to the development, validation, and launch of a continental framework for priority setting for Africa, as well as two guidance documents on institutionalizing evidence-informed priority setting more broadly and in the context of epidemic preparedness and responses. Thus, Africa has taken steps to develop contextually relevant evidence-informed priority setting, which will guide implementation across countries, and harmonize partner support for countries. Such implementation, guided by country experiences in the region, is crucial to ensuring that priority setting does not, indeed, become only an academic exercise.

The development of the continental framework has benefited from earlier work by the International Decision Support Initiative, the Disease Control Priorities Project, the World Health Organization's WHO-CHOICE, and others. This volume, *Country-Led Priority Setting for Health*—which covers the overall lessons in defining and implementing universal health coverage benefits packages and country-specific lessons synthesized from the experiences of many countries—could greatly contribute to facilitating learning across countries. Such experiences remind us that a one-size-fits-all approach to priority setting does not solve problems; it rather compounds them. Although it is helpful to use lessons from one context for another, it is more important to not simply pluck and plant but to ensure that country context plays a key role in designing or redesigning solutions.

Whether it relates to developing or revising health benefits packages or informing introduction or scaling-up decisions, priority setting should focus not only on the decision-making process but also on the postdecision implementation period and eventually the health outcomes affected by the decision. Thus, countries should ensure that their prioritized essential lists of health services can be implemented and should commit to addressing the health system constraints and regularly monitor progress and adjust along the way.

In the current discourse of global health, it is common to limit the role of priority setting to country decision-making. However, priority setting is essential also for regional and global decision-making, including decision-making by development partners within and across countries. Priority setting should not be limited to government decision-making alone. For example, in global health financing, how do we apply the concept of priority setting to determine what, when, and how global health institutions (such as the Global Fund to Fight AIDS, Tuberculosis and Malaria; Gavi, The Vaccine Alliance; and the Pandemic Fund) decide on allocating scarce resources to critical health interventions? Are these decisions informed by a systematic, transparent priority-setting process? Assessing the processes for priority setting is critical, as is assessing the impact of priority setting on health outcomes.

The collaborations and learning with researchers and policy makers among countries demonstrated by the various chapters presented in this volume are commendable, and I believe this will enhance the relevance and impact of the lessons learned.

Justice Nonvignon
Foundation Head
Division of Health Economics and Financing
Africa Centres for Disease Control and Prevention
African Union Commission
Addis Ababa, Ethiopia

Foreword by Juan Pablo Uribe

The world is facing an era marked by complex and overlapping challenges. At the country level, health systems face new threats—shrinking fiscal space for health, changes in disease burdens, and climate change and fragility and demographic shifts—that significantly impact access to quality, affordable health services for all. However, such complexities also bring unique opportunities to rethink, innovate, and chart a course that leads us closer to achieving universal health coverage (UHC). This pursuit, grounded not in naive optimism but in an unwavering commitment to evidence and pragmatism, is what shapes the spirit of the fourth edition of the *Disease Control Priorities Project (DCP4)*.

The journey that began over three decades ago with the 1993 World Bank report *Investing in Health*—a pivotal work that effectively became the first edition of *DCP*—laid the groundwork for using economic evaluation to inform health priority setting and the creation of cost-effective health benefits packages. This first edition provided the impetus for reimagining health investments as a vehicle for economic growth and equity, particularly in low- and middle-income countries. Since then, subsequent editions of *DCP* have progressively expanded both the scope and depth of evidence, widening our understanding of prioritizing diseases, interventions, and health system strategies.

As we launch Volume 1 of *DCP4*, which is dedicated to country- and economy-led priority setting, we recognize the profound advancements that have emerged over the past 30 years. *DCP4* is uniquely positioned to serve as a critical reference for implementing country- and economy-driven, locally tailored strategies to improve health outcomes. The emphasis in this volume uniquely lies in real-world case studies where countries have successfully adopted priority-setting practices.

The fourth edition is timely, as it responds to growing questions about the so-called "know-do gap." There is a recognized need for faster dissemination of knowledge and more streamlined paths to implementation. By focusing on concrete country and economy experiences, this volume highlights actionable strategies for integrating priority setting into national health agendas. This is in line with the World Bank country-led model and its approach to knowledge, along with the strong focus on country leadership and ownership of the Global Financing Facility for Women, Children and Adolescents (GFF).

The work presented in *DCP4* also underscores the value of a systemwide approach. As countries and economies seek to achieve UHC, they are increasingly learning from the successes and limitations of single-disease, vertical programs that were initially funded through off-budget grant financing. The integration of these vertical programs into broader primary health care systems offers lessons in building sustainable systems that deliver essential high-quality services that are accessible to all. These efforts, when aligned with deliberate design of health benefit packages, remain a promising pathway to UHC.

In sum: this volume is more than an academic compendium. It is a guide for policy makers, health professionals, and advocates dedicated to creating sustainable and impactful change. With strong political and technical leadership at the country level, and by leveraging critical knowledge, we can work together to create a world where every health need is met.

Juan Pablo Uribe
Global Director for Health, Nutrition and Population
World Bank
Washington, DC

Foreword by Dr. Bruce Aylward

Fundamental to the Sustainable Development Goal agenda is the achievement of universal health coverage (UHC), part of Sustainable Development Goal 3, by 2030. That goal requires ensuring that all people, everywhere, can receive quality health services, when and where needed, without incurring financial hardship. Since 2000, many low-income countries and lower-middle-income countries have made substantial improvements in their coverage of essential services, although out-of-pocket expenditure has risen at the same time (WHO and World Bank 2023).

With just over five years remaining to 2030, the world remains off track to achieve UHC. The proportion of the global population not covered by essential health services has stagnated, and impoverishment due to ill health is increasing (WHO and World Bank 2023). Ensuring adequate health financing is critical to reverse this trend and to protect populations from high levels of out-of-pocket expenditure and from having to make the difficult choice between poverty and health. Unfortunately, providing an essential package of high-quality health services remains unaffordable for many countries within current levels of health expenditure (Hailu et al. 2021; Stenberg et al. 2019). Globally, the challenges of increasing health needs, together with new technological development and aging populations, are placing considerable financial pressure on the health sector.

Financing UHC is increasingly challenging. Many countries are grappling with a lack of access to concessional financing to invest in health service expansion, managing aid volatility, and navigating competing needs to adapt to the changing climate and prepare for future pandemics, while maintaining essential health services. Ensuring that any financing available is spent well is a critical health policy challenge globally. Against this backdrop, there are early signs of reductions in public spending on health: since 2021, health spending has reduced in several countries where data are available (WHO 2023).

Disease Control Priorities (DCP) has a long track record as a global public good informing decision-makers as they define essential packages of health services. This fourth edition of DCP *(DCP4)* includes a welcome and timely shift to supporting country-level processes using DCP and other evidence, and the implementation of packages. *DCP4*'s Volume 1 presents an impressive compendium of country-led actions over recent years to ensure health sector resources are spent well. This is no easy task—it requires locally relevant evidence on what works, an understanding of value for money, and institutionalizing structures for stakeholders and social participation. At the World Health Organization, we are pleased to have contributed to this effort, working with countries, organizing our clinical guidance to align with priority setting, producing global evidence on costs and cost-effectiveness, and providing guidance on effective ways to institutionalize priority setting.

DCP4 demonstrates that, even in the most resource-constrained settings, countries have been able to successfully define their pathway to UHC. Achieving UHC will require implementation of these priorities—as well as links with health financing and delivery systems—to ensure impact on the ground. We look forward to our continued partnership with DCP, working together to accelerate progress toward UHC.

Dr. Bruce Aylward
Assistant Director-General
Universal Health Coverage, Life Course
World Health Organization
Geneva, Switzerland

REFERENCES

Hailu, A., G. T. Eregata, K. Stenberg, and O. F. Norheim. 2021. "Is Universal Health Coverage Affordable? Estimated Costs and Fiscal Space Analysis for the Ethiopian Essential Health Services Package." *Health Systems & Reform* 7 (1): e1870061. https://doi.org/10.1080/23288604.2020.1870061.

Stenberg, K., O. Hanssen, M. Bertram, C. Brindley, A. Meshreky, S. Barkley, and T. Tan-Torres Edejer. 2019. "Guide Posts for Investment in Primary Health Care and Projected Resource Needs in 67 Low-Income and Middle-Income Countries: A Modelling Study." *The Lancet Global Health* 7 (11): e1500–10. https://doi.org/10.1016/S2214-109X(19)30416-4.

WHO (World Health Organization). 2023. *Global Spending on Health: Coping with the Pandemic.* Geneva: WHO. https://www.who.int/publications/i/item/9789240086746.

WHO (World Health Organization) and World Bank. 2023. *Tracking Universal Health Coverage: 2023 Global Monitoring Report.* Geneva: WHO and Washington, DC: World Bank. https://www.who.int/publications/i/item/9789240080379.

Main Messages from Volume 1

This volume presents and critically discusses how selected low- and middle-income countries have translated available evidence into priority setting and the processes they have followed in designing and implementing essential health service packages within the framework of universal health coverage (UHC). Many countries are implementing reforms to move them closer to UHC, with an essential package of health services (EPHS) serving as one of the key policy tools for achieving this goal. EPHSs define which services are covered in the context of limited resources, the proportion of health care costs financed through various schemes, and who is eligible to receive these services. Drawing cross-cutting lessons from the country experiences detailed in this volume and from an in-depth evaluation of selected programmatic areas (modules), such as school health and nutrition, essential surgery, and essential noncommunicable diseases, we highlight 12 main conclusions.

1. Substantial improvement has been observed in laying foundational work for EPHS design.

Significant improvement has been observed compared to earlier efforts in terms of laying the foundational work for evidence-informed priority setting, such as stakeholder engagement; evidence synthesis; EPHS design processes and institutional capacity building, particularly in evidence generation and synthesis; economic analysis; and decision-making.

However, experience in various countries has also identified significant weaknesses in the design and implementation of UHC packages, including issues related to feasibility, affordability, alignment with service delivery, financing, and health system readiness. These weaknesses can impede meaningful progress.

2. High-level leadership is essential for ensuring the success of an EPHS revision and its implementation.

A fundamental lesson learned is that the design and revision of an EPHS must be led and owned by the respective country's high-level leadership. Packages developed without sufficient involvement from national authorities are less likely to lead to successful implementation. Achieving success requires sustained high-level political commitment, active involvement of key stakeholders, health system preparedness, affordability, secured funding, and strong leadership for implementation. Government leadership is therefore essential, and early engagement of the planning and finance actors (and subnational authorities in decentralized systems) is crucial for success.

3. Open and inclusive decision-making processes are needed.

Our review of decision-making processes finds that countries generally follow a stepwise process for EPHS revision, though the implementation of specific steps varies. Fair process is promoted through stakeholder involvement but does not always include patient and community representatives. Key recommendations for countries include ensuring meaningful early key stakeholder engagement and enhancing transparency in the decision-making process, both of which are crucial for fairness. Additionally, countries should continue to take steps toward institutionalizing their EPHS revision process to support regular revision and sustainability.

4. Despite improved evidence and thorough policy processes, there is lack of implementation.

EPHSs have an impact only when they are implemented, yet a significant implementation gap remains in many countries. The failure to incorporate delivery considerations already at the prioritization and design stage can result in packages that undermine the goals countries have for service delivery. Furthermore, developing a health service package without considering health system constraints, such as well-trained human resources, infrastructure, and financing, undermines its potential value.

Critical translational work is needed to move from criteria-driven formulations to packages designed to support implementation. Package design elements that can strengthen implementation include the use of a common taxonomy of interventions, entries expressed as services rather than diseases, specification of local delivery platforms with assignment of services to platforms, and visualizing the link to burden of disease.

To ensure sustainability, countries need to develop affordable and feasible EPHSs, along with implementation plans that address health system constraints.

5. There is a weak link between priority setting, financing, and budgets.

The link between EPHS design and health financing mechanisms is weak. Our review of country experiences found that using EPHSs to directly leverage funds for health has rarely been effective. Furthermore, empirical evidence is limited regarding the role of EPHSs in mobilizing resources. This inability to mobilize resources may be due to a lack of strategic and solid high-level government leadership and poor alignment to financing mechanisms throughout the design process. Improved dialogue between health policy makers, public finance authorities, and higher-level political leaders, such as the president's or prime minister's office, can help link additional public spending to progress on UHC indicators.

EPHS development has been more successful in facilitating resource pooling across different financing schemes. It aids in assessing the performance of coverage schemes, which can lead to a harmonization of UHC interventions and identification of gaps between financing and service delivery. Developing and revising EPHSs is also crucial for strategic purchasing as countries build health technology assessment capacity.

High-level political leaders' and public finance authorities' commitment is critical to link EPHSs to raising new revenue. Furthermore, the design of EPHSs should be based on realistic projections of fiscal space for health and must be aligned with purchasing arrangements and public financing management systems.

6. Countries may benefit from using standardized methods and tools while localizing economic evidence.

For the analytical methods and tools used for UHC health benefit package design, we find that countries have used cost-effectiveness evidence as a core criterion for EPHS design. Yet most countries rely on published cost-effectiveness studies from other settings, despite the known limitations of this approach. Additionally, EPHS costing exercises have usually been done by international consultants rather than by local health economists, and the costing has not been linked to budgeting or financing arrangements, hindering its implementation. We identify two needs relating to EPHS analysis. First, the methods have varied widely across country projects, so analysts would benefit from international guidance, including on how to do an EPHS costing exercise, and how to extrapolate cost-effectiveness evidence from the literature when local data are lacking. Improvements in tools like the Integrated Health Tool and DCP FairChoices Analytics Tool could also help bridge these gaps. Second, development partners need to invest more in local analytical capacity, including both formal training programs to increase the number of local health economists and short courses for practitioners already working in government. Addressing these needs is essential to ensuring that the EPHS is locally owned and led.

7. The role of the private sector has been ignored.

The role of the private sector in delivering EPHSs has largely been ignored. The private sector—although a major provider of health services in many low- and middle-income countries—frequently operates on self-guided and market-oriented objectives and does not align with public sector goals, including UHC. In health systems where the private health sector provides a major part of essential health services, implementing EPHSs without involving the private sector is unrealistic. Despite growing guidance on developing UHC packages of health services, the role of the private sector in implementing these packages is generally missing. Addressing this gap is critical for the transition from package design to effective implementation. Governments need to address key barriers related to governance, regulation, accountability, and quality of services, guided by existing evidence and international experience.

8. A comprehensive monitoring and evaluation plan should be an integral part of EPHS design and implementation.

Monitoring and evaluation plans for EPHS implementation should be integrated into the UHC policy process from the very beginning. The EPHS monitoring and evaluation process, although focused narrowly on the implementation of EPHSs themselves, should align with the global monitoring framework for UHC and the Sustainable Development Goals indicators on service coverage and catastrophic expenditures. Evaluation activities should focus on changes in service coverage and financing of high-priority health services that can serve as "tracer measures."

9. Although a remarkable neglect of research on school-age children ages 5–14 years persists, a transformation has started.

Global interest in school-based health and nutrition interventions to promote cognitive skills and education outcomes has grown since the World Bank's *World Development Report 1993: Investing in Health* and throughout the *Disease Control Priorities* (*DCP*) series. Countries have increasingly recognized this area as an investment in human capital, with momentum accelerated by two major social shocks: the 2008 food, fuel, and financial crisis that initiated a global recession and the 2020 COVID-19 pandemic.

Health and education and well-being and learning all benefit if they work together. Substantial evidence now shows that investment in the whole 8,000-day period of development is a necessary contribution to the creation of human capital. Investment after the first 1,000 days (the next 7,000 days of life) offers returns not only to health and education but also to many other important sectors. Evidence increasingly supports the relevance and effectiveness of the school health package proposed in *DCP3* and encourages the inclusion of additional components. Coverage of programs worldwide has seen sustained increases, with even greater momentum spurred by the COVID-19 pandemic.

10. Access to essential surgery remains low in low- and middle-income countries.

Regarding essential surgery, DCP finds that country commitment to increasing availability of essential surgery remains low in developing countries despite the compelling investment case presented in earlier DCP publications and the Lancet Commission on Global Surgery. Experts involved in programs to advance surgical care in low- and middle-income countries point to the need to use language that policy makers can better understand and to partner with in-country organizations and champions in disseminating findings. Greater dissemination of the information in *DCP3 Essential Surgery* to several audiences (for example, policy makers, academics, and professional communities) also is needed.

11. Expanding noncommunicable disease interventions in low- and middle-income countries is a major challenge.

To respond to demographic and epidemiological changes, countries need to expand programs and services to include more noncommunicable disease (NCD) interventions. Previous editions of DCP have been influential in the international NCD discourse and in specific country projects. However, much more needs to be done on NCDs, and these DCP country collaborations have given us crucial insights into the gaps in the existing evidence. For example, DCP has been effective at identifying and promoting a handful of "best buys," but these have covered a relatively small number of specific NCD conditions, and countries also benefit from guidance on the "worst buys." Digital tools to support priority setting for NCDs have shown promise, and we can learn from these experiences as we continue to develop the DCP FairChoices Analytics Tool. Because many of the specific actions on NCDs take place outside the health sector, it will also be important to consider intersectoral interventions (for example, tobacco taxes) and to engage other stakeholders within government (for example, finance ministries). It is also important to engage nongovernment stakeholders, including civil society organizations, persons with lived experience, and local researchers. Fostering durable multisector coalitions can help ensure that political commitment to NCDs translates into financial commitment, implementation, and impact.

12. New tools and platforms are becoming available for sharing evidence.

The scientific and technical community is clearly moving more into the digital and online space with each passing year. Printed books and Excel spreadsheets have extremely limited use in the setting of rapid growth in research and evidence in low- and middle-income countries. The DCP4 team will use alternative ways to disseminate findings by producing continuously updated online content and open-access online analytical tools that can incorporate local data.

Abbreviations

AB-HWC	Ayushman Bharat Health and Wellness Center (India)
ACEi	angiotensin-converting enzyme inhibitors
ASHA	Accredited Social Health Activist (India)
BCEPS	Bergen Center for Ethics and Priority Setting
BHCPF	Basic Health Care Provision Fund (Nigeria)
BMPHS	Basic Minimum Package of Health Services (Nigeria)
BPHS	Basic Package of Health Services (Afghanistan)
BRICS	Brazil, Russian Federation, India, China, and South Africa
CABCT	Comisión Asesora de Beneficios, Costos y Tarifas (Colombia)
CAUSES	Catálogo Universal de Intervenciones Esenciales en Salud (Mexico)
CEA	cost-effectiveness analysis
CHE	current health expenditure
CHSI	Costing of Health Services in India
CI	confidence interval
CNSSS	National Social Security Council in Health (Colombia)
CPHC	comprehensive primary health care
CR	contributory regime
CRES	Health Regulation Commission, or Comisión de Regulación en Salud (Colombia)
CSO	civil society organization
DALY	disability-adjusted life year
DCP	*Disease Control Priorities*
DCP1	*Disease Control Priorities*, first edition
DCP2	*Disease Control Priorities*, second edition
DCP3	*Disease Control Priorities*, third edition
DCP4	*Disease Control Priorities*, fourth edition
DHIS2	District Health Information System 2
DRBCTAS	Dirección de Regulación de Beneficios, Costos y Tarifas del Aseguramiento en Salud (Colombia)
DTP	diphtheria, tetanus, pertussis

ECD	early childhood development
EHCP	essential health care package (Zanzibar)
EHP	Essential Health Package (Malawi)
EHP-TWG	EHP Technical Working Group (Malawi)
EMRO	Eastern Mediterranean Regional Office (of World Health Organization)
EPHS	essential package of health services
EUHC	essential universal health coverage
FAO	Food and Agriculture Organization of the United Nations
FMoH	Federal Ministry of Health (Nigeria, Sudan)
FPGC	Catastrophic Spending Protection Fund, or Fondo de Protección para Gastos Catastróficos (Colombia)
FPP	Family Physician Program (Islamic Republic of Iran)
FRP	financial risk protection
FSSHIP	Formal Sector Social Insurance Programme (Nigeria)
GBD	Global Burden of Disease
GCEA	generalized cost-effectiveness analysis
GDP	gross domestic product
GFF	Global Financing Facility for Women, Children and Adolescents
GGHE	general government health expenditure
GHPs	General Health Policies (Islamic Republic of Iran)
GP	general practitioner
GPE	Global Partnership for Education
HBP	Health Benefits Package (Nigeria)
HCI	Human Capital Index
HIPtool	Health Interventions Prioritization tool
HMIS	health management information system
HPV	human papillomavirus
HRC	Healthcare Reform Committee (Nigeria)
HSSP	Health Sector Strategic Plan (Malawi)
HTA	Health Technology Assessment (Islamic Republic of Iran)
HTP	Health Transformation Plan (Colombia, Islamic Republic of Iran)
IETS	Instituto de Evaluación Tecnológica en Salud (Colombia)
IMSS	Mexican Institute of Social Security, or Instituto Mexicano del Seguro Social
INSABI	National Institute of Health for Well-Being, or Instituto de Salud para el Bienestar (Colombia)
INVIMO	Instituto Nacional de Vigilancia de Medicamentos y Alimentos (Colombia)
IPEHS	Integrated Package of Essential Health Services (Afghanistan)
kg	kilogram
km	kilometer
LAYS	learning-adjusted years of schooling
LiST	Lives Saved Tool
LMICs	low- and middle-income countries
LNC	Lancet Nigeria Commission

M&E	monitoring and evaluation
MIPRES	Mi Prescripción
MoF	Ministry of Finance
MoH	Ministry of Health
MoHFW	Ministry of Health and Family Welfare (India)
MoHME	Ministry of Health and Medical Education (Islamic Republic of Iran)
MoHSP	Ministry of Health and Social Protection (Colombia)
MoNHSR&C	Ministry of National Health Services, Regulations & Coordination (Pakistan)
MoPH	Ministry of Public Health (Afghanistan)
NCD	noncommunicable disease
NCDI	noncommunicable diseases and injuries
NGO	nongovernmental organization
NHA	National Health Authority (India)
NHIA	National Health Insurance Authority (Nigeria)
NHIF	National Health Insurance Fund (Sudan)
NHIS	National Health Insurance Scheme (Nigeria)
NHM	National Health Mission (India)
NHP	National Health Policy (India)
NHV	Natonal Health Vision (Pakistan)
NITI Aayog	National Institution for Transforming India
NPHCDA	National Primary Healthcare Development Agency (Nigeria)
NSHDP	National Strategic Health Development Plan (Nigeria)
NSOAP	national surgical, obstetric, and anesthesia plans
NTD	neglected tropical disease
OHT	OneHealth Tool
OOP	out of pocket
ORS	oral rehydration solution
PAC	Program for Extension of Coverage, or Programa de Ampliación de Cobertura (Mexico)
PHC	primary health care
PHS	private health sector
PM-JAY	Pradhan Mantri Jan Arogya Yojana (India)
POS	Mandatory Health Plan, or Plan Obligatorio de Salud (Colombia)
POS-S	Mandatory Health Plan–Subsidized, or Plan Obligatorio de Salud–Subsidiado (Colombia)
PPP	public-private partnership
RAF	Resource Allocation Formula (Malawi)
RE-AIM	Reach, Effectiveness, Adoption, Implementation, and Maintenance (framework)
REDCap	Research Electronic Data Capture
RMNCAH	reproductive, maternal, newborn, child, and adolescent health
RMNCH	reproductive, maternal, newborn, and child health
SABER	Systems Approach for Better Education Result

SaLTS	Saving Lives through Safe Surgery
SCHI	Supreme Council of Health Insurance (Islamic Republic of Iran)
SCI	service coverage index
SDG	Sustainable Development Goal
SHA	state health agency (India)
SHI	social health insurance
SORMAS	Surveillance Outbreak Response Management and Analysis System
SP	Seguro Popular (Mexico)
SPDI	Service Planning, Delivery, and Implementation
SR	subsidized regime
SSA	Sub-Saharan Africa
STI	sexually transmitted infection
TaRL	Teaching at the Right Level
TB	tuberculosis
TD	tetanus-diphtheria
THE	total health expenditure
TWG	Technical Working Group
UHC	universal health coverage
UN	United Nations
UNESCO	United Nations Educational, Scientific and Cultural Organization
UPC	Unidad de Pago por Capitación (Colombia)
USAID	United States Agency for International Development
VIA	visual inspection with acetic acid
WFP	World Food Programme
WHO	World Health Organization
WHO-CHOICE	World Health Organization Choosing Interventions That Are Cost-Effective
ZEHCP	Zanzibar essential health care package

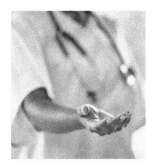

1

Translating Evidence to Practice: Defining and Implementing Universal Health Coverage Health Benefits Packages across Contexts

Ala Alwan and Ole F. Norheim

ABSTRACT

This chapter explores how various countries have translated available evidence into priority setting and the processes they have followed in designing and implementing essential health service packages within the framework of universal health coverage. It draws on cross-cutting lessons from the experiences detailed in this volume and from an in-depth evaluation of the *Disease Control Priorities*, third edition (DCP3) Country Translation Project. The chapter highlights both successes and failures and discusses the necessary actions for transitioning from package design to effective implementation.

INTRODUCTION

More than 75 years ago, the constitution of the World Health Organization (WHO) defined health as a "state of complete physical, mental, and social well-being" (WHO 1946). The constitution envisaged the highest attainable standard of health as a fundamental human right of every human being. Since then, multiple declarations and resolutions have been endorsed by the United Nations to translate that right into concrete actions and ensure health for all. More recently, in September 2015, all United Nations Member States adopted the 2030 Sustainable Development Goals (SDGs) as an integrated global agenda to chart a new era for development and poverty reduction. One of the key targets in the health goal, SDG Target 3.8, requires all countries to achieve universal health coverage (UHC) by 2030 (UN General Assembly 2015).

Translating Evidence to Practice: Defining and Implementing Universal Health Coverage Health Benefits Packages across Contexts

1

UHC means that all people and communities have access to the full range of quality health services they need, when and where they need them, without financial hardship (WHO 2023). It covers the full continuum of essential health services, from health promotion to prevention, treatment, rehabilitation, and palliative health care. The ultimate responsibility of a country's health system lies with the government, and key aspects of this responsibility are to provide at least the minimum essential health services, reduce financial risk, and protect against catastrophic expenditures from out-of-pocket (OOP) health spending (WHO 2000). The type of essential health services covered and the pathway to UHC vary across countries, shaped by the health needs of their populations, health system capacity, and available resources.

Although all countries endorsed the UHC target in 2015, effective action has generally been slow and fragmented (WHO and World Bank 2023). As of 2023, the global UHC service coverage index was 68 out of 100, with about 13.5 percent of households facing catastrophic health expenditure—that is, OOP expenditure greater than 10 percent of household budget (consumption or income). At current rates of progress for both service coverage and financial hardship, as of 2023, only an estimated 270 million of the 1 billion people targeted to benefit from UHC by WHO's Thirteenth General Programme of Work 2019–2023 (WHO 2019) were covered by essential health services without risk of catastrophic OOP health spending—a shortfall of about 730 million people.

Translating declared commitments into effective action requires political leadership at the highest level. In September 2019, four years after the endorsement of the SDGs and the UHC target, heads of state and government convened a high-level meeting at the United Nations General Assembly and committed to scaling up efforts to achieve SDG Target 3.8, adopting the most effective, evidence-based, high-impact, and quality-assured interventions and using public spending as the main driver (UN General Assembly 2019). Four years later, in September 2023, a second high-level meeting was convened to reinvigorate global action on UHC. However, the resulting political declaration does not appear to contain a different approach to achieve a breakthrough (UN 2023).

Strengthening health systems through strong primary health care is essential for attaining the UHC target. Countries need to redouble their efforts in improving access to, and delivery of, evidence-informed essential health services. Defining and implementing an affordable package of essential health services are at the center of health reforms leading to UHC. In this respect, most countries will need to reinforce their technical capacity in the areas of setting priorities and designing, financing, implementing, and monitoring UHC packages and related health service delivery reforms.

This volume presents country experience in translating available evidence into priority setting and defining and implementing essential packages of health services (EPHSs) or health benefits packages[1] in the context of UHC (part 1). The volume also extracts cross-cutting lessons learned from those country experiences and seeks to identify both successes and failures (part 2). Although the review of experiences covered in this volume focuses primarily on the countries involved in the country translation initiative set out in the previous edition, the volume includes other countries as case studies in priority setting: Colombia, India, the Islamic Republic of Iran, Malawi, Mexico, and Nigeria. The key challenges, lessons learned, and conclusions presented in this chapter are highly relevant to the situation in most low- and lower-middle-income countries.

DISEASE CONTROL PRIORITIES AND UHC

UHC consists of three fundamental dimensions: (1) expanding coverage to the whole population, (2) reducing financial risk, and (3) extending the range of essential services. Initiatives to accelerate progress on UHC need to address all three dimensions (figure 1.1).

Figure 1.1 The Three UHC Dimensions

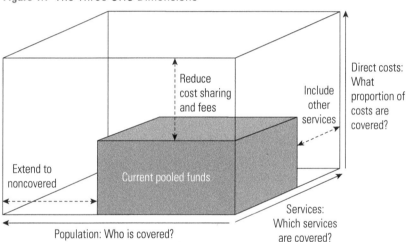

Source: Boerma et al. 2014.
Note: UHC = universal health coverage.

To scale up UHC, countries need to define priority services and incrementally expand the range of services offered to noncovered populations; at the same time, they need to reduce cost sharing and financial risk through resource mobilization, revenue generation, resource pooling, and strategic purchasing. Defining priority services will not work without action to improve access and clear links to health financing mechanisms. One strategic framework used by an increasing number of countries to identify the services to be prioritized for public subsidy consists of the evidence provided and the approach adopted by the third edition of *Disease Control Priorities* (*DCP3*) and its model service packages (Jamison, Gelband, et al. 2018; Watkins et al. 2018). *DCP3* provides a systematic review of the evidence, including cost-effectiveness, of a wide range of health services to support policy makers in decision-making on the highest-impact investments in the context of limited resources.

Based on the *DCP3* evidence, two generic model UHC packages of essential health services were launched in December 2017 as a starting point for evidence-informed country-specific analysis of priorities that countries can consider in designing their packages and charting the road map to UHC (Jamison, Alwan, et al. 2018). Health services were selected for inclusion in the model packages using the following criteria: evidence of impact, cost-effectiveness, financial risk protection, equity, and feasibility of implementation (Jamison, Gelband, et al. 2018). The essential UHC package includes 218 health sector interventions for lower-middle-income countries, with a subset of interventions distilled into a highest-priority package of 108 interventions recommended for low-income countries. In addition to its focus on investing in high-priority interventions, DCP3 also addresses the three UHC dimensions. A properly designed package of essential health interventions, funded publicly or through mandatory prepayment schemes, can reach all people, improve access to these services, and reduce financial risk.

For low- and lower-middle-income countries, the *DCP3* approach recommends implementing the package in a stepwise manner through a progressive universalism approach (Jamison et al. 2013). In that way, those countries can design the package to initially provide highly cost-effective health services, particularly for diseases that disproportionately affect the disadvantaged. As health resources and health system readiness grow, countries can expand the package to include a wider range of interventions and a higher level of coverage.

The *DCP3* and other model packages cannot be uniformly applied to any given context. They should be contextualized by countries' disease burden, health care needs, health system capacity, health policy objectives, and available financial resources. Many countries have recently used the *DCP3* evidence and approach to develop and implement their own EPHS (Alwan, Jallah, et al. 2023; Alwan, Siddiqi, et al. 2023; Alwan, Yamey, and Soucat 2023; Blanchet et al. 2020; Eregata et al. 2020; NHSRC, WHO, and the DCP3 Secretariat 2019; Somalia, Ministry of Health and Human Services 2021). Some of those countries have received technical support from the DCP3 Country Translation Project.[2] The project also reviewed the experience of six of those countries—Afghanistan, Ethiopia, Pakistan, Somalia, Sudan, and Zanzibar—in priority setting and designing their own packages to identify strengths and challenges and to update technical guidance for other countries (Alwan, Yamey, and Soucat 2023). Liberia was subsequently added to this group of countries (Alwan, Jallah, et al. 2023).

The review process involved a knowledge network of experts, seven groups of professionals addressing specific areas of EPHS development, and three review meetings organized in Geneva and London. The outcome of the review, which includes lessons learned, resulted in the publication of an editorial and seven papers in January–May 2023 (Alwan, Majdzadeh, et al. 2023; Alwan, Yamey, and Soucat 2023; Baltussen, Mwalim, et al. 2023; Danforth et al. 2023; Reynolds et al. 2023; Siddiqi et al. 2023; Soucat, Tandon, and Gonzales Pier 2023). Another series of papers covering the experience in Pakistan was subsequently published in 2023 and

2024 (Alwan et al. 2024; Alwan, Siddiqi, et al. 2023; Baltussen, Jansen, et al. 2023; Huda et al. 2023; Raza et al. 2024; Torres-Rueda et al. 2024). Some of those papers, which guided the writing of this chapter, have been revised and reprinted as chapters 2–6, 14–15, and 17–19 in this volume.

COUNTRY AND ECONOMY EXPERIENCES

The six countries and one economy participating in the review are classified by the World Bank as either lower-middle-income (Pakistan and Zanzibar, a semiautonomous region of Tanzania) or low-income (the remaining five). This section provides a brief outline of the findings and conclusions of the review. Several published articles present a more elaborate account of the different aspects of the package design process (Alwan et al. 2024; Alwan, Jallah, et al. 2023; Alwan, Yamey, and Soucat 2023), as do the official websites of the relevant ministries of health and several chapters in this volume.

General information on the health and health financing indicators in the six countries and one economy appears in table 1.1, which was adapted and updated from an earlier publication (Alwan, Majdzadeh, et al. 2023). The six countries and one economy have a low service coverage index, ranging from 27 to 45, and health care financing environments characterized by limited funding and major resource gaps and challenges. They have low per capita current health expenditure, ranging from US$23.4 to US$80.3, and government per capita spending as low as US$6.00. Apart from Zanzibar, the countries have very high OOP expenditure, reaching 75 percent of total health expenditure in Afghanistan. All have defined their own packages as a key milestone for the realization of UHC.

Table 1.1 Selected Health System Indicators in the Six Focus Countries and One Economy

	Afghanistan	Ethiopia	Liberia	Pakistan	Somalia	Sudan	Zanzibar
UHC Service Coverage Index (2021)	41	35	45	45[b]	27	44	43
Incidence of catastrophic health expenditure as % of households paying >10% (year)[a]	23.8 (2016)	2.1 (2015)	6.7 (2016)	5.4 (2015)	—	18.4 (2009)	4.3 (2018)
Current health expenditure per capita, US$ (2020)	80.3	28.7	56.7	38.2	—	23.4	39.3
Domestic general government health expenditure as % of gross domestic product (2020)	1.2	0.98	1.6	1.0	—	1.0	1.6
Government spending for health per capita, US$ (2020)	6.1	8.1	9.5	13.4	—	8.0	16.8
Domestic general government health expenditure as % of general government expenditure (2020)	4.2	6.8	4.5	5.12	2.0	9.6	9.4
Out-of-pocket expenditure as % of current health expenditure (2020)	74.8	33.0	46.9	55.4	—	53.0	23.1

Sources: Based on data from the World Health Organization's Global Health Observatory, https://www.who.int/data/gho/data/indicators (accessed July 19, 2024), and Global Health Expenditure Database, https://apps.who.int/nha/database (accessed July 19, 2024).

Note: UHC = universal health coverage; — = not available.

a. Data from WHO and World Bank 2021.

b. WHO Global Health Observatory data, which differ from the UHC Service Coverage Index of 49.9 reported in 2020 by Pakistan's Ministry of National Health Services Regulations and Coordination.

Table 1.2 provides an overview of the characteristics of the EPHS in each of the seven focus countries and economy. Five already had a package, and the current EPHS in those countries and economy represents a revised and expanded version. Only two countries, Ethiopia and Sudan, developed their packages for the first time. All used *DCP3* evidence to guide the prioritization of essential health services, but two countries, Ethiopia and Sudan, used additional sources of evidence, such as WHO's UHC Compendium.[3] The time required to design the packages, including evidence-informed prioritization and costing, ranged from eight months to three years. Prioritization covered five health service delivery platforms (community, health center, first-level hospital, tertiary care, and population-based interventions), but two countries, Liberia and Pakistan, decided to focus initially on a primary care package designed according to the structures of their own health systems. Liberia's core package covers community, clinic, health center, and first-level hospital platforms; Pakistan's final package covers community, health center, and first-level hospital platforms.

As mentioned earlier, all six countries and one economy faced a major challenge of limited fiscal space for public expenditure on health. They adopted different approaches to address that challenge, with decisions on package financing varying across them. Depending on their national vision, those endorsing a primary health care package (Liberia and Pakistan) decided to publicly finance the core or high-priority services, whereas the remaining four countries and one economy adopted financing mechanisms that included other prepayment schemes, including health insurance schemes, combined with user fees and donor funding.

Table 1.2 Main Characteristics of the EPHS in the Six Focus Countries and One Economy

	Afghanistan	Ethiopia	Liberia	Pakistan	Somalia	Sudan	Zanzibar
Year package completed	2021	2019	2022	2020 (generic EPHS), 2021 (6 provincial EPHSs)	2020	2022	2022
Time to construct the package	2 years	1–2 years	8 months	2 years	1–2 years	2 years	3 years
Main source of evidence adopted	*DCP3*	*DCP3* expanded with the UHC Compendium	*DCP3*	*DCP3*	*DCP3* and UHC Compendium	*DCP3*	*DCP3*
New package or revision of a previous package	Revision and expansion	Revision and expansion	Revision and updating	New package[a]	Revision and expansion	New package	Revision and updating
Delivery platforms targeted by the package	All delivery platforms[b]	All delivery platforms	Primary health care platforms[c]	District-level platforms[d]	All delivery platforms	All delivery platforms	All delivery platforms
First year cost of the core package in US$/person[e]	6.90	40.0	14.18; 6.93 cost to the government[f]	13.00 for the federal EPHS[g]	8.00	23.30	37.00

table continues next page

Table 1.2 Main Characteristics of the EPHS in the Six Focus Countries and One Economy (continued)

	Afghanistan	Ethiopia	Liberia	Pakistan	Somalia	Sudan	Zanzibar
Number of interventions in the final package	158	1,018	128 (78 core; 50 complementary)	88	412	824	314
Position of the country on the source of financing the final package	Prepayment schemes and donor funding	Public finance, donor funding, and user fees	Public finance and donor funding for core subpackage[h]	Public finance with gap filling from donor funding	Public finance, donor funding, and user fees	Public finance, prepayment, donor funding, and user fees	Public finance, public health insurance, prepayment, donor funding, and user fees

Source: Adapted from Alwan, Majdzadeh, et al. 2023.

Note: DCP3 = Disease Control Priorities, third edition; EPHS = essential package of health services; UHC = universal health coverage.

a. A rudimentary EPHS existed in two provinces focusing on a few programs.

b. DCP3 delivery platforms are community, health center, first-level hospital, referral and specialty hospitals, and population-based interventions.

c. Liberia's UHC package consists of a core subpackage, which includes interventions at the primary health care level, and a complementary subpackage, which includes health center and district, county, and tertiary hospital interventions.

d. The government prioritized and costed all five delivery platforms but decided to initially implement the three district-level platforms.

e. All packages will have increasing coverage along the timeline of Sustainable Development Goal Target 3.8; the projected costs will be considerably higher and require an increase in health allocation.

f. The total cost of the complementary package is US$13.82, with a cost to the government of US$5.35. The total cost of the core and complementary subpackages is US$28.00, with a total cost to the government of US$12.28.

g. The EPHS in each province/area has a different set of interventions and a different unit cost.

h. The complementary subpackage will be financed through the Liberian Ministry of Health's cost-sharing program.

As partly evident in tables 1.1 and 1.2, the review of the country and economy experience highlights critical challenges at different stages of EPHS development. Some of those challenges relate directly to the processes and methodologies used, including gaps in preparedness and readiness; other challenges are inherent in the capacity, resources, and performance of the health system. The challenges were compounded by the timing of the package design process in some of the countries and the economy, which coincided with the height of the COVID-19 (coronavirus) pandemic.

National efforts in prioritizing essential services to achieve UHC succeed only when the selected services become accessible to all population groups. Many countries designing EPHSs face major challenges in transitioning from design to implementation. Those challenges often stem from limited financing and health system gaps resulting from a disconnect between benefit package design (including the processes, methodologies, feasibility, and affordability) and health system reforms, which policy makers often struggle to address. Therefore, the assessment of country experiences in this chapter distinguishes clearly between two phases of successful priority setting: (1) evidence to policy and (2) policy to practice (refer to figure 1.2).

Figure 1.2 Two Phases of Designing and Implementing Essential Packages of Health Services

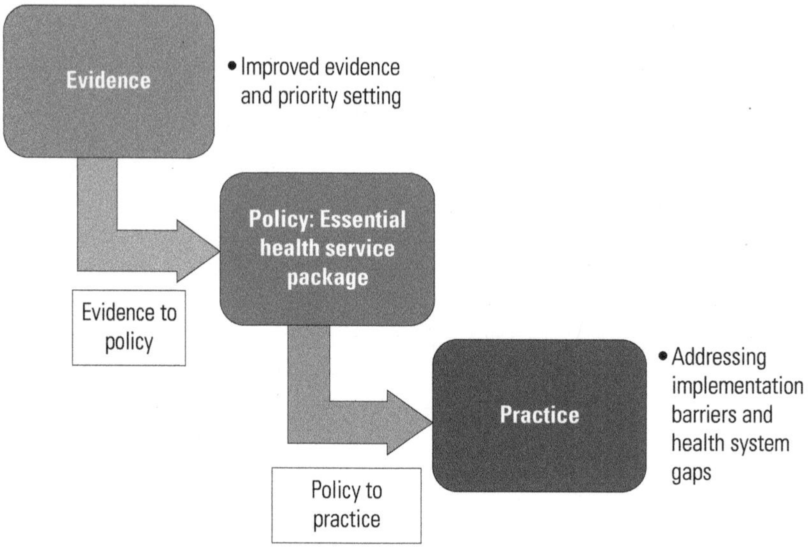

Source: Original figure created for this publication.

The next sections of the chapter focus on the lessons learned, with special emphasis on key messages for policy makers regarding (1) the phase of evidence to policy (that is, defining or revising an implementable EPHS) and (2) the phase of policy to practice (that is, actually implementing the EPHS). At a general level, although many of the country case studies document substantial improvements compared to earlier efforts in terms of evidence synthesis and the processes adopted to move from evidence to policy, most countries experience a large implementation gap in moving from policy to practice.

FROM EVIDENCE TO POLICY AND SUBSEQUENT ACTION

Investing in designing an evidence-informed EPHS has little value if the process does not lead to high-level government endorsement and subsequent action (Alwan, Majdzadeh, et al. 2023). Achieving a successful outcome requires meeting specific prerequisites, principles, and standards. The country translation review examined existing experience in the appropriate design of UHC packages and recommended a framework outlining the essential requirements for the transition from package design to implementation and improved access to services (Alwan, Majdzadeh, et al. 2023). Box 1.1 summarizes the key components of the framework.

A Framework for Action on Country and Economy Readiness and Prerequisites for the Successful Design and Implementation of a UHC EPHS

Evidence to policy

Defining and agreeing on the objectives of an essential package of health services (EPHS) design and securing political commitment

- Reaching consensus on the justification and objectives of designing an evidence-informed EPHS
- Securing sustained commitment and a clear government position on universal health coverage (UHC) in the national health vision and strategic plans, including serious engagement of the finance and planning sectors
- Securing commitment at the level of parliament
- Securing commitment at the subnational level, particularly in decentralized/federal systems.

Engaging key stakeholders

- Conducting stakeholder analysis of key national players
- Ensuring early, meaningful, open, and inclusive engagement of key stakeholders
- Building national consensus and conducting public dialogue on health service priority setting
- Mobilizing multilateral agencies and key development partners (where relevant).

Assessing health system readiness and performance and financing mechanisms

- Conducting an in-depth assessment of the health system, including governance structure, delivery arrangements, health workforce, and supplies, including medicines
- Assessing the fiscal space, health financing mechanisms, sustainability of health financing, and the level of public funds provided to finance the package
- Mapping the health services currently provided against prioritized health services covered by UHC model packages.

Developing and implementing a road map for the EPHS design process

- Developing a road map that comprehensively describes the entire design process
- Agreeing on principles of the design process: national ownership, transparency, data-driven decision-making, and focus on feasibility and affordability
- Building the capacity of the technical core team and key stakeholders
- Setting a governance structure for dialogue and deliberation
- Agreeing on decision criteria for prioritization of health services
- Defining the scope of the EPHS, including health delivery platforms targeted
- Prioritizing and costing interventions based on agreed decision criteria and linking costing to budgeting and financing mechanisms.

box continues next page

Policy to practice

Securing a successful transition to sustainable implementation

- Developing an implementation plan that addresses health system constraints
- Ensuring affordable and sustainable financing of the EPHS
- Aligning the packaging of EPHS with the service delivery
- Establishing a monitoring framework and revising the package accordingly
- Institutionalizing technical capacity and skills within the Ministry of Health and ensuring regular EPHS revision
- Addressing the risks of instability in fragile and politically unstable contexts, and instituting risk-mitigation measures with stakeholders.

Source: Adapted from Alwan, Majzadeh, et al. 2023.

FROM EVIDENCE TO POLICY: PREREQUISITES FOR THE SUCCESSFUL DESIGN OF THE EPHS

This section of the chapter provides a brief outline of the key elements of the framework with special emphasis on the first phase—evidence to policy.

Defining the Objectives of EPHS Design

A key factor affecting the success of EPHS design is establishing a good understanding of why the EPHS is required and its intended goals. Such clarity beforehand could help streamline the approach, improve communication, and clarify stakeholder expectations, thus increasing the likelihood of creating a feasible package. The objectives may vary depending on whether the EPHS is being developed for the first time or is a revision. If the budget space has limited room for growth, the design could prioritize enhancing the transparency, explicitness, affordability, efficiency, and fairness of the current package. If an increase in fiscal space for health is projected, additional focus could be placed on expanding the EPHS by including underfunded interventions.

Securing Sustained Political Commitment and Leadership

Political commitment to UHC and the resolve to improve access to essential health services are key prerequisites for the successful design and implementation of UHC packages. Such commitment should be translated into full endorsement of the UHC target by the government in its national health vision and strategies and should come with adequate financing. Early and serious engagement of government planning and finance sectors is an essential part of this commitment to address the fiscal space for health. The critical challenges of health system strengthening and adequate financing often require the political backing of the parliament, ministerial cabinet, and subnational governments (in the case of a decentralized system). Only two countries reported some engagement of parliamentarians at certain stages of the package development process, but even those parliamentarians made no formal decisions or resolutions on UHC or the EPHS. Priority setting and package design are major undertakings that require considerable technical resources and capacity strengthening. Making such an investment in the absence of sustained high-level government decisions is unlikely to result in a significant impact.

Although all countries reviewed in this volume illustrated an initial political commitment to develop and implement the EPHS, the sustainability of that commitment in implementing the EPHS represents a major challenge, particularly in countries facing political instability. Afghanistan, Ethiopia, Pakistan, Somalia, and Sudan consistently have high global rankings in terms of their vulnerability to political instability or politically motivated violence. Since defining their packages, Afghanistan underwent a regime change; Pakistan, Somalia, and Sudan experienced shifts in government; and Ethiopia and Sudan have been in civil war. Such instability is commonly associated with economic constraints and a restricted budget for health and social services.

Engaging Key Stakeholders

As mentioned earlier, national ownership of the process and its outcome requires engaging key internal and external stakeholders throughout the design process. Thus, conducting a comprehensive stakeholder analysis and developing key engagement plans are essential; however, the types of stakeholders, modalities, and depth of engagement vary by country. Table 1.3 provides a list of the main stakeholders involved in the *DCP3* country translation review.

Table 1.3 Stakeholder Involvement in the EPHS Process in the Six Focus Countries and One Economy

	Number of countries (Total = 7)
Countries and economy conducting stakeholder analysis	2
Countries and economy engaging key national stakeholders	
Parliament	2
Finance	2
Planning	4
Community and patients groups	1
Private sector	2
National academia	4
Countries and economy engaging multilateral organizations and development partners[a]	
World Health Organization	7
United Nations Children's Fund	5
United Nations Population Fund	3

table continues next page

Table 1.3 Stakeholder Involvement in the EPHS Process in the Six Focus Countries and One Economy (continued)

	Number of countries (Total = 7)
United Nations Development Programme	0
Bill & Melinda Gates Foundation	4
US Agency for International Development	4
World Bank	4
Engagement of international academic institutions or consultancy firms	6

Source: Adapted from Alwan, Majdzadeh, et al. 2023.

a. Additional partners for Ethiopia included the World Food Programme, United Nations (UN) International Organization for Migration, UN health and nutrition cluster, and the countries of Canada, Finland, Germany, Italy, Norway, Sweden, Switzerland, and the United Kingdom. For Liberia, they included the German Agency for International Cooperation and Last Mile Health through the Technical Working Groups. For Pakistan, they included the Global Fund; GAVI, the Vaccine Alliance; and the UK Foreign, Commonwealth and Development Office. For Somalia, they included the European Union. For Sudan, they included the European Union, GAVI, the Global Fund, and the countries of Canada, Germany, Italy, Sweden, Switzerland, and the United Kingdom.

Although all stakeholders engaged in the countries covered by the DCP3 review are important, civil society dialogue and engagement among community groups play a critical role, particularly in understanding and considering priority health needs. Only one country has partly acknowledged this requirement, and no country has engaged in serious interaction with people's representatives.

Assessing Health System Readiness and Financing Mechanisms

A key prerequisite for developing a properly designed and feasibly implemented UHC package is to conduct reliable assessments of the health system and financing mechanisms. The assessments should aim to identify gaps that impede access to essential services across the different building blocks of the health system. All the countries reviewed have considerable weaknesses in their health systems, but the experiences documented in this volume indicate that most countries did not conduct a comprehensive review. When countries did conduct such a review, the assessment tended to underestimate or even ignore the gaps, thus undermining the transition from package design to implementation.

Experience shows that mapping the availability and coverage levels of services already provided by the public health sector constitutes another important part of the assessment. It provides the necessary information on baseline offerings in terms of health services and on missing essential interventions that the prioritization phase should include. The Technical Working Groups—made up of experienced health professionals in health systems, reproductive and maternal and child health, communicable diseases, and noncommunicable diseases—play a central role in this task, particularly in analyzing existing services against the contents of model packages like the DCP3 essential UHC, the DCP3 highest-priority package, and the menu of health services in the WHO UHC Compendium. This step will help determine the total number of interventions (existing and proposed) that will be submitted for the evidence-based prioritization process (Alwan, Jallah, et al. 2023; Alwan, Siddiqi, et al. 2023).

Another essential component of health system assessments is a detailed analysis of existing financing mechanisms and fiscal space for health to guide the EPHS design process and to ensure the affordability of the recommended package along the SDG timeline. Adequate funding should not only cover initial implementation but should also account for population growth in some countries; the progressive increase in the coverage of interventions along the UHC timeline will result in rising costs that will far exceed the current expenditure for health and any forecasted economic growth. Ideally, part of the fiscal space assessment should involve exploring the potential for increasing health allocations based on projections for economic growth and government funding and on objective forecasts of partner and donor funding.

Developing and Implementing a Road Map for EPHS Design

Several of the review countries and economy developed an operational plan and road map at the outset. Those road maps cover the EPHS's scope, objectives, process, and required actions, and a timeline for the different steps in EPHS development. In their road maps, countries have included the establishment of a special unit within the Ministry of Health and a comprehensive governance structure covering roles and responsibilities of the key actors and stakeholders. The governance structure included the formation of Technical Working Groups to lead the work in prioritizing essential health interventions. The following subsections briefly discuss the critical components of the road map.

Prioritization of Essential Health Services A starting point for the prioritization process involves reaching consensus on the decision-making criteria the country will adopt to select interventions or services. This undertaking presents challenges because stakeholders need to agree on the principles and criteria and because the selection of criteria must be evidence-informed and participatory. Benchmarking global experience, reviewing the sector's existing values and principles in health policies and strategies, and conducting transparent deliberations could help in identifying the criteria and reaching consensus. Countries considered the following key criteria: (1) burden of disease, (2) effectiveness, (3) cost-effectiveness, (4) financial risk protection, (5) quality of evidence, (6) equity and targeting vulnerable populations. (7) feasibility of implementation, and (8) budget impact. Several publications, as well as other chapters in this volume, cover the definitions and additional information on the decision criteria adopted by some countries (refer to Alwan, Jallah, et al. 2023; Alwan, Siddiqi, et al. 2023; Baltussen, Mwalim, et al. 2023).

Evidence Synthesis and Analytics The identification and ranking of candidate health interventions for priority setting require the gathering and synthesizing of various data and evidence. Experience shows that collecting and collating evidence on the decision-making criteria are challenging and time-consuming given the frequently weak health information systems, inadequate capacity, and scarcity of locally generated accurate data in many countries. Decision-makers should make every effort to use the most locally relevant evidence. When countries did not have available local evidence, often the case for cost-effectiveness evidence, they consulted regional and international data sources and recommendations. All the reviewed countries and economy in this chapter used multiple sources, such as the Institute for Health Metrics' Global Burden of Disease, DCP3, the WHO UHC Compendium, and the Tufts Cost-Effectiveness Analysis Registry, as well as local expert opinion when data were not available.

Getting data on the equity and financial risk protection impacts of interventions also presented challenges. Even with available data, however, trade-offs among multiple criteria can make priority-setting decisions difficult. To overcome such challenges, countries apply deliberative decision-making, highlighting the importance of decision-facilitating analytics tools. Some tools commonly used in EPHS design include the FairChoices DCP Analytics Tool, the Health Interventions Prioritization Tool, the OneHealth Tool, and the UHC Service Package Delivery and Implementation Tool.

Costing and Fiscal Space All health interventions set for prioritization will require economic evaluation and costing to assess their budget impact. Costing interventions and estimating the budget impact of the whole EPHS are challenging, and results may be indicative rather than accurate. Gaudin et al. (2023) conducted a survey to review the EPHS costing experience in five countries as part of the DCP3 country translation review (refer to chapter 16 in this volume). The review shows a wide variation in the application of costing methodologies and interpretation of terminology, particularly regarding common health system–related costs and capacity constraints in low- and lower-middle-income countries. That variation calls for more systematic guidance and standard ways to implement economic evaluation methods.

The results and conclusions of the survey suggest that the usefulness of costing depends entirely on the availability and accuracy of costing data (chapter 16). Reporting ranges of uncertainty, conducting sensitivity analysis, and ensuring transparency in the methods and assumptions used could improve trust, policy relevance, and the use of costing estimates in decision-making. The study strongly recommends routine gathering of costing data and training to properly collect and use those data. It also notes the critical importance of ensuring that the package is properly designed and integrated into a country's budget cycle. The survey found that none of the DCP3 review countries had explicitly linked costing with the budgeting process, which is essential for implementation. Finally, the study recommends engaging in long-term capacity building in costing as an integral part of institutionalizing the EPHS design process.

Prioritization of costed health interventions is based on the agreed decision criteria, with serious consideration of the funding envelope agreed to finance the EPHS. When the cost of the recommended high-priority interventions exceeds the available fiscal space for public expenditure, countries may need a subsequent round of prioritization to develop another version of the EPHS that aligns with the government resource envelope. For instance, both Liberia and Pakistan needed a second phase of prioritization. In Liberia, the government decided to split the initially recommended package into two subpackages, proposing a core, publicly financed package of high-priority primary health care interventions and a second package to be implemented through a cost-sharing program (Alwan, Jallah, et al. 2023). In Pakistan, the outcome of the second phase was an implementation package endorsed for immediate rollout. Pakistan approved the full national EPHS with a larger number of interventions for implementation if and when the country could increase health allocations (Alwan, Siddiqi, et al. 2023). In both countries, the final EPHS was endorsed at the highest level of the health sector.

Overall Assessment

Despite several shortcomings, many of the country and economy case studies reported in this chapter show the possibility and feasibility of building on existing evidence to develop a policy-relevant EPHS. The case studies show the substantial efforts made to synthesize evidence on the costs and effectiveness of health interventions. National capacity exists (even if it is scarce) to conduct all or part of the technical work, sometimes with support from international partners (WHO, World Bank, development agencies, academic institutions, and—perhaps too often—consultants). Countries often have road maps and governance structures in place, and the processes of translating evidence into policy have improved, with broader stakeholder involvement, even if none of the processes can be said to be fully open and inclusive. Few of these efforts, however, have translated from policy to practice, as discussed in the next section. Several of the chapters in part 2 of this volume also discuss these efforts.

FROM POLICY TO PRACTICE: SECURING A SUCCESSFUL TRANSITION TO SUSTAINABLE IMPLEMENTATION

Many countries had developed EPHSs before the SDG era, but not all successfully implemented them (Glassman, Giedion, and Smith 2017; Shekh Mohamed et al. 2022; Wright and Holtz 2017). Some crisis countries established EPHSs as part of donor funding programs, whereas others aimed to secure the delivery of a minimum set of basic primary health care services delivered by the private sector or nongovernmental organizations. Most of the packages discussed in this volume were developed mainly as part of national efforts to achieve UHC. Almost all of the packages have significant challenges in the transition to implementation for several reasons: some are unaffordable, cannot be implemented because of unattended or ignored health system weaknesses, have no clear implementation and monitoring plan, and, in certain situations, were designed without securing government ownership and high-level engagement. It is therefore crucial to ensure that those impediments are addressed during package design by securing national commitment and ownership; by ensuring feasibility, affordability, and sustainable financing of high-priority health services; and by identifying and addressing key health system gaps as part of the design process.

Implementation Plan

The crucial step of developing a comprehensive EPHS implementation plan requires extensive dialogue and deliberation. The plan should focus on communicating the package to various stakeholders, organizing the package by service delivery platforms, identifying additional investment needs (such as infrastructure, human resources, and supply chain management), mobilizing additional revenue, enhancing strategic purchasing, and monitoring. To guide implementation, the EPHS should be linked to other national strategies, guidelines, initiatives, and reforms, including budgeting, provider payment mechanisms, human resources development and management, service delivery platforms, infrastructure investment, standard treatment guidelines, essential drug lists, medical equipment lists, and monitoring and evaluation. Four of the seven DCP3 country translation–supported countries and economies—Ethiopia, Pakistan, Somalia, and Zanzibar—developed implementation plans (Alwan, Majdzadeh, et al. 2023). Each plan's development, however, involved limited stakeholder engagement, making the implementation plan less likely to address the health system constraints that impede EPHS rollout.

Aligning EPHSs to Health System Delivery

One of the key challenges in implementing an EPHS is the weak link between the way health interventions are organized within the package and the way the health system is organized to deliver services. Most EPHSs are organized by diseases or specific interventions, but implementing them requires mapping to the platform that best addresses them and mapping interdependent services and platforms. Interdependent interventions must be reviewed and prioritized together, which often does not happen. In addition, the interventions should be mapped to the input required for the health system to deliver them. Countries face substantial challenges aligning disease- or intervention-specific priority lists to the capacity-building, human and material resources, and organizational and financing elements needed to get services to people. Thus, service delivery considerations should be integrated into package development and critical translational work done to regroup the packages by service type from the intervention- or disease-focused package lists and align them with health system input needs.

Aligning an EPHS with Health Financing Mechanisms

The EPHS can serve as a tool for advocating for and mobilizing more revenue, reducing fragmentation of financing, reinforcing pooling, and enhancing efficiency through strong strategic purchasing. Attaining those goals depends on the clarity of the design objectives and the process followed. Experience from the low- and lower-middle-income countries' EPHS revisions shows a significant disconnect between the EPHS and health-financing strategies and plans, especially in revenue raising. In most of the countries reviewed, the EPHS has not resulted in a significant increase in the allocation of resources to health (Soucat, Tandon, and Gonzales Pier 2023). That situation could be mainly due to an unaffordable package and unrealistic fiscal space projections, leading to an imbalance between the available budget space and the aspirational package, and inadequate engagement and commitment of political leaders. Aspirational packages developed without adequate participation of key political leaders are less likely to be implemented. Therefore, development needs to include a thorough and transparent discussion about the affordability of the package, the financing sources and mechanisms, and securing political endorsement during the design phase.

Although most countries reported some involvement of the finance and planning sectors, the level and timing of their engagement were not convincingly effective. It is important to ensure the ownership and commitment of beyond-line ministries, such as at high levels like the president or prime minister, parliament, ministerial cabinet, and subnational leaders. The gap in securing an adequate level of engagement and commitment from high-level decision-makers in resource allocation is likely a major cause of the weak link between the EPHS design and the adequate allocation of public funds for package financing.

Furthermore, countries can use EPHS design as an opportunity to consider the introduction of fiscal measures such as taxing unhealthy products like alcohol, tobacco, and sugar-sweetened beverages, which have the double benefit of increasing fiscal space (with the possibility of increasing the health budget) and reducing disease burden. Removing subsidies or taxing fossil fuels—recommended as measures to address both health and climate issues—will require further exploration of the unintended impacts of such measures, especially in low-income settings, and of mitigation measures needed before implementing such reforms. The EPHS is a crucial document for harmonizing benefits, pooling funds, and guiding purchasing agencies on what, how, and from whom to purchase; and it links high-priority services to tailored payment mechanisms for health providers at different levels. Nevertheless, EPHSs are only rarely aligned with ongoing financial reforms in the case study countries, highlighting the importance of guiding budget mechanisms that explicitly allocate funds to priority health services and establish purchase incentives that support service delivery objectives, limit cost escalation, and promote efficiency and quality.

Private Sector Engagement

The private sector plays a substantial role in the provision of health services in many low- and lower-middle-income countries. It has limited engagement, however, in the development and implementation of health policies such as EPHSs, indicating untapped potential. For instance, the private health sector was involved in package design in only two out of the seven countries reviewed in this chapter. The private for-profit sector often operates on self-guided and market-oriented objectives that do not align with public sector goals, including UHC, because of the limited enabling environment, participation, incentives, and regulation. When the private health sector plays a major role in essential health services delivery, implementing the EPHS without involving the private sector is unrealistic (Siddiqi et al. 2023). Thus, governments need to comprehensively map the extensive and heterogeneous private sectors by their characteristics (such as nonprofit versus for-profit, service domain, level and type of specialty, geographical distribution interest, and power dynamics) and define the roles they can play in EPHS design and implementation. Identifying and providing key incentives to gear private sector objectives and interests toward UHC are key, as are addressing key barriers related to governance, regulation, accountability, contracting, performance monitoring, and quality of services. This process should be guided by existing evidence and local and international experiences and lessons.

Monitoring and Evaluation

A monitoring and evaluation (M&E) framework that aligns with the existing national health information system is essential for evaluating progress and making timely revisions to an EPHS. The UHC policy process needs to incorporate M&E plans right from the start. Those plans should also align with the global monitoring framework for UHC building from SDG indicators 3.8.1 and 3.8.2 on service coverage and catastrophic expenditures, respectively. The M&E framework should include a combination of those two global indicators and a set of dynamic, country-specific indicators that assess EPHS implementation along the timeline of SDG Target 3.8 (Alwan, Yamey, and Soucat 2023). The country-specific indicators can measure policy availability, resource availability, health system preparedness, service availability, coverage, equity, efficiency, and financial hardship in accessing health care. Some of the countries reviewed in this chapter developed an M&E plan by integrating it into the overall M&E system, but with differences in the types of indicators and the data source. For example, the M&E framework in Ethiopia relies heavily on population-level surveys, whereas other countries use routine data-based monitoring (Danforth et al. 2023).

Institutionalization

Revising a health benefits package is a dynamic process that changes over time with varying demand, health system capacity, and fiscal space. Thus, countries need to put in place a system for institutionalizing regular revision of the EPHS as a whole or in part. The institutionalization process requires interventions such as establishing and strengthening institutions and governance platforms, developing a legal framework and guiding documents, generating routine evidence and analytics, developing a robust knowledge management system, and securing funds. Despite efforts by the focus countries to establish political will and commitment, a governance structure, an accountable body, a road map to guide the design process, and a method for documenting the process, they still need to do more to establish a legitimate, transparent, and regular revision of their EPHS.

CONCLUSION AND KEY MESSAGES

In general, substantial improvement has been observed compared to earlier efforts in terms of laying the foundational work for priority setting, stakeholder engagement, evidence synthesis, technical capacity, and EPHS design processes. However, experiences in countries also reveal significant weaknesses in the design and implementation of UHC packages (such as feasibility, affordability, alignment with service delivery, financing, and health system readiness), which can unfortunately impede any meaningful progress to their implementation. Despite countries' limited experience in implementing an EPHS, a successfully designed package will generally address the main causes of failure to move to package rollout and will facilitate implementation. Addressing weaknesses and gaps by meeting the requirements and prerequisites covered in the framework for action presented in box 1.1 will provide better prospects for implementation and accelerated progress to UHC. Two of the five components of the framework relate to the initial situation analysis, including the level of political commitment and the state of the country's health system. The remaining components focus on other areas of the package development process and implementation, particularly those related to the requirements necessary for the transition from package design to implementation.

These areas are also covered in the following key messages emerging from the DCP3 country translation review and addressed to policy makers in low- and lower-middle-income countries:

- Countries must execute and own the process of setting and revising an EPHS. Packages developed without adequate engagement of national authorities are less likely to be implemented.
- Requirements for a successful outcome are sustained high-level political commitment, effective engagement of key stakeholders, health system readiness, affordability, committed funding, and strong leadership for implementation.
- Early, committed engagement of the government's planning and finance sectors is essential—investing in package development has limited value without a realistic financing plan.
- Even a perfectly designed, affordable package has no major impact without adequate and well-trained human resources to deliver effective services, including a clear role for the private sector.

- Sustainability for implementing UHC packages requires leadership, political stability, sustained resources, and institutionalization of technical and managerial capacity.
- Low- and lower-middle-income countries need reinforced technical assistance in UHC-related programs, including through regional institutions.

ACKNOWLEDGMENTS

We are grateful for many colleagues who have made extremely valuable contributions to the DCP3 country translation work over the past five years. Many of these colleagues have also been actively involved in authoring the different chapters in this volume and in engaging the different stages of the country work reported in this chapter. We express great appreciation to Dean T. Jamison, who led the development of the third edition of the DCP, and for his continued engagement and support to the DCP3 Country Translation Project in several countries. We also appreciate the contributions of the following colleagues: Wafa Aftab, Rob Baltussen, Karl Blanchet, Manuel Carballo, Sylvestre Gaudin, Ina Gudumac, Alemayehu Hailu, George Jacob, Mohamed Jama, Kjell Arne Johansson, Francis Kateh, Mizan Kiros, Reza Majdzadeh, Awad Mataria, Omar Mwalim, Teri Reynolds, Malik Safi, Sameen Siddiqi, Jolene Skordis, Agnès Soucat, Pakwanja Desiree Twea, Anna Vassal, David A. Watkins, David Wilson, Gavin Yamey, Raza Zaidi, and other co-authors of the country translation papers published in special supplements of *BMJ Global Health* and the *International Journal of Health Policy Management* and in relevant chapters in this volume. We are indebted to the Bill & Melinda Gates Foundation for supporting and funding the DCP3 Country Translation and Disease Control Priorities–Ethiopia projects.

NOTES

1. This chapter uses *EPHS* and *health benefits package* interchangeably.
2. University of Washington, Department of Global Health, "DCP3 Country Translation Project," https://www.dcp-3.org/translation (accessed August 20, 2023).
3. WHO, "UHC Compendium" (database), https://www.who.int/universal-health-coverage /compendium (accessed August 22, 2023).

REFERENCES

Alwan, Ala, Wilhemina Jallah, Rob Baltussen, Manuel Carballo, Ernest Gonyon, Ina Gudumac, Hassan Haghparast-Bigoli, et al. 2023. "Designing an Evidence Informed Package of Essential Health Services for Universal Health Coverage: Lessons Learned and Challenges to Implementation in Liberia." *BMJ Global Health*. https://gh.bmj.com /content/9/6/e014904.

Alwan, Ala, Dean T. Jamison, Sameen Siddiqi, and Anna Vassall. 2024. "Pakistan's Progress on Universal Health Coverage: Lessons Learned in Priority Setting and Challenges Ahead in Reinforcing Primary Healthcare." *International Journal of Health Policy and Management* 13 (8450). https://doi.org/10.34172/ijhpm.2024.8450.

Alwan, Ala, Reza Majdzadeh, Gavin Yamey, Karl Blanchet, Alemayehu Hailu, Mohamed Jama, Kjell Arne Johansson, et al. 2023. "Country Readiness and Prerequisites for Successful Design and Transition to Implementation of Essential Packages of Health Services: Experience from Six Countries." *BMJ Global Health* 8 (Suppl 1): e010720. https://doi.org/10.1136/bmjgh-2022-010720.

Alwan, Ala, Sameen Siddiqi, Malik Safi, Raza Zaidi, Muhammad Khalid, Rob Baltussen, Ina Gudumac, et al. 2023. "Addressing the UHC Challenge Using the Disease Control Priorities 3 Approach: Lessons Learned and an Overview of the Pakistan Experience." *International Journal of Health Policy and Management* 12 (December): 8003. https://doi.org/10.34172/ijhpm.2023.8003.

Alwan, Ala, Gavin Yamey, and Agnès Soucat. 2023. "Essential Packages of Health Services in Low-Income and Lower-Middle-Income Countries: What Have We Learnt?" *BMJ Global Health* 8: e010724. https://doi.org/10.1136/bmjgh-2022-010724.

Baltussen, Rob, Maarten Jansen, Syeda Shehirbano Akhtar, Leon Bijlmakers, Sergio Torres-Rueda, Muhammad Khalid, Wajeeha Raza, et al. 2023. "The Use of Evidence-Informed Deliberative Processes for Designing the Essential Package of Health Services in Pakistan." *International Journal of Health Policy and Management* 12: 8004. https://doi.org/10.34172/ijhpm.2023.8004.

Baltussen, Rob, Omar Mwalim, Karl Blanchet, Manuel Carballo, Getachew Teshome Eregata, Alemayehu Hailu, Maryam Huda, et al. 2023. "Decision-Making Processes for Essential Packages of Health Services: Experience from Six Countries." *BMJ Global Health* 8 (Suppl 1): e010704. https://doi.org/10.1136/bmjgh-2022-010704.

Blanchet, Karl, Ala Alwan, Caroline Antoine, Marion Jane Cros, Ferozuddin Feroz, Tseguaneh Amsalu Guracha, Oystein Haaland, et al. 2020. "Protecting Essential Health Services in Low-Income and Middle-Income Countries and Humanitarian Settings while Responding to the COVID-19 Pandemic." *BMJ Global Health* 5 (10): 1–9. https://doi.org/10.1136/bmjgh-2020-003675.

Boerma, Ties, Patrick Eoenou, David Evans, Tim Evans, Marie-Paule Kieny, and Adam Wagstaff. 2014. "Monitoring Progress towards Universal Health Coverage at Country and Global Levels." *PLoS Med* 11 (9): e1001731. https://doi.org/10.1371/journal.pmed.1001731.

Danforth, Kristen, Ahsan Maqbool Ahmad, Karl Blanchet, Muhammad Khalid, Arianna Rubin Means, and Solomon Tessema Memirie. 2023. "Monitoring and Evaluating the Implementation of Essential Packages of Health Services." *BMJ Global Health* 8 (Suppl 1): e010726. https://doi.org/10.1136/bmjgh-2022-010726.

Eregata, Getachew Teshome, Alemayehu Hailu, Zelalem Adugna Geletu, Solomon Tessema Memirie, Kjell Arne Johansson, Karin Stenberg, Melanie Y. Bertram, et al. 2020. "Revision of the Ethiopian Essential Health Service Package: An Explication of the Process and Methods Used." *Health Systems and Reform* 6 (1): e1829313. https://doi.org/10.1080/23288604.2020.1829313.

Gaudin, Sylvestre, Wajeeha Raza, Jolene Skordis, Agnès Soucat, Karin Stenberg, and Ala Alwan. 2023. "Using Costing to Facilitate Policy Making towards Universal Health Coverage: Findings and Recommendations from Country-Level Experiences." *BMJ Global Health* 8 (Suppl 1): e010735. https://doi.org/10.1136/bmjgh-2022-010735.

Glassman, Amanda, Ursula Giedion, and Peter C. Smith. 2017. *What's in, What's out? Designing Benefits for Universal Health Coverage*. Washington, DC: Center for Global Development. https://www.cgdev.org/publication/whats-in-whats-out-designing-benefits-universal-health-coverage.

Huda, Maryam, Nichola Kitson, Nuru Saadi, Saira Kanwal, Urooj Gul, Maarten Jansen, Sergio Torres-Rueda, et al. 2023. "Assessing Global Evidence on Cost-Effectiveness to Inform Development of Pakistan's Essential Package of Health Services." *International Journal of Health Policy and Management* 13 (8005). https://doi.org/10.34172/ijhpm.2023.8005.

Jamison, Dean T., Ala Alwan, Charles N. Mock, Rachel Nugent, David Watkins, Olusoji Adeyi, Shuchi Anand, et al. 2018. "Universal Health Coverage and Intersectoral Action for Health: Key Messages from *Disease Control Priorities*, 3rd Edition." *The Lancet* 391 (10125): 1108–20. https://www.thelancet.com/journals/lancet/article/PIIS0140 -6736(17)32906-9/abstract.

Jamison, Dean T., Hellen Gelband, Susan Horton, Prabhat Jha, Ramanan Laxminarayan, and Charles N. Mock, eds. 2018. *Disease Control Priorities* (third edition), Volume 9, *Disease Control Priorities: Improving Health and Reducing Poverty*. Washington, DC: World Bank. https://documents.worldbank.org/en/publication/documents-reports/docum entdetail/527531512569346552/disease-control-priorities-improving-health-and-reducing -poverty.

Jamison, Dean T., Lawrence H. Summers, George Alleyne, Kenneth J. Arrow, Seth Berkley, Agnes Binagwaho, Flavia Bustreo, et al. 2013. "Global Health 2035: A World Converging within a Generation." *The Lancet* 382 (9908): 1898–955. https://doi.org/10.1016/S0140- 6736(13)62105-4.

NHSRC (Pakistan, Ministry of National Health Services Regulation and Coordination), WHO (World Health Organization), and DCP3 Secretariat. 2019. "Review of Essential Health Services in Pakistan Based on Disease Control Priorities 3." NHSRC, Islamabad. https:// www.dcp-3.org/sites/default/files/resources/Review%20of%20Essential%20Health%20 Services%20Pakistan%20based%20on%20DCP3%20WHO%202019_web.pdf.

Raza, Wajeeha, Wahaj Zulfiqar, Mashal Murad Shah, Maryam Huda, Syeda Shehirbano Akhtar, Urooj Aqeel, Saira Kanwal, et al. 2024. "Costing Interventions for Developing an Essential Package of Health Services: Application of a Rapid Method and Results from Pakistan." *International Journal of Health Policy and Management* 13 (8006). https://doi .org/10.34172/ijhpm.2023.8006.

Reynolds, Teri, Thomas Wilkinson, Melanie Y. Bertram, Matthew Jowett, Rob Baltussen, Awad Mataria, Ferozuddin Feroz, and Mohamed Jama. 2023. "Building Implementable Packages for Universal Health Coverage." *BMJ Global Health* 8 (Suppl 1): e010807. https://doi.org/10.1136/bmjgh-2022-010807.

Shekh Mohamed, Idil, Jasmine Sprague Hepburn, Björn Ekman, and Jesper Sundewall. 2022. "Inclusion of Essential Universal Health Coverage Services in Essential Packages of Health Services: A Review of 45 Low- and Lower- Middle Income Countries." *Health Systems and Reform* 8 (1). https://doi.org/10.1080/23288604.2021.2006587.

Siddiqi, Sameen, Wafa Aftab, A. Venkat Raman, Agnès Soucat, and Ala Alwan. 2023. "The Role of the Private Sector in Delivering Essential Packages of Health Services: Lessons from Country Experiences." *BMJ Global Health* 8: e010742. https://doi .org/10.1136/bmjgh-2022-010742.

Somalia, Ministry of Health and Human Services. 2021. "Essential Package of Health Services (EPHS) Somalia 2020." Federal Government of Somalia. https://reliefweb.int/report /somalia/essential-package-health-services-ephs-somalia-2020.

Soucat, Agnès, Ajay Tandon, and Eduardo Gonzales Pier. 2023. "From Universal Health Coverage Services Packages to Budget Appropriation: The Long Journey to Implementation." *BMJ Global Health* 8: e010755. https://doi.org/10.1136/bmjgh-2022 -010755.

Torres-Rueda, Sergio, Anna Vassall, Raza Zaidi, Nichola Kitson, Muhammad Khalid, Wahaj Zulfiqar, and Ala Alwan. 2024. "The Use of Evidence to Design an Essential Package of Health Services in Pakistan: A Review and Analysis of Prioritisation Decisions at Different Stages of the Appraisal Process." *International Journal of Health Policy and Management* 13 (8043).

UN (United Nations) General Assembly. 2015. *Transforming Our World: The 2030 Agenda for Sustainable Development*. New York: United Nations. https://sdgs.un.org/publications /transforming-our-world-2030-agenda-sustainable-development-17981.

UN (United Nations) General Assembly. 2019. "Political Declaration of the High-Level Meeting on Universal Health Coverage." Resolution A/RES/74/2 adopted October 10, 2019, United Nations, New York. https://documents.un.org/doc/undoc/gen/n19/311/84/pdf/n1931184.pdf?token=c98Nhz6vwIm4Je1kJ5&fe=true.

UN (United Nations) General Assembly. 2023. "Universal Health Coverage: Expanding Our Ambition for Health and Well-Being in a Post-COVID World." Political Declaration of the High-Level Meeting on Universal Health Coverage. https://www.un.org/pga/77/wp-content/uploads/sites/105/2023/09/UHC-Final-Text.pdf.

Watkins, David, Dean T. Jamison, Anne Mills, Rifat Atun, Kristen Danforth, Amanda Glassman, Susan Horton, et al. 2018. "Annex 3C. Essential Universal Health Coverage: Interventions and Platforms." In *Disease Control Priorities* (3rd edition), Volume 9, *Disease Control Priorities: Improving Health and Reducing Poverty,* edited by D. T. Jamison, H. Gelband, S. Horton, P. Jha, R. Laxminarayan, C. N. Mock, and R. Nugent. Washington, DC: World Bank.

WHO (World Health Organization). 1946. "Constitution of the World Health Organization." Adopted by the International Health Conference, New York, July 22, 1946. https://apps.who.int/gb/bd/PDF/bd47/EN/constitution-en.pdf?ua=1.

WHO (World Health Organization). 2000. *World Health Report 2000: Health Systems: Improving Performance.* Geneva: WHO. https://apps.who.int/iris/handle/10665/42281.

WHO (World Health Organization). 2019. "Thirteenth General Programme of Work 2019–2023." WHO, Geneva. https://www.who.int/about/general-programme-of-work/thirteenth.

WHO (World Health Organization). 2023. "Universal Health Coverage (UHC)." Fact sheet, October 5, 2023, World Health Organization, Geneva. https://www.who.int/news-room/fact-sheets/detail/universal-health-coverage-(uhc).

WHO (World Health Organization) and World Bank. 2021. *Global Monitoring Report on Financial Protection in Health 2021.* Geneva: World Health Organization and Washington, DC: World Bank. https://www.who.int/publications/i/item/9789240040953.

WHO (World Health Organization) and World Bank. 2023. *Tracking Universal Health Coverage: 2023 Global Monitoring Report.* Geneva: World Health Organization and Washington, DC: World Bank. https://www.who.int/publications/i/item/9789240080379.

Wright, Jenna, and Jenna Holtz. 2017. "Essential Packages of Health Services in 24 Countries: Findings from a Cross-Country Analysis." Health Finance and Governance Project, Bethesda, MD. https://www.hfgproject.org/ephs-cross-country-analysis/.

Part 1

Experience in Selected Countries and Economies

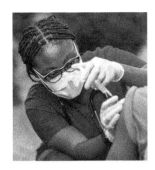

2

Lessons from the Revision Process of Ethiopia's Essential Health Services Package

Alemayehu Hailu, Getachew Teshome Eregata, Zelalem Adugna Geletu, Solomon Tessema Memirie, Wubaye Walelgne, Amanuel Yigezu, Mieraf Taddesse, Kjell Arne Johansson, Karin Stenberg, Melanie Y. Bertram, Amir Aman, Lia Tadesse Gebremedhin, and Ole F. Norheim

ABSTRACT

This chapter discusses Ethiopia's revision of its essential health services package in 2019 to achieve universal health coverage. The revision process involved 35 consultative workshops with experts and the public. It employed seven prioritization criteria, including disease burden, cost-effectiveness, and public acceptability. The process identified 1,018 relevant health interventions from an initial list of 1,749; further evaluation and ranking resulted in a package of 594 high-priority interventions (58 percent) assigned to health care delivery platforms and linked to financing mechanisms. The discussion in this chapter concludes that the process was participatory, inclusive, and evidence-based, leading to a comprehensive essential health services package.

INTRODUCTION

In 2015, Ethiopia signed on to the Sustainable Development Goals (SDGs), of which SDG target 3.8 relates explicitly to achieving universal health coverage (UHC) for all population segments.[1] With that commitment, the Ethiopian Ministry of Health (MoH) needed to define the essential health services it would deliver to the population without incurring financial risk. Which services coverage should it scale up first? For which services should the government reduce direct costs?

How could it expand the range of services to be delivered in the future? (Refer to Glassman et al. 2016; Hogan et al. 2018; Reich 2016; Rieger, Wagner, and Bedi 2017; Wagstaff and Neelsen 2020.)

Ethiopia determined in 2018 that its essential health services package (EHSP), first defined in 2005, needed revision for three primary reasons. First, the country needed a package that matched the current disease burden. The 2005 EHSP constituted about 120 interventions focused on reproductive, maternal, newborn, and child health and on preventing and controlling major communicable and vaccine-preventable diseases (MoH 2005). In the first two decades of the twenty-first century, however, the disease burden profile of the country changed substantially. With the rise of injuries and noncommunicable diseases as important causes of mortality and morbidity, the 2005 EHSP no longer adequately addressed the current situation (Misganaw et al. 2017). Second, the country needed a package that matched the current population's health care demand. Because of economic growth, increased health literacy due to the expansion of health extension programs also markedly increased the demand for health services in Ethiopia. Third, the country needed to institutionalize a clear, transparent, and deliberative priority-setting process. Since the 2005 EHSP, several new interventions had been introduced to the (publicly funded) health care delivery system without proper cost-benefit and cost-effectiveness evaluation (MoH 2015).

Therefore, in May 2018, the MoH executive council decided to revise the Ethiopian EHSP. It launched the revision process immediately in June 2018 and launched the final EHSP document in November 2019 (MoH 2018, 2019). This chapter describes the rationales, objectives, scope, process, methods, context, and challenges of Ethiopia's EHSP revision process, emphasizing the use of evidence from the third edition of *Disease Control Priorities* (DCP3). In addition, it discusses the relevance of Ethiopia's process for similar work in other countries.

ELEMENTS OF THE PRIORITY-SETTING PROCESSES

The priority-setting process for Ethiopia's EHSP was meticulously designed to ensure inclusiveness, transparency, and evidence-based decision-making. This section outlines the key components and steps involved in the process, highlighting the collaborative efforts and structured methodologies that guided the revision of the EHSP. It covers ownership and governance, scope and content, criteria used, and accountability and transparency measures.

Ownership and Governance

Ethiopia designed its EHSP revision process to be participatory and inclusive, and to follow an evidence-based prioritization process. The MoH leadership approved a detailed road map of the revision process and the methods to be used from June 2018 to November 2019 (figure 2.1).

Figure 2.1 Road Map for the Revision of Ethiopia's EHSP

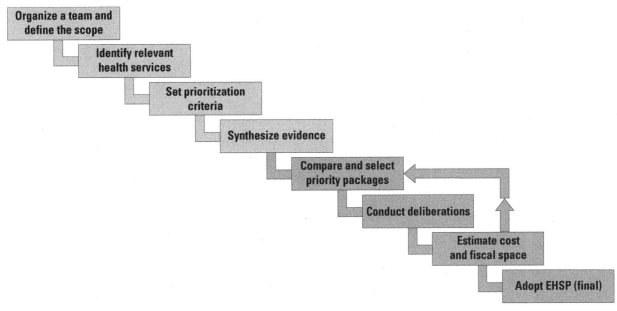

Source: MoH 2019.
Note: EHSP = essential health services package.

The MoH initiated the revision of the EHSP, holding eight inception meetings from June to August 2018 to outline the detailed revision plan, define the revision road map, and determine the scope and objectives of the revised EHSP (MoH 2018). It applied the existing MoH governance structure for decision-making and involved directorates at the MoH and representatives of all Regional Health Bureaus throughout the process to ensure inclusiveness and transparency. Additionally, national and international experts (that is, the World Health Organization [WHO] and Disease Control Priorities–Ethiopia) provided technical support throughout the process. The minister organized an EHSP core coordinating team comprising a health economist and a health systems specialist. The core team's role was to facilitate the development of the entire package, including developing a prioritization protocol, collating data, synthesizing evidence, engaging stakeholders, and conducting costing and fiscal space analysis. A Technical Working Group was established, comprising 30 senior experts on various health system dimensions. It supported the core team in preparing the revision road map, which helped develop a shared understanding of the steps necessary to achieve an evidence-based package revision.

Scope and Content

The primary objective of the revised EHSP is to reduce the burden of disease in Ethiopia by making high-priority interventions available and affordable. It also aims to protect people from catastrophic health expenditures, increase equitable access to health services, improve the efficiency of the health system, and increase public participation and transparency in decision-making in the health sector. The scope of the revised EHSP reflects the national health policy and the country's SDG UHC commitments while considering the constraints of resource availability and economic growth. The EHSP has four fundamental features: (1) it was designed to address the health needs of the Ethiopian population across the whole life course regardless of income, gender, or place of residence (that is, urban or rural); (2) it was designed to be delivered at all service levels (that is, primary, secondary, and tertiary); (3) it was intended to serve for five years (2020–25); and (4) it includes promotive, preventive, curative, and rehabilitative interventions.

Criteria Used

The prioritization criteria arose from a review of the literature, national health policy documents, and relevant strategic health sector documents. The process also considered the criteria for the prioritization of health services recommended by WHO's Consultative Group on Equity and Universal Health Coverage, which include maximizing the total health gains for a given investment, giving priority to health services that target or benefit the less fortunate, and providing financial risk protection (FRP), particularly to the poor (WHO 2014). Broadly, such a prioritization approach is based on data, dialogue, and decisions (Terwindt, Rajan, and Soucat 2016). Ten consultations and deliberative meetings on the proposed criteria took place with the participation of global and local experts, public representatives, and professional associations.

Finally, the priority-setting process resulted in the selection of seven prioritization criteria: disease burden, cost-effectiveness, equity, FRP, budget impact, public acceptability, and political acceptability. Disease burden was used to identify the relevant conditions and risk factors of particular importance in the Ethiopian context. The cost-effectiveness criterion was used to rank and compare health interventions quantitatively according to the health gains they would yield per dollar spent. The equity and FRP criteria were used to compare health interventions further and give higher value to health benefits for the less fortunate and interventions that protect against catastrophic out-of-pocket health expenditures. In addition, the public and political acceptability of the interventions was considered through a qualitative deliberative process and dialogue with policy makers (figure 2.2).

Figure 2.2 Priority-Setting Criteria for Ethiopia's EHSP

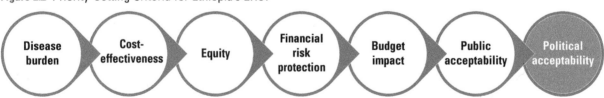

Source: MoH 2019.

Note: EHSP = essential health services package.

Accountability and Transparency Measures

The EHSP's acceptability and legitimacy depend not only on the type and quality of evidence used in defining the package but also on the transparency and deliberativeness of the process. Legitimacy and trust crucially depend on a deliberative process that involves stakeholders (Daniels and Sabin 2008). Ethiopia actively engaged stakeholders from a wide range of groups in matters ranging from setting prioritization criteria and identifying health interventions to prioritizing and ranking the interventions. The stakeholders included local experts, such as primary health care practitioners, doctors, and specialists, and public representatives, including a women's association, a youth association, and various professional associations. Thirty-five consultative workshops were convened with experts and the public to define the EHSP.

The core team undertaking the evaluation presented the full results to policy makers at the MoH for review, discussing whether to include or exclude specific interventions, and for their approval. The MoH executive council, the higher-level decision-making body in the sector, made the final decision.

ANALYSIS AND TOOLS

This section delves into the methodologies and resources used in the revision of Ethiopia's EHSP. It covers the comprehensive data sources, analytical tools, and processes employed to ensure a robust and evidence-based approach. The detailed analysis includes cost-effectiveness evaluations, equity and FRP assessments, and the integration of expert opinions to prioritize health interventions.

Data Sources and Tools

The revision process involved an exhaustive search of the Ethiopian health sector's plans, strategies, and national publications along with reviews of international resources such as the volumes of DCP3[2] and various WHO documents, including a draft version of the WHO UHC intervention compendium.[3] At a subsequent two-day workshop, 80 experts from various program areas—including primary health care practitioners, doctors, and specialists—came together to identify additional interventions. They jointly identified and proposed an extensive list of health services relevant to the Ethiopian context.

The 2019 EHSP has a total of 1,018 interventions. Cost-effectiveness was estimated using various methods, including a new context-specific analysis and a literature review. For 159 interventions, average cost-effectiveness ratios were calculated using the generalized cost-effectiveness analysis method and local input data (Eregata et al. 2021). The cost-effectiveness of 393 interventions was analyzed using evidence from the literature—such as DCP3, the Tufts Global Health Cost Effectiveness Analysis Registry,[4] and peer-reviewed articles—after the application of appropriate contextualization to Ethiopia by using general transferability criteria based on the Consolidated Health Economic Evaluation Reporting Standards (Husereau et al. 2013a). Searches for articles used keywords constructed with a combination of the intervention's name, the study location (with priority given to studies done in Ethiopia or another low-income setting), and time (prioritizing recent studies). Two independent reviewers appraised the studies. Those studies deemed to meet a minimum quality standard were accepted for inclusion in the evidence base. For the rest of the interventions, expert opinions were applied. The health system perspective was taken for the cost-effectiveness analysis, using only data transferable to the Ethiopian context (Hailu, Eregata, Yigezu, et al. 2021).

When a cost-effectiveness estimation found in the literature applied to a different setting, the currency difference was adjusted using the appropriate exchange rate and inflated to 2019 US dollars using a gross domestic product deflator. All costs were discounted at 3 percent per year. A study's reported health effects were analyzed and compared with the Ethiopian epidemiological context, with adjustments made as necessary. Primary health outcome measures—discounted at 3 percent per year—included healthy life years gained, disability-adjusted life years averted, and quality-adjusted life years gained (Drummond et al. 2009; Husereau et al. 2013b).

Equity and FRP scores were generated using the Delphi process involving four key steps: (1) defining the equity framework (established on the basis of local social values and policy commitments, prioritizing interventions for the socioeconomically disadvantaged, pregnant mothers, people in remote areas, and children under five years); (2) recruiting experts (a diverse panel of 30 experts from the MoH, academia, professional associations, and civil societies ensured a broad representation of expertise); conducting a Delphi workshop (in April 2019, involving individual scoring, group discussions, and validation) and two rounds of scoring to allow for adjustments based on feedback; and (4) feedback and validation (that is, analysis of scores using descriptive statistics, with summary results shared for further discussion and validation). Final equity and FRP scores, generated using the mean of individual scores, ranged from 1 (lowest) to 5 (highest), with 1 indicating no equity impact/no financial risk and 5 suggesting that not including the intervention would be inequitable and that people would pay large sums out of pocket. Equity and FRP estimates varied widely and were sensitive to the guiding framework of the Delphi process.

The interventions were first ranked according to cost-effectiveness. Next, the ranking was adjusted to account for interventions with high equity and FRP scores. Thus, all the interventions were ranked in descending order by their priority score; cost-effective, equitable, and financially protective health interventions were classified accordingly and included in the EHSP as high-, medium-, and low-priority interventions (MoH 2019).

The gap between aspirational targets and available financial and physical resources constitutes a rate-limiting factor in implementing EHSPs in many low-income countries. The expected available budget determined the set of services to be provided, which made conducting a costing exercise for the EHSP an important step. Figure 2.3 presents the conceptual framework linking costs, available resources, and financial gap analysis. The costing exercise used the OneHealth Tool,[5] for which the default setup included 438 of the 1,018 interventions. The costs of the remaining 580 interventions in the EHSP were manually updated using an Excel spreadsheet. The OneHealth Tool's default data on the cost of drugs and supplies and Ethiopia's default population model were updated with local country-level data.[6]

Budget impact, and the number of interventions the health system needs and can provide, depends on the number of individuals in need and the intervention coverage. The population in need was estimated from the total number of individuals affected by a condition and the proportion of those affected who needed the appropriate intervention. The estimation used prevalence and incidence data estimates from national-level estimates and employed baseline UHC coverage data published by Eregata et al. (2019), supplemented by expert judgments when necessary.

Figure 2.3 Conceptual Framework of the Study, Linking Costs, Available Resources, and Financial Gap Analysis

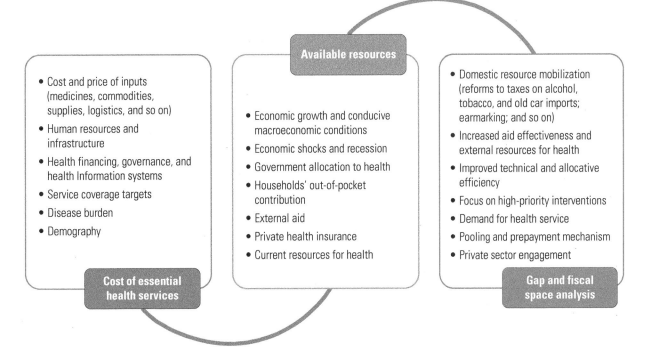

Source: Hailu, Eregata, Stenberg, and Norheim 2021.

Summary of Analysis Findings

The first comprehensive list included 1,749 interventions for consideration. That initial list was then revised to avoid duplication and merged into 1,442 interventions. Various directorates of the MoH then commented on the intervention list. Interventions were further compared to the magnitude of the disease burden or the targeted risk factor. Removing interventions unmatched by the burden of disease or not relevant in the Ethiopian setting reduced the number of interventions to 1,223. Finally, regrouping and reorganizing health interventions yielded 1,018 interventions ready for evaluation and comparison based on the other criteria. Panel a of figure 2.4 presents the interventions by major program area.

Compared with the 2005 Ethiopian EHSP, the revised EHSP includes a wide range of interventions in mental health, neurological disorders, emergency care, noncommunicable diseases, and injuries. For instance, it includes screening and treatment of cervical cancer, cardiac surgery for valvular heart disease, and the diagnosis and management of epilepsy.

Level of priority. The MoH decided to make all 1,018 interventions in the EHSP available. Using the agreed criteria, 594 (58 percent) of the interventions were categorized as high-priority, 213 (21 percent) as medium-priority, and 211 (21 percent) as low-priority interventions (figure 2.4, panel b).

Cost of the EHSP compared to the budget constraint. Figure 2.5 presents the estimated cost per capita of delivering the EHSP interventions. Implementing the EHSP would require estimated per capita costs of US$67, US$94, and US$132 for the low-, medium-, and high-coverage scenarios, respectively, in 2030. The resource needs steadily increase over the projection period. For example, the required resources for the medium-coverage scenario in 2030 (US$94) would cost more than twice as much as in 2020 (US$40).

The projected available resources in a business-as-usual scenario increase from US$40 in 2020 to US$63 in 2030, a resource gap ranging from 1 percent in 2020 to 33 percent in 2030. In general, the estimated required resources are comparable with DCP3, WHO, and Chatham House cost estimates for delivering essential UHC services in a low-income country. The DCP3 projections, using 2016 US dollars, range from US$60 to US$110 per capita (Watkins et al. 2020). WHO estimates indicate a range of US$92 to US$114 total per capita spending in 2014 US dollars, whereas the Chatham House report estimates US$86 per capita in 2012 US dollars (McIntyre and Meheus 2014; Stenberg et al. 2017).

Figure 2.4 Share of EHSP Interventions in Ethiopia, by Major Program Area and Priority Level

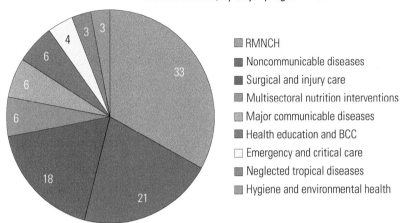

a. Interventions, by major program area

- RMNCH
- Noncommunicable diseases
- Surgical and injury care
- Multisectoral nutrition interventions
- Major communicable diseases
- Health education and BCC
- Emergency and critical care
- Neglected tropical diseases
- Hygiene and environmental health

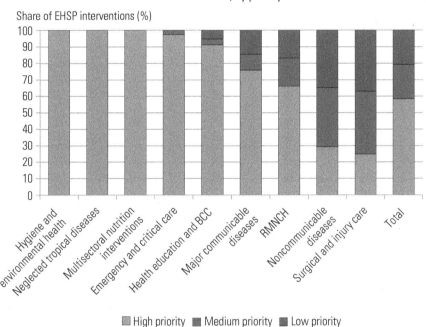

b. Interventions, by priority level

Share of EHSP interventions (%)

- High priority
- Medium priority
- Low priority

Source: MoH 2019.

Note: BCC = behavioral change communication; EHSP = essential health services package; RMNCH = reproductive, maternal, newborn, and child health.

Figure 2.5 Required Resources for Implementation of Ethiopia's EHSP, by Scenario, 2020–30

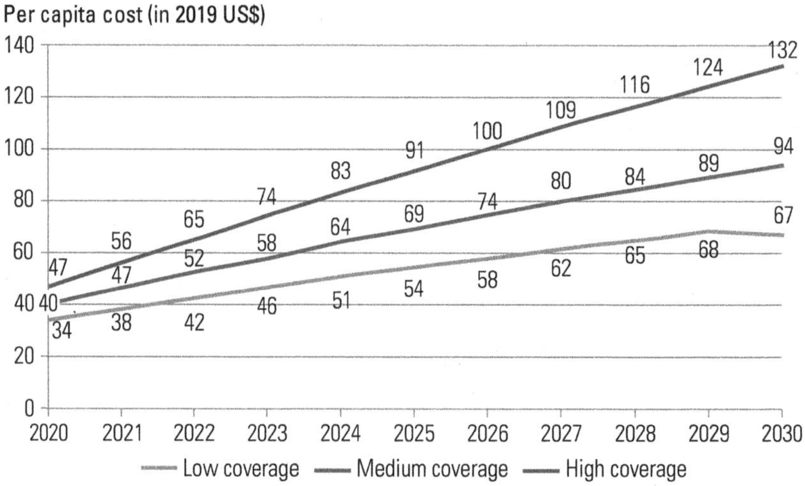

Per capita cost (in 2019 US$)

Source: Hailu, Eregata, Stenberg, and Norheim 2021.

EHSP IMPLEMENTATION PLANS

About 60 percent of the 1,018 interventions can be delivered through primary care (that is, community-based interventions, health posts, health centers, and primary hospitals), about 20 percent at the secondary level of care, and about 20 percent at the tertiary level hospitals (figure 2.6, panel b). When interventions are disaggregated by program area, 70 percent of the reproductive, maternal, newborn, and child health interventions can be delivered at the primary care level. In comparison, only 30 percent should be provided at the secondary or tertiary level of care. In all, 84 percent of the interventions for hygiene and environmental health, and 86 percent of interventions for health education and promotion, can be delivered at the primary care level. By contrast, 53 percent of the more advanced noncommunicable disease and surgical interventions should be delivered at secondary and tertiary hospitals.

According to the revised EHSP, the MoH would provide 570 of the 1,018 interventions (56 percent) free of charge. The remaining services would come with cost-sharing (38 percent) and cost-recovery (6 percent) mechanisms (figure 2.6, panel a). All interventions under the multisectoral and health education program should be provided free of charge, whereas all emergency and critical care interventions should be provided with cost-sharing arrangements. Work is ongoing to practically implement insurance mechanisms that allow for sustainable financing and guaranteed access to these services.

The ability to take corrective action during implementation and to document the lessons learned in implementation will require linking the implementation, monitoring, and evaluation system with the theory of change (Norheim 2018). Launched in November 2019, the revised EHSP serves as a policy goal for the health sector. So far, the country has used the revised EHSP as the basis for the health sector transformation plan (2020) and the human resources for health plan

(2020), and to inform the optimization of the health extension program (2021) and the primary care planning process.

A well-designed EHSP can help decision-makers better organize the health care system in terms of delivery platforms and payment mechanisms (MoH 2015; Glassman, Giedion, Smith 2017). Interventions in the EHSP are linked to clearly defined levels within the current service delivery platform, and the prioritization process informs funding needs and financing arrangements.

Figure 2.6 EHSP Interventions in Ethiopia, by Payment Mechanism and Delivery Platform

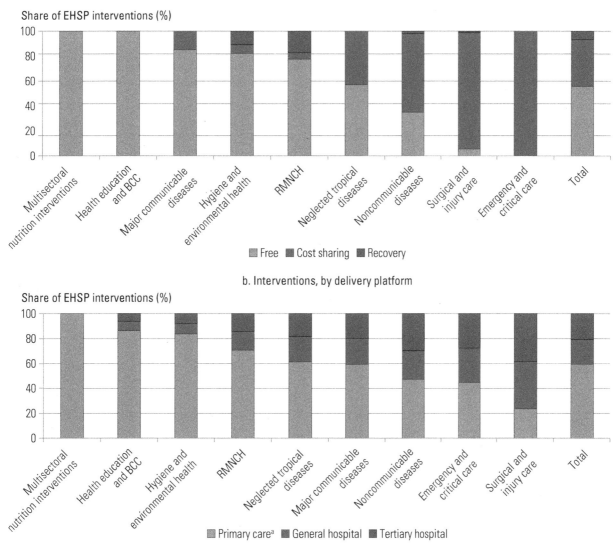

a. Interventions, by payment mechanism

Share of EHSP interventions (%)

Free   Cost sharing   Recovery

b. Interventions, by delivery platform

Share of EHSP interventions (%)

Primary care[a]   General hospital   Tertiary hospital

Source: MoH 2019.

Note: BCC = behavioral change communication; EHSP = essential health services package; RMNCH = reproductive, maternal, newborn, and child health.

a. Primary care includes community-based interventions, health posts, health centers, and primary hospitals.

LIMITATIONS AND FUTURE DIRECTIONS

Data availability represented the most critical challenge in revising the EHSP. A Delphi technique, using expert opinions, was applied to systematically generate equity and FRP scores. That approach can synthesize expert opinions when other data are not available. Although the Delphi technique provided the opportunity to explore equity impact and FRP from a broader perspective (that is, by including socioeconomics, geography, gender, age, and so on), it is prone to various types of biases—highlighting the need to conduct more studies on equity impact and FRP.

Furthermore, method development could advance the Delphi method and other nominal group techniques to better estimate interventions' equity and FRP impacts. In addition, despite the availability of cost-effectiveness information for most of the interventions from peer-reviewed articles of good quality and a comprehensive systematic review provided by DCP3 and others, the transferability and standardization of the results remain imperfect because of factors including inconsistent design (discounting, perspective, currency, and so on) and irregular and nontransparent reporting. More relevant evidence would have been available if more cost-effectiveness analyses were published.

The other significant challenge related to the general approach to EHSP design. Of the three approaches to defining an EHSP—positive listing, negative listing, and a mix of the two techniques—Ethiopia's process applied a positive listing approach. The existence of significant data limitations on the cost and impact of several interventions might have suggested the use of a hybrid system. A negative list could include high-cost interventions with modest health impacts (for example, new immunotherapies for cancer) based on evidence from high-income countries and could have informed decision-makers about what not to invest in (Tangcharoensathien 2019). Because health needs, disease patterns, and health care technology change quickly over time, the MoH has started preparing a road map to institutionalize a health technology assessment mechanism to continuously review new technologies and update the list of interventions in the EHSP on an ongoing basis.

The fiscal space analysis on the Ethiopian EHSP indicates relatively high package costs and the need for substantial additional resources. Linking the EHSP plan with the health care financing strategy will leverage implementation of the package at national and regional levels. Therefore, domestic and external resource mobilization should remain vital components of the EHSP implementation strategy (Hailu, Eregata, Stenberg, and Norheim 2021). The ongoing work of revising the health benefits package for social health insurance and mandatory community-based health insurance provides another example of such an effort to narrow the gap between what the EHSP promises and what it can deliver within existing financial resource constraints.

Finally, overall limited expertise in health economics and the lack of a formal health technology assessment agency in the country present another challenge. The capacity-building activities in the Disease Control Priorities–Ethiopia project have played an important role. Continuous capacity strengthening through the training of health economists is crucial to supporting the use of evidence in strategic purchasing for UHC in Ethiopia (Evans and Palu 2016).

LESSONS LEARNED

In principle, the priority-setting approach for designing an EHSP should employ evidence-based, open, deliberative, participatory decision-making processes. Comparing the approach of the Ethiopian EHSP revision process with normative recommendations offers some lessons for similar future work in Ethiopia or other low- and middle-income countries (Chalkidou et al. 2016; Daniels 2000; Glassman, Giedion, and Smith 2017; Kieslich et al. 2016; Norheim et al. 2014; WHO 2014).

Ensure political commitment. Involving policy makers of all levels from the beginning is essential. Exemplary political commitment and country ownership in Ethiopia drove the revision of the EHSP, which was well embedded in the existing governance system and structure of the MoH. The MoH leadership was actively engaged from the top to medium and even low levels.

Have a road map for the revision. Road map preparation for revising the EHSP was crucial in shaping the process. Starting by preparing a road map for a revision makes the process more transparent and robust. In Ethiopia, the road map included the scope, objective, expected outcomes, methodological details, timeline, governance structure, communication plan, and roles and responsibilities of various stakeholders.

Ensure timeliness. The timeliness of the revision is an essential factor for the uptake of an EHSP. An EHSP should be prepared ahead of national strategic plans (for example, the health sector transformation plan in Ethiopia). The revision of the Ethiopian EHSP aligned with the national health sector transformation plan. Participants should have a clear understanding of the time needed for the revision. Although Ethiopia's road map proposed an initial timeline of 6 months for the revision, the whole process took 18 months (from May 2018 to November 2019).

Design a participatory process. Ethiopia's EHSP revision process was open, participatory, and inclusive (Daniels 2000). It allowed many internal and external stakeholders to actively engage from the inception to the finalization of the EHSP. Five workshops involved health sector policy makers at regional and federal levels, including ministers, state ministers, director generals, directors, technical experts, and regional health bureau heads and deputy heads. Those individuals, responsible for technical and policy decision-making in the health sector, discussed and defined the scope and goal of the revised EHSP, the selection criteria, the proposed payment mechanism, the level of health care delivery, and the budget impact of the package. The same group approved the final, prioritized list of interventions (MoH 2019).

Aim for a comprehensive package. The Ethiopian EHSP was defined comprehensively. Some countries have prepared separate packages for primary and tertiary health care, whereas other countries have separated the noncommunicable diseases package from the reproductive, maternal, newborn, and child health package. Having a single comprehensive package, like Ethiopia's, that encompasses all levels of care and all types of diseases and health conditions is vital for various reasons, such as allocating the available resources for the health sector. Therefore, it is recommended that other countries aim and work toward a more comprehensive package.

Use multicriteria decision-making. Many countries have long used cost-effectiveness as the most commonly applied prioritization criterion in defining EHSP decision-making processes (Blumstein 1997; Jamison et al. 1993). Recently, however, using multiple criteria, as in Ethiopia's EHSP revision, has become a widely accepted approach because of the recognition that UHC is about more than maximizing health (Baltussen and Niessen 2006). The process must also consider FRP, equity and budget impacts, and public and political acceptability. However, using a multiple-criteria approach for priority-setting decisions presents certain challenges. For instance, Ethiopia's design process did not assign specific weights to each criterion but instead employed the criteria holistically. Furthermore, it was difficult to obtain precise data regarding the number of interventions that were either included or excluded because of specific criteria or because of applying a single criterion.

Account for local values. Prioritization criteria should be defined by country context rather than by using generic criteria. Every country decides on national policy goals and the criteria for defining its essential health services. A legitimate, fair decision-making process begins with transparent and inclusive identification of local values, and the criteria-selection process should include all appropriate stakeholders.

ACKNOWLEDGMENTS

The Bill & Melinda Gates Foundation through the Disease Control Priority–Ethiopia project (OPP1162384), as well as the Trond Mohn Foundation and the Norwegian Agency for Development Cooperation through Bergen Centre for Ethics and Priority Setting, funded this study. The funders had no role in the study design, data collection and analysis, decision to publish, or manuscript preparation. The authors gratefully acknowledge the Ministry of Health of Ethiopia for providing the data for this study and thank Stéphane Verguet (Harvard T. H. Chan School of Public Health) for critical feedback.

NOTES

1. United Nations Department of Economic and Social Affairs, "The 17 Goals," https://sdgs.un.org/goals; World Health Organization, "What Is Universal Health Coverage?" https://www.who.int/news-room/questions-and-answers/item/what-is-universal-health-coverage.
2. University of Washington, Department of Global Health, "DCP3 Country Translation," https://www.dcp-3.org (accessed March 30, 2020).
3. WHO, "UHC Compendium" (database), https://www.who.int/universal-health-coverage/compendium (accessed September 29, 2022).
4. Tufts Medical Center, Center for the Evaluation of Value and Risk in Health, "GH CEA Registry," https://cevr.tuftsmedicalcenter.org/databases/gh-cea-registry (accessed March 25, 2020).
5. Avenir Health, "OneHealth Tool," https://www.avenirhealth.org/software-onehealth.
6. University of Washington, Department of Global Health, "DCP3 Country Translation."

REFERENCES

Baltussen, R., and L. Niessen. 2006. "Priority Setting of Health Interventions: The Need for Multi-criteria Decision Analysis." *Cost Effectiveness and Resource Allocation* 4 (14): 14.

Blumstein, J. F. 1997. "The Oregon Experiment: The Role of Cost-Benefit Analysis in the Allocation of Medicaid Funds." *Social Science & Medicine* 45 (4): 545–54.

Chalkidou, K., A. Glassman, R. Marten, J. Vega, Y. Teerawattananon, N. Tritasavat, M. Gyansa-Lutterodt, et al. 2016. "Priority-Setting for Achieving Universal Health Coverage." *Bulletin of the World Health Organization* 94 (6): 462–67.

Daniels, N. 2000. "Accountability for Reasonableness." *BMJ* 321 (7272): 1300–01.

Daniels, N., and J. E. Sabin. 2008. *Setting Limits Fairly: Can We Learn to Share Medical Resources?* Second edition. Oxford: Oxford University Press.

Drummond, M., M. Barbieri, J. Cook, H. A. Glick, J. Lis, F. Malik, S. D. Reed, et al. 2009. "Transferability of Economic Evaluations across Jurisdictions: ISPOR Good Research Practices Task Force Report." *Value in Health* 12 (4): 409–18.

Eregata, G. T., A. Hailu, S. T. Memirie, and O. F. Norheim. 2019. "Measuring Progress towards Universal Health Coverage: National and Subnational Analysis in Ethiopia." *BMJ Global Health* 4 (6): e001843.

Eregata, G. T., A. Hailu, K. Stenberg, K. A. Johansson, O. F. Norheim, and M. Y. Bertram. 2021. "Generalised Cost-Effectiveness Analysis of 159 Health Interventions for the Ethiopian Essential Health Service Package." *Cost Effectiveness and Resource Allocation* 19 (1): 2.

Evans, T. G., and T. Palu. 2016. "Setting Priorities, Building Prosperity through Universal Health Coverage." *Health Systems & Reform* 2 (1): 21–22.

Glassman, A., U. Giedion, Y. Sakuma, and P. C. Smith. 2016. "Defining a Health Benefits Package: What Are the Necessary Processes?" *Health Systems & Reform* 2 (1): 39-50.

Glassman, A., U. Giedion, and P. C. Smith, eds. 2017. *What's In, What's Out? Designing Benefits for Universal Health Coverage.* Washington, DC: Center for Global Development.

Hailu, A., G. T. Eregata, K. Stenberg, and O. F. Norheim. 2021. "Is Universal Health Coverage Affordable? Estimated Costs and Fiscal Space Analysis for the Ethiopian Essential Health Services Package." *Health Systems & Reform* 7 (1): e1870061.

Hailu, A., G. T. Eregata, A. Yigezu, M. Y. Bertram, K. A. Johansson, and O. F. Norheim. 2021. "Contextualization of Cost-Effectiveness Evidence from Literature for 382 Health Interventions for the Ethiopian Essential Health Services Package Revision." *Cost Effectiveness and Resource Allocation* 19 (1): 58.

Hogan, D. R., G. A. Stevens, A. R. Hosseinpoor, and T. Boerma. 2018. "Monitoring Universal Health Coverage within the Sustainable Development Goals: Development and Baseline Data for an Index of Essential Health Services." *The Lancet Global Health* 6 (2): e152–68.

Husereau, D., M. Drummond, S. Petrou, J. Mauskopf, and E. Loder. 2013a. "Consolidated Health Economic Evaluation Reporting Standards (CHEERS) Statement." *Value in Health* 16 (2): e1–e5.

Husereau, D., M. Drummond, S. Petrou, J. Mauskopf, and E. Loder. 2013b. "Consolidated Health Economic Evaluation Reporting Standards (CHEERS)—Explanation and Elaboration: A Report of the ISPOR Health Economic Evaluation Publication Guidelines Good Reporting Practices Task Force." *Value in Health* 16 (2): 231–50.

Jamison, D. T., W. H. Mosley, A. R. Measham, and J. L. Bobadilla. 1993. *Disease Control Priorities in Developing Countries.* New York: Oxford University Press.

Kieslich, K., J. B. Bump, O. F. Norheim, S. Tantivess, and P. Littlejohns. 2016. "Accounting for Technical, Ethical, and Political Factors in Priority Setting." *Health Systems & Reform* 2 (1): 51–60.

McIntyre, D., and F. Meheus. 2014. *Fiscal Space for Domestic Funding of Health and Other Social Services.* London: Chatham House, Centre on Global Health Security.

Misganaw, A., T. N. Haregu, K. Deribe, G. A. Tessema, A. Deribew, Y. A. Melaku, A. T. Amare, et al. 2017. "National Mortality Burden Due to Communicable, Non-communicable, and Other Diseases in Ethiopia, 1990–2015: Findings from the Global Burden of Disease Study 2015." *Population Health Metrics* 15: 29.

MoH (Ministry of Health of Ethiopia). 2005. *Ethiopian Essential Health Service Package 2005.* Addis Ababa: Government of Ethiopia.

MoH (Ministry of Health of Ethiopia). 2015. *Health Sector Transformation Plan 2008–2012 EFY.* Addis Ababa: Government of Ethiopia.

MoH (Ministry of Health of Ethiopia). 2018. *Roadmap for the Revision of Essential Health Service Package for Ethiopia.* Addis Ababa: Government of Ethiopia.

MoH (Ministry of Health of Ethiopia). 2019. *Essential Health Services Package of Ethiopia 2019.* Addis Ababa: Government of Ethiopia.

Norheim, O. F. 2018. "Disease Control Priorities Third Edition Is Published: A Theory of Change Is Needed for Translating Evidence to Health Policy." *International Journal of Health Policy and Management* 2018; 7(9): 771–77.

Norheim, O. F., R. Baltussen, M. Johri, D. Chisholm, E. Nord, D. W. Brock, P. Carlsson, et al. 2014. "Guidance on Priority Setting in Health Care (GPS-Health): The Inclusion of Equity Criteria Not Captured by Cost-Effectiveness Analysis." *Cost Effectiveness and Resource Allocation* 12 (1): 18.

Reich, M. R. 2016. "Introduction to the PMAC 2016 Special Issue: 'Priority Setting for Universal Health Coverage.'" *Health Systems & Reform* 2 (1): 1–4.

Rieger, M., N. Wagner, and A. S. Bedi. 2017. "Universal Health Coverage at the Macro Level: Synthetic Control Evidence from Thailand." *Social Science & Medicine* 172: 46–55.

Stenberg, K., O. Hanssen, T. Tan-Torres Edejer, M. Bertram, C. Brindley, A. Meshreky, J. E. Rosen, et al. 2017. "Financing Transformative Health Systems towards Achievement of the Health Sustainable Development Goals: A Model for Projected Resource Needs in 67 Low-Income and Middle-Income Countries." *The Lancet Global Health* 5 (9): e875–87.

Tangcharoensathien, V., W. Patcharanarumol, W. Suwanwela, S. Supangul, W. Panichkriangkrai, H. Kosiyaporn, and W. Witthayapipopsakul. 2019. "Defining the Benefit Package of Thailand Universal Coverage Scheme: From Pragmatism to Sophistication." *International Journal of Health Policy and Management* 9 (4): 133–37.

Terwindt, F., D. Rajan, and A. Soucat. 2016. "Priority-Setting for National Health Policies, Strategies and Plans." In *Strategizing National Health in the 21st Century: A Handbook*, edited by G. Schmets, D. Rajan, and S. Kadandale. Geneva: World Health Organization.

Wagstaff, A., and S. A. Neelsen. 2020. "Comprehensive Assessment of Universal Health Coverage in 111 Countries: A Retrospective Observational Study." *The Lancet Global Health* 8 (1): e39–e49.

Watkins, D. A., J. Qi, Y. Kawakatsu, S. J. Pickersgill, S. E. Horton, and D. T. Jamison. 2020. "Resource Requirements for Essential Universal Health Coverage: A Modelling Study Based on Findings from Disease Control Priorities, 3rd edition." *The Lancet Global Health* 8 (6): e829–39.

WHO (World Health Organization). 2014. *Making Fair Choices on the Path to Universal Health Coverage: Final Report of the WHO Consultative Group on Equity and Universal Health Coverage.* Geneva: World Health Organization, 2014.

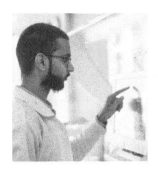

3

Using Evidence-Informed Deliberative Processes to Design Pakistan's Essential Package of Health Services

Sameen Siddiqi, Raza Zaidi, Maryam Huda, Ina Gudumac, and Ala Alwan

ABSTRACT

Pakistan developed its first evidence-informed essential package of health services using evidence from the third edition of *Disease Control Priorities* (Jamison et al. 2018) as a key component of universal health coverage reforms. The final package focuses on primary health care and comprises 88 publicly financed and 12 population-level interventions. The design followed an evidence-informed deliberative process to develop affordable services that represent good value for money and address a major part of the country's disease burden. This chapter describes Pakistan's experience in developing the package, focusing on the processes used to prioritize services, the policy decisions adopted, and the gaps and lessons learned in designing the package.

INTRODUCTION

As part of the United Nations (UN) Sustainable Development Goals (SDGs), Pakistan along with other Member States committed in 2015 to achieve universal health coverage (UHC) by 2030 (Tangcharoensathien, Mills, and Palu 2015). Global commitment to UHC was reinforced, in 2019, in a special high-level meeting of the UN General Assembly on UHC when heads of state and government pledged to scale up efforts in improving access to essential health services (Rodi et al. 2022; UN General Assembly 2019). Despite that commitment, significant challenges remain. For instance, the global UHC service coverage index of 68 reported in 2023 means that one-third of the world's population lacks access to essential health services (WHO and World Bank 2023). In addition, at least 1.4 billion people face impoverishing health spending (WHO and World Bank 2021). The situation in Pakistan is no different: almost half of the population lacks access to essential services, and over 13 percent of households incurred catastrophic health expenditure in 2018–19 (Bashir, Kishwar, and Salman 2021).

A key step in the road map to UHC is for countries to develop an essential package of health services (EPHS) that is evidence informed, feasible, of high impact, and accessible to all. The first chapter of this volume describes the principles of UHC, its three fundamental dimensions, and the strategic directions adopted by Pakistan for designing the EPHS. Despite several past efforts to develop an EPHS for Pakistan, none applied the UHC principles and strategic directions. For instance, the package of services offered in the provinces by the Sehat Sahulat Program, a social health insurance initiative, is for inpatients only, and there are concerns about whether it is evidence informed (Khan, Cresswell, and Sheikh 2022).

The initiative published by the World Bank in its third edition of *Disease Control Priorities* (DCP3) provides an up-to-date review of priority health interventions for low- and lower-middle-income countries through a systematic appraisal of evidence, new economic analyses, and expert judgment across 21 health areas, with the goal of influencing resource allocation at the country level (Jamison 2018). DCP3 proposes two generic packages: an essential UHC (EUHC) package for lower-middle-income countries that has 218 interventions, and a highest-priority package that includes 108 interventions to serve the immediate needs of low-income countries with severely constrained fiscal space (Jamison 2018).

In 2018, a DCP3 Country Translation Project was established to support pilot countries in using the DCP3 evidence to guide the development of their national UHC benefit package (EPHS and intersectoral policy actions). Pakistan was among the first countries to adopt the DCP3 evidence and approach in its effort to accelerate progress toward UHC and develop a national EPHS. Its experience has been extensively documented in an editorial and five papers published in a special supplement on Pakistan by the *International Journal of Health Policy and Management* in 2023–24 (Alwan, Jamison, et al. 2024; Alwan, Siddiqi, et al. 2024; Baltussen et al. 2023; Huda et al. 2023; Raza et al. 2024; Torres-Rueda et al. 2024). Chapters 1 and 15 of this volume review specific aspects of the Pakistan experience published in that supplement.

This chapter provides a bird's-eye view of Pakistan's health care system; the process of developing the EPHS, including the methodological aspects; the final package endorsed by the government; and the challenges encountered. It concludes by presenting the lessons learned for the benefit of other low- and lower-middle-income countries. The special supplement provides a more elaborate review of the experience and an overview of the lessons learned.[1]

PAKISTAN'S HEALTH CARE SYSTEM: CONTEXT AND CHALLENGES

Pakistan is the world's fifth most populous country, with a projected population of over 250 million people in 2024—including the regions of Azad Jammu and Kashmir, and Gilgit Baltistan. Pakistan's population is predominantly young, with 40 percent under the age of 15 and 19 percent ages 15–25 years. Relatedly, 56 percent of the total population falls in the productive age group (15–65 years), and only 4.2 percent is 65 years and above.[2] In addition, Pakistan has been hosting more than 1.4 million registered Afghan refugees for over four decades.[3]

Pakistan, a lower-middle income country, had a gross domestic product of US$383 billion in 2021–22, which translates to per capita income of US$1,798 (Pakistan, Ministry of Finance 2021). According to a 2019 government report, nearly 37 percent of Pakistanis live in multidimensional poverty (Planning Commission of Pakistan and UNDP 2019). Urban areas have a poverty rate of 32.1 percent and rural areas of 39.3 percent.

According to National Health Accounts data, Pakistan has low total per capita health expenditure from all sources, at US$52 (Pakistan Bureau of Statistics 2017). By comparison, such spending averages US$135 in other lower-middle-income countries, US$477 in upper-middle-income countries, and US$3,135 in high-income countries.[4] Pakistan's low health spending can be attributed to the relatively small share of total government spending on health, a level that cannot adequately support universal coverage with essential quality health services. Pakistan's 2020–21 public expenditure on health—PRe 657 billion, equivalent to US$4.1 billion (Pakistan, Ministry of Finance 2021)—represented less than 6 percent of total government spending, compared to an average of 10 percent in developing countries and 15 percent in high-income countries.

Pakistan's low government spending could also reflect the limited capacity to mobilize revenues. Government efforts to raise taxes consistently fall short at 9.4 percent of gross domestic product (base year 2016) in 2021,[5] compared to a minimum threshold of 15 percent identified by the International Monetary Fund as critical to engender sustained, inclusive growth (World Bank 2019). Low levels of domestic government financing mean that a substantial gap currently exists between available resources and the costs of financing an essential package of quality health services for everyone. Filling that gap will require good economic growth, along with political stability and strong commitment for efficient and effective health reforms.

Because of the low levels of government spending, out-of-pocket payments constitute a large share of health spending in Pakistan—51.9 percent of the total health expenditure (Pakistan Bureau of Statistics 2017). By comparison, the global average for out-of-pocket spending is about 15 percent. Such payments prevent some people from using needed essential health services, and push others into poverty.

Pakistan's health care delivery system consists of a mix of public and private sector providers. According to Pakistan's Constitution, provision of health is mainly the responsibility of provincial governments, but with some federal health function mentioned in Federal Legislative Lists I and II (National Assembly of Pakistan 1973). The public sector provides health care at multiple levels, including community health workers, primary health care (PHC) centers, first-level hospitals, and tertiary hospitals (MoNHSR&C 2018b). In addition, vaccinators and environmental and infectious diseases field staff provide outreach services. However, the core of the PHC system in the public sector consists of Health Houses (community-based Lady Health Workers), Basic Health Units, Community Health Centres (or 24/7 Basic Health Units), and Rural Health Centres. Referral services are supposed to be provided for acute, ambulatory, and inpatient care through the Tehsil/Taluka Headquarter Hospitals and District Headquarter Hospitals supported by tertiary care and teaching hospitals (table 3.1). Promotive and preventive services are augmented through public health programs (moving gradually toward horizontal integration) and through population-level interventions.

Table 3.1 Number of Public Sector Health Care Facilities in Pakistan, by Type

Type of facility	Number
Hospitals (secondary and tertiary)	1,276
Rural Health Centres	736
Basic Health Units	5,558
Dispensaries	5,802
Maternal and Child Health Centres	780
Tuberculosis Centres	416
Health Houses (Lady Health Workers)	89,240

Source: Pakistan, Ministry of Finance 2021.

The private sector is also active at all five levels of the health care delivery system, with community-based organizations and workers at the community level, clinics of general practitioners and nursing homes at the PHC center level, first-level hospitals with more and fewer than 50 beds, tertiary or specialized hospitals, and population-level interventions.

By the end of 2021, Pakistan had an estimated 120,334 hospital beds in the public sector and 112,841 in the private sector, for a total of 233,175 beds. Overall, the hospital bed density (both public and private) was only 10 hospital beds per 10,000 people, against the desired minimum threshold of 18 beds (MoNHSR&C, DCP3, and WHO 2022).

According to the National Health Vision (NHV) 2016–25, workforce constraints represent the most critical factor in the provision of quality preventive, promotive, and curative services (MoNHSR&C 2016). The health sector faces an imbalance in the number, skill mix, and deployment of human resources for health as well as inadequate resource allocation across the different levels of health care. Other pressing issues include maldistribution of human resources, retention issues, and low workplace satisfaction levels, which result in significant brain drain across all levels. Adequate quantity, quality, and performance of health workers are crucial for the effective functioning of health systems. Considering its production capacity, Pakistan can achieve the target of an adequate number of physicians by 2030. Achieving the required numbers of nurses, Lady Health Workers, and Community Midwives by 2030, however, continues to present a major challenge (table 3.2).

Table 3.2 Pakistan's Essential Health Workforce, 2030 Target and Current Status

Type of worker	2030 target	Current status (registered as of end-2021)
Number of physicians	314,170	270,168
Number of nurses, Lady Health Workers, and Community Midwives	942,511	138,107

Source: MoNHSR&C 2022.

In 2016, the Ministry of National Health Services Regulations and Coordination (MoNHSR&C) and provincial authorities agreed on the NHV 2016–25. The NHV strives to provide a unified direction to overcome the key health challenges by "providing universal access to affordable, quality, essential health services which are delivered through a resilient and responsive health system, capable of attaining the Sustainable Development Goals and fulfilling its other global health responsibilities" (MoNHSR&C 2016).

The NHV and its eight thematic pillars have the support of all provincial governments, and the next generation of health strategies for provinces/federating areas align with the NHV. Localization of health-related SDGs in Pakistan offered a monitoring framework for the NHV, setting the UHC service coverage index (SCI) as one of the main outcome indicators (SDG indicator 3.8.1) along with reduction in catastrophic health expenditures (SDG indicator 3.8.2). The baseline value for the UHC SCI was estimated at 40 percent in 2015 for Pakistan, lower than the corresponding value of 42 percent for Sub-Saharan Africa for the same year (WHO and World Bank 2017).

Accordingly, MoNHSR&C and the Provincial Health Departments started several UHC-related reforms to improve coverage, along with improvements in data quality for measuring progress. MoNHSR&C regularly collates and analyzes UHC-related data not only at the national and provincial levels but also at the district level (MoNHSR&C 2022). Table 3.3 provides a summary of Pakistan's progress on the UHC SCI. Despite a positive trajectory, Pakistan has made very slow progress and seems unlikely to achieve the national target of 65 percent by 2030 set for the UHC SCI. Figure 3.1 illustrates the trends in catastrophic health expenditures.

Table 3.3 Trends in Pakistan's UHC SCI, National and by Province and Area, 2015–21

Province/Area	UHC service coverage index (0–100)							% change
	2015	2016	2017	2018	2019	2020	2021	
Islamabad	44.7	47.7	48.9	48.5	51.3	56.0	56.3	+25.9
Punjab	40.6	42.8	45.6	47.3	48.2	52.0	53.8	+32.5
Azad Jammu and Kashmir	39.0	40.7	43.6	46.2	47.9	49.8	50.2	+28.8
Khyber Pakhtunkhwa	36.2	40.7	45.8	47.3	47.6	50.3	49.8	+37.5
Sindh	37.6	40.6	43.9	45.0	46.7	48.6	48.0	+27.6
Balochistan	27.1	29.3	32.3	33.5	35.0	35.2	35.7	+31.7
Pakistan	**39.7**	**42.1**	**45.3**	**46.3**	**47.1**	**49.9**	**52.0**	**+30.9**

Source: MoNHSR&C 2022.

Note: SCI = service coverage index; UHC = universal health coverage.

Figure 3.1 Trends in Catastrophic Health Expenditure in Pakistan, 2000–18

Catastrophic health expenditure (> 10% of HH income, percent)

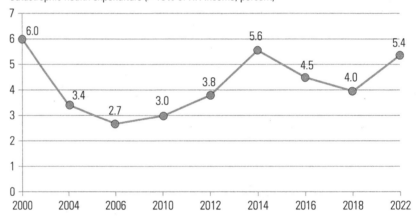

Source: Pakistan Bureau of Statistics data, 2000–22. https://www.pbs.gov.pk/publication/national-health-accounts-pakistan-2021-22

Note: Catastrophic health expenditure represents the share of households spending more than 10 percent of their income on health. HH = household.

EPHS/UHC BENEFIT PACKAGE DEVELOPMENT PROCESS AND THE METHODOLOGY ADOPTED

The government of Pakistan has committed to UHC and to achieving equitable access to essential health care as clearly stated in the NHV 2016–25. The 12th Five-Year Plan (health chapter) and National Action Plan 2019–23 also underscore the provision of essential health services (MoNHSR&C 2018a, 2018b). To translate the government's commitment into action, MoNHSR&C established a collaboration with the DCP3 Country Translation Project and the World Health Organization (WHO) to develop an EPHS based on localized evidence and considering the interventions recommended by DCP3.

The effort was launched in 2018 during an international workshop held in Islamabad and organized by the government of Pakistan, DCP3, and WHO. Participants from countries of the Eastern Mediterranean were sensitized to the concept and the evidence on cost-effective interventions for low- and lower-middle-income countries described in the nine DCP3 volumes and model packages (Jamison et al. 2018). The workshop recommended that Pakistan develop an evidence-informed EPHS and an intersectoral action plan based on the DCP3 global recommendations. The Inter-Ministerial Health and Population Council subsequently endorsed that recommendation. A formal request was then submitted to the DCP3 secretariat to provide technical assistance for adapting the DCP3 evidence to develop the EPHS/UHC benefit package for Pakistan.

A road map for the development of Pakistan's EPHS/UHC benefit package was developed following a joint DCP3 and WHO mission in January 2019. Around the same time, MoNHSR&C initiated a process to map Pakistan's existing essential health services. The assessment revealed that only 135 (or 62 percent) of the 218 DCP3 EUHC interventions were being implemented in facilities (not withstanding service quality). Of those interventions, 42 (31 percent) were generally available and 93 (69 percent) had limited availability. As shown in table 3.4, only 16 of the 45 (35 percent) EUHC interventions were available in the noncommunicable diseases (NCDs) and injuries cluster (MoNHSR&C, WHO, and DCP3 2019).

Table 3.4 Mapping of Pakistan's Available DCP3 EUHC Health Interventions, by Cluster

Cluster[a]	No. of EUHC interventions	No. of available interventions	General availability	Limited availability
RMNCAH	67	50	22 (44%)	28 (56%)
Communicable diseases	52	32	10 (31%)	22 (69%)
NCDs and injuries	45	16	6 (37.5%)	10 (62.5%)
Health services	54	37	4 (11%)	33 (89%)
Total	**218**	**135**	**42 (31%)**	**93 (69%)**

Source: Alwan, Siddiqi, et al. 2024.

Note: DCP3 = *Disease Control Priorities*, third edition; EUHC = essential universal health coverage; NCDs = noncommunicable diseases; RMNCAH = reproductive, maternal, newborn, child, and adolescent health.

a. Clusters matching definitions from DCP3.

The mapping exercise demonstrated major gaps in accessing essential services across all four clusters proposed by the DCP3 model package. Following that exercise, an initial list of 193 out of the 218 EUHC interventions was recommended for formal assessment and prioritization. Concurrently, four National Technical Working Groups (TWGs)—one for each cluster—were established, and workshops were organized covering communicable diseases; NCDs and injuries; reproductive, maternal, newborn, child, and adolescent health; and health system services.

The DCP3 Country Translation Project for Pakistan was formally established in July 2019 during the joint DCP3 and WHO Mission. The Health Planning, System

Strengthening and Information Analysis Unit of MoNHSR&C; the Department of Community Health Sciences of Aga Khan University; the Health Services Academy; WHO; and the DCP3 Country Translation Project based at the London School of Hygiene & Tropical Medicine agreed on a partnership. MoNHSR&C and DCP3 also signed a formal memorandum of understanding.

The process of developing the package was guided by a set of key principles: transparency and inclusivity, national ownership and execution, a focus on ensuring the affordability of the package and feasibility of its implementation, and engagement of public sector institutions, nongovernmental stakeholders, and development partners. The approach to arrive at the package included robust governance and institutional arrangements, engaging a wide range of stakeholders, and conducting an evidence-based appraisal and prioritization process. The governance structure was put in place by instituting a secretariat within MoNHSR&C, with technical support from the DCP3 Country Translation Project (figure 3.2).

Figure 3.2 Governance Structure for the Development of Pakistan's UHC EPHS

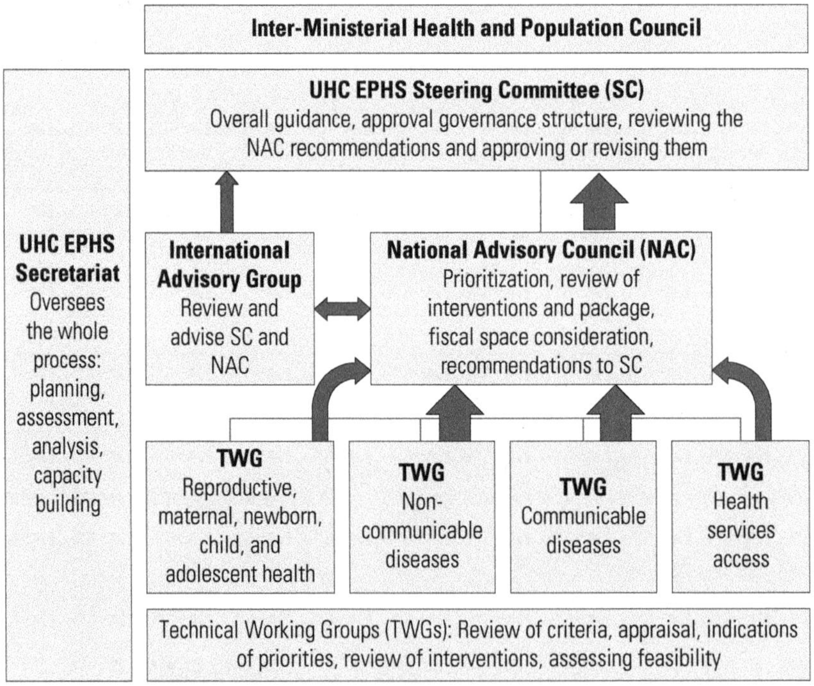

Source: Alwan, Siddiqi, et al. 2024.

Note: Arrows represent the flow of information. Larger arrows represent reporting obligations. EPHS = essential package of health services; UHC = universal health coverage.

The decision-making forums included (1) four TWGs, with membership representing a range of public health, health system, and clinical professions; (2) the National Advisory Committee; (3) the UHC EPHS Steering Committee, chaired by the federal Minister of Health; and (4) the Inter-Ministerial Health and Population Council, which includes the federal and provincial ministers of health and population. In addition, an International Advisory Group, comprising experts and DCP3 authors, reviewed the process and methodologies and provided extensive input to successive versions of the EPHS.

A survey was conducted among all TWG members to identify criteria that would facilitate the prioritization process. The initially proposed criteria included avoidable burden of disease, cost-effectiveness, financial risk protection, budget impact, equity, feasibility, and socioeconomic impact. The assessment process considered three criteria using quantitative evidence: burden of disease, budget impact, and cost-effectiveness. The TWGs considered and discussed other criteria identified by the survey, but data on those criteria were insufficient to make a quantitative assessment.

For burden of disease, the most recent evidence was obtained from the Institute for Health Metrics and Evaluation's 2017 Global Burden of Disease study (2019 data for provincial/federating areas' EPHS).[6] Evidence on cost-effectiveness, a critical step in the choice of interventions, came primarily from the Tufts Medical Center Global Health Cost-Effectiveness Analysis Registry,[7] which compiles incremental cost-effectiveness ratio data on many interventions. The remaining incremental cost-effectiveness ratio data came from the DCP3 database. Applicability of global cost-effectiveness evidence to the country context was systematically assessed using general and specific knockout criteria.

For evidence on budgetary impact, a context-specific, normative, ingredients-based rapid method was developed to estimate the unit costs of the DCP3 EUHC interventions. Costing, undertaken from a provider's perspective, used a one-year time frame. A bottom-up approach to costing was applied to community, health center, and hospital platforms, whereas a top-down approach was used for population-based interventions. The approach followed the principles set out in the Global Health Costing Consortium reference case, largely considered the gold standard for costing health interventions in lower-middle-income countries (Vassall et al. 2017). Unit costs per beneficiary for each intervention were calculated in 2019 US dollars.

For each of the 170 shortlisted and costed DCP3 EUHC interventions, the evidence on decision criteria was reported to the TWGs and the National Advisory Committee using a combination of intervention descriptions and evidence summary sheets. The intervention descriptions sheets contained details on the delivery platform, process, providers, medicines, supplies, equipment, health information tools, supervision, availability of in-service training curriculum, and reference documents. The evidence summary sheets included information on burden of disease, cost-effectiveness and rank order, quality of cost-effectiveness evidence, and budget impact for each intervention. Total costs, disability-adjusted life years averted, and a bookshelf of interventions were also presented, using a combination of the Health Interventions Prioritization tool (HIPtool) and bespoke analyses.

Prioritization of the shortlisted DCP3 EUHC interventions was initially conducted through meetings held by the TWGs and using the agreed-upon decision criteria. The interventions were initially prioritized and costed for community, health center, first-level hospital, tertiary/referral hospital, and population-level platforms. A district-level package of 117 interventions covering three platforms (community, health center, and first-level hospital) was designed, with an overall per capita cost of US$29.70.

As highlighted earlier, affordability and feasibility of implementation of the EPHS are key principles adopted for the design process. Because the cost of the district package exceeded the fiscal space for public health expenditure, a second prioritization process was necessary (Alwan, Siddiqi, et al. 2024). Estimating that about 60 percent of public health expenditure goes to the district level, MoNHSR&C arrived at a limit of US$13 per capita for a package of interventions for immediate implementation. It aimed to develop an affordable and feasible package for immediate implementation until health allocations increased to match the costs of the full district-level EPHS. The National Advisory Committee decided to recommend a more limited immediate implementation package of district-level interventions, covering the community, health center, and first-level hospital platforms.

The International Advisory Group and MoNHSR&C's various departments and programs subsequently reviewed the immediate implementation package. In October 2020, the UHC-EPHS Steering Committee and the Inter-Ministerial Health and Population Council approved a final package of 88 district-level interventions and 12 population-level interventions.

The Inter-Ministerial Health and Population Council further decided to localize scientific evidence at the province/federating area level and produce EPHS documents specific to the province/federating area. That exercise was done in 2021 by the Health Planning, System Strengthening and Information Analysis Unit using the national description of interventions, incremental cost-effectiveness ratio, and costing of each intervention, except with minor adjustments to salaries using values specific to the province/area. The remaining evidence was specific to the province/federating area, including burden of disease data (2019), targeted population, budget impact, estimates for health system cost, unit cost per intervention and per capita, and disability-adjusted life years averted.

PAKISTAN'S ESSENTIAL PACKAGE OF HEALTH SERVICES

Developed and approved at the national level, the final district-level EPHS comprised a total of 88 health care interventions across three levels of care: community, PHC centers, and first-level hospitals. It reflected evidence gathered on the burden of disease, cost-effectiveness, budget impact, feasibility, financial risk protection, equity, and social context of Pakistan. On initial implementation, that district-level EPHS would cost an estimated US$12.98 per person per year (table 3.5).

Table 3.5 Distribution and Cost of Pakistan's EPHS Interventions, by Cluster and Platform

| Platform | Initially prioritized | Finally selected | Distribution by clusters | | | | Unit cost ($)/ person/year |
			RMNCAH	Infectious diseases	NCDs and injuries	Health services	
Community	28	19	15	3	1	0	2.92
PHC center	43	37	13	7	9	8	4.40
First-level hospital	46	32	14	2	3	13	5.66
District	117	88	42	12	13	21	12.98

Source: Health Planning, System Strengthening and Information Analysis Unit, Pakistan Ministry of National Health Services Regulations and Coordination.

Note: EPHS = essential package of health services; NCDs = noncommunicable diseases; PHC = primary health care; RMNCAH = reproductive, maternal, newborn, child, and adolescent health.

The EPHS has 19 interventions at the community level, mainly provided through Lady Health Workers and Community Midwives; 37 interventions at the PHC level, to be offered through Basic Health Units, Rural Health Centres, and dispensaries; and 32 interventions at first-level hospitals—that is, Tehsil Headquarter and District Headquarter Hospitals in the respective districts. The reproductive, maternal, newborn, child, and adolescent health cluster accounts for almost half of the interventions (42), with the other half divided among the remaining three clusters: 12 in infectious diseases, 13 in NCDs and injuries, and 21 in health system services (table 3.5).

DEVELOPMENT OF THE EPHS FOR PROVINCES/FEDERATING AREAS

After the development of the generic EPHS for Pakistan, adapting the package was a critical step before rolling it out across the provinces/federating areas. Each province is unique with respect to health system dynamics, prioritized interventions, health service delivery, and barriers to accessible health care. As such, to streamline interventions and maximize impact and population health outcomes, it is crucial that each province consider the local context and evidence in adapting the EPHS. Each province/area carried out a separate exercise and prioritized interventions for its EPHS. The total number of interventions across five platforms varied from 132 to 153 (compared to a range of 90 to 104 for the district-level EPHS), costing US$15.82 and averting almost 15.32 million disability-adjusted life years on average. Like the outcome of the EPHS design process at the national level, the total cost of the district-level package exceeds the available fiscal space in most provinces and a second prioritization process may therefore be required. A comprehensive report published by MoNHSR&C and the DCP3 secretariat provides a more elaborate description of the provincial packages (MoNHSR&C et al. 2023).

MOVING TO EPHS IMPLEMENTATION

The development of DCP3-based packages in Pakistan has made an important contribution to strengthening national capacities in evidence-informed priority setting while ensuring an inclusive consultative process. The DCP3-based packages have also influenced subsector strategies and plans in Pakistan, such as the National NCD and Mental Health Action Framework 2021–30, the Lady Health Workers' Strategic Plan (2022–28), the UHC Investment Case, health system reforms related to polio eradication in 40 high-risk union councils, and the Health-Related Inter-sectoral Interventions Action Plan 2022–30. MoNHSR&C is considering how to use the scientific evidence and package for future reforms in the Global Fund to Fight AIDS, Tuberculosis and Malaria investments in infectious diseases.

Pakistan's EPHS development process was based on sound advocacy and secured commitment from the highest level, including the Cabinet, Inter-Ministerial Health and Population Council, Ministry of Planning, and Provincial Health Departments. That commitment at the design stage is being currently translated into financial commitments not only from the governments at the national and provincial levels but also through additional support from development partners. A National Health Support Programme was established in collaboration with the World Bank to facilitate the pilot implementation of the UHC package. The program has initial funding through a World Bank loan of US$300 million and grants of US$132 million from some development partners (Bill and Melinda Gates Foundation; Global Financing Facility; Global Fund to Fight AIDS, Tuberculosis and Malaria; and Gavi, The Vaccine Alliance).

GAPS AND CHALLENGES

Overall, the DCP3 Country Translation Project in Pakistan is a success story. However, the EPHS design process identified several gaps and challenges that will have implications at the time of implementation. The following paragraphs highlight some of the challenges.

Apart from the unprecedented crisis caused by the COVID-19 pandemic, which coincided with the EPHS development processes, several important challenges arose. One significant constraint involved the scarcity of local data encountered during the health system assessment and prioritization processes. As in most low- and lower-middle-income countries, the reduced capacity to collect, analyze, and generate data, particularly lack of evidence on the cost-effectiveness of interventions, had to be addressed using regionally generated data and global databases despite limitations in the relevance and applicability of such evidence.

Effective monitoring during EPHS implementation will require backup support such as by strengthening health information systems or through periodic surveys that provide progress on measures such as service coverage index, catastrophic health expenditure, economic rate of return, and health outcomes.

Health system assessments and reviews of existing financial schemes are critical components of EPHS development. Although a comprehensive assessment was conducted following package design, it would have been more effective if such a review had been systematically conducted early on as part of the preparatory assessment or at least concurrently with the prioritization process.

A key feature has been the additional cost of health system strengthening and capital investment needed for infrastructure development for EPHS implementation. Although the overall cost of the package factors in the cost of health system strengthening, it does not factor in the cost of infrastructure development. Thus, substantial investment in infrastructure will be needed during package implementation.

The package also needs to provide for greater flexibility and an institutional mechanism for including interventions that address newly emerging diseases (for example, COVID-19) and developing technologies (for example, COVID-19 and malaria vaccines), and mandates such as International Health Regulations within the package.

LESSONS LEARNED IN THE UHC EPHS PROCESS

This section provides a summary of the key lessons learned in Pakistan. The DCP3 Country Translation Project has published a more elaborate review of the experience of six countries, including Pakistan, in developing their own EPHSs (Alwan, Yamey, and Soucat 2023).

The lack of institutional capacity in priority setting and design of the EPHS was an initial challenge but was later effectively addressed by the intensive joint work and partnership with international experts, the DCP3 secretariat, Aga Khan University, and a committed team in MoNHSR&C. Nevertheless, capacity building in those areas and in health financing will still need to be reinforced at the federal and provincial levels. The transition from package design to implementation will also require major efforts in reinforcing capacity in several health system areas (Alwan, Jamison, et al. 2024).

Although donors have shown interest in the implementation of EPHS, there is a need for greater harmonization among donors through better integration across programs for greater value for money. At the same time, enhanced donor coordination will require greater leadership by and synergy among ministries of health, finance, and planning.

Considering the current worsening political and economic situation in Pakistan (such as its high inflation rate), maintaining a high level of government commitment and financial sustainability of the EPHS presents a constant challenge.

The Pakistan experience also highlights important gaps regarding package design. First, it did not involve a robust process of societal dialogue and community engagement. Community engagement would have helped in determining public perception of the top priority health needs and in gaining public support for the health reforms. Experiences in Thailand and Tunisia provide good practices in participatory governance (Ben Mesmia, Chtioui, and Ben Rejeb 2020; Rajan et al. 2019).

Second, stronger engagement of the planning and finance sectors, which control the public purse, would have resulted in a more rigorous understanding of current and future opportunities and the extent to which domestic financing could be made available to implement the package across the SDG timeline. Early engagement of the Ministry of Finance is also essential for a robust assessment of fiscal space and realistic planning for options of increased health allocation.

Third, as previously mentioned, work on assessing the health system should be undertaken concurrently with package development activities to avoid producing an unrealistic package that is not immediately implementable or does not meet the minimum quality standards. Low-quality care has a demonstrated high cost and can undermine efforts to achieve UHC (Ben Mesmia, Chtioui, and Ben Rejeb 2020). The EPHS can be bolstered by examining geospatial effective coverage cascades to best understand the need, use, and quality of health services across the population.

Fourth, there is a strong need for institutionalization of the process in Pakistan and for continued capacity building. The DCP3 Country Translation Project, given its timebound nature, placed particular emphasis on building analytical capacity within MoNHSR&C in priority setting, economic evaluation, and setting and revising EPHSs. A positive spinoff was the successful adaptation of the national EPHS to develop provincial packages, primarily done by national staff trained during the development of the national EPHS. Similar successes could be enjoyed in additional areas relevant to universal effective coverage, for example in building capacity in implementation science and quality improvement methodology to gain even greater efficiencies within health service delivery.

Finally, efforts to estimate the fiscal space for health should inevitably be tied to the macroeconomic situation and assessment of the country's prospects for economic growth. Given the current economic forecast and the effects of the COVID-19 pandemic in Pakistan, it was not considered feasible to rely on macroeconomic growth to generate new resources. In such a situation, other options that demanded consideration were to (1) enhance the efficient use of available resources at least partly by implementing an evidence-informed EPHS; (2) generate new health sector-specific resources through earmarked public health taxes on tobacco and unhealthy foods and beverages, and through other innovative means; (3) increase health allocation by reprioritizing the government budget; (4) mobilize additional resources through external financing; and (5) build implementation and improvement capacity to deliver health services with greater efficiency.

Additionally, Pakistan's experience offers important lessons that should be considered in updating the DCP3 model packages. The EUHC model package is a valuable tool and a good starting point to guide country work, but experience indicates the need for a better-defined and more specific definition of interventions, mainly because some are currently too generic or have multiple components requiring several clinical actions. Although the scope of the proposed interventions covers a wide range of essential services needed in lower-middle-income countries, some critical interventions are missing, notably in the areas of emergency medical services and pandemic preparedness and response. In addition, the review of EPHS design in countries using the DCP3 evidence in recent years has shown that the cost of the DCP3 EUHC interventions is significantly higher than what Pakistan and many other lower-middle-income countries can realistically afford given their limited public health spending (Alwan, Siddiqi, et al. 2024; Gaudin et al. 2023). That challenge is likely to be true even of the more limited DCP3 highest-priority package of 108 interventions. In general, package development is a dynamic exercise that needs to be revisited at regular intervals to respond to changes in disease burden and to emerging health challenges.

CONCLUSION

The development of the EPHS has been at the center of UHC-related health reforms in Pakistan. High-level government commitment and continued support, sustained engagement of national stakeholders and development partners, and highly effective collaboration with the DCP3 Country Translation Project have contributed to a successful outcome. The next challenge, however, is for the government and all stakeholders and partners to move systematically and confidently to ensure an equally promising transition to implementation. The Pakistan experience in designing the UHC EPHS offers important lessons learned for other countries committed to accelerating progress toward UHC. Doing so will require strengthening the health system to the level that allows for effective EPHS implementation, ensuring affordable financing of the EPHS, and reinforcing and institutionalizing technical capacity in priority setting and health reforms within ministries of health.

ACKNOWLEDGMENTS

The contributions made by the following are gratefully acknowledged: Muhammad Khalid; Rob Baltussen; Nichola Kitson; Nuru Saadi, Leon Bijlmakers, Maryam Huda, Maarten Jansen, Wajeeha Raza, Mashal Shah, Sergio Torres-Rueda, Wahaj Zulfiqar, and Anna Vassall.

The development of the Pakistan EPHS was part of the collaboration between the government of Pakistan and the DCP3 Country Translation Project. The engagement of and the input provided by well over 100 national experts from across the country and representatives of development partners is gratefully acknowledged. The support received from the Bill & Melinda Gates Foundation and the WHO in the EPHS process was pivotal to its development.

NOTES

1. For the full list of articles, refer to the *International Journal of Health Policy and Management* web page for the special issue, https://www.ijhpm.com/issue_723_725.html.
2. Pakistan Bureau of Statistics, "7th Population and Housing Census: Detailed Results," https://www.pbs.gov.pk/digital-census/detailed-results.
3. United Nations High Commissioner for Refugees, "Afghan Refugees in Pakistan by Province," https://data.unhcr.org/en/country/pak.
4. World Bank Open Data (database), https://data.worldbank.org/.
5. World Bank Open Data.
6. Institute for Health Metrics and Evaluation, "Global Burden of Disease Study 2017 (GBD 2017) Data Resources," https://ghdx.healthdata.org/gbd-2017; refer also to Institute for Health Metrics and Evaluation, "Global Burden of Disease Study 2019 (GBD 2019) Data Resources, https://ghdx.healthdata.org/gbd-2019.
7. Tufts Medical Center, Center for the Evaluation of Value and Risk in Health, "GH CEA Registry," https://cevr.tuftsmedicalcenter.org/databases/gh-cea-registry.

REFERENCES

Alwan, Ala, Dean T. Jamison, Sameen Siddiqi, and Anna Vassall. 2024. "Pakistan's Progress on Universal Health Coverage: Lessons Learned in Priority Setting and Challenges Ahead in Reinforcing Primary Healthcare." *International Journal of Health Policy and Management* 13 (Special Issue): 1–5. https://doi.org/10.34172/ijhpm.2024.8450.

Alwan, Ala, Sameen Siddiqi, Malik Safi, Raza Zaidi, Muhammad Khalid, Rob Baltussen, Ina Gudumac, et al. 2024. "Addressing the UHC Challenge Using the Disease Control Priorities 3 Approach: Experience from Pakistan and Lessons Learned." *International Journal of Health Policy and Management* 12: 8003. https://doi.org/10.34172/ijhpm.2023.8003.

Alwan, Ala, Gavin Yamey, and Agnès Soucat. 2023. "Essential Packages of Health Services in Low-Income and Lower-Middle-Income Countries: What Have We Learnt?" *BMJ Global Health* 8: e010724. https://doi.org/10.1136/bmjgh-2022-010724.

Baltussen, Rob, Maarten Jansen, Syeda Shehirbano Akhtar, Leon Bijlmakers, Sergio Torres-Rueda, Muhammad Khalid, Wajeeha Raza, et al. 2023. "The Use of Evidence-Informed Deliberative Processes for Designing the Universal Health Coverage Benefit Package in Pakistan." *International Journal of Health Policy and Management* 12: 8004.

Bashir, S., S. Kishwar, and Salman. 2021. "Incidence and Determinants of Catastrophic Health Expenditures and Impoverishment in Pakistan." *Public Health* 197. https://doi.org/10.1016/j.puhe.2021.06.006.

Ben Mesmia, H., R. Chtioui, and M. Ben Rejeb. 2020. "The Tunisian Societal Dialogue for Health Reform (a Qualitative Study)." *European Journal of Public Health* 30 (Supplement_5). https://doi.org/10.1093/eurpub/ckaa166.1393.

Gaudin, Sylvestre, Wajeeha Raza, Jolene Skordis, Agnès Soucat, Karin Stenberg, and Ala Alwan. 2023. "Using Costing to Facilitate Policy Making towards Universal Health Coverage: Findings and Recommendations from Country-Level Experiences." *BMJ Global Health* 8 (Suppl 1): e010735. https://gh.bmj.com/content/8/Suppl_1/e010735.

Huda, Maryam, Nichola Kitson, Nuru Saadi, Saira Kanwal, Urooj Gul, Maarten Jansen, Sergio Torres-Rueda, et al. 2023. "Assessing Global Evidence on Cost-Effectiveness to Inform Development of Pakistan's Essential Package of Health Services." *International Journal of Health Policy and Management* 13 (8005). https://doi.org/10.34172/ijhpm.2023.8005.

Jamison, Dean T. 2018. "*Disease Control Priorities*, Third Edition: Improving Health and Reducing Poverty." *The Lancet* 391 (10125). https://doi.org/10.1016/S0140-6736(15)60097-6.

Jamison, Dean T., Hellen Gelband, Susan Horton, Prabhat Jha, Ramanan Laxminarayan, Charles N. Mock, and Rachel Nugent, eds. 2018. *Disease Control Priorities* (third edition), Volume 9, *Disease Control Priorities: Improving Health and Reducing Poverty*. Washington, DC: World Bank. https://documents.worldbank.org/en/publication/documents-reports /documentdetail/527531512569346552/disease-control-priorities-improving-health-and -reducing-poverty.

Khan, Sheraz Ahmad, Kathrin Cresswell, and Aziz Sheikh. 2022. "Contextualising Sehat Sehulat Programme in the Drive towards Universal Health Coverage in Khyber Pakhtunkhwa, Pakistan." *Khyber Medical University Journal* 14 (1): 63–70. https://doi .org/10.35845/kmuj.2022.21481.

MoNHSR&C (Pakistan, Ministry of National Health Services Regulations and Coordination). 2016. "National Health Vision of Pakistan 2016–2025." Government of Pakistan, Islamabad. https://extranet.who.int/countryplanningcycles/sites/default/files/planning _cycle_repository/pakistan/national_health_vision_2016-25_30-08-2016.pdf.

MoNHSR&C (Pakistan, Ministry of National Health Services Regulations and Coordination). 2018a. "12th Five Year Plan." Government of Pakistan, Islamabad.

MoNHSR&C (Pakistan, Ministry of National Health Services Regulations and Coordination). 2018b. "Action Plan National Health Services, Regulations & Coordination Division (2019–23)." Government of Pakistan, Islamabad.

MoNHSR&C (Pakistan, Ministry of National Health Services Regulations and Coordination). 2022. "Pakistan 2022 UHC Monitoring Report." Government of Pakistan, Islamabad.

MoNHSR&C (Pakistan, Ministry of National Health Services Regulations and Coordination), DCP3 (Disease Control Priorities 3 Country Translation Project), and WHO (World Health Organization). 2022. "Universal Health Coverage Benefit Package of Pakistan: Essential Package of Health Services with Localized Evidence." https://dcp-3.org/resources /universal-health-coverage-benefit-package-pakistan-essential-package-health-services.

MoNHSR&C (Pakistan, Ministry of National Health Services Regulations and Coordination), Disease Control Priorities 3 Country Translation Project, World Health Organization, Aga Khan University, and Radboud University. 2023. "Report on the Priority Setting and Development of the Pakistan Universal Health Coverage Essential Package of Health Services." https://www.dcp-3.org/sites/default/files/resources/Report on development of the Pakistan EPHS for UHC.pdf.

MoNHSR&C (Pakistan, Ministry of National Health Services Regulations and Coordination), WHO (World Health Organization), and DCP3 (Disease Control Priorities 3). 2019. "Review of Essential Health Services in Pakistan Based on Disease Control Priorities 3." http://dcp-3.org/sites/default/files/resources/Review of Essential Health Services Pakistan based on DCP3 WHO 2019_web.pdf.

National Assembly of Pakistan. 1973. *Constitution of the Islamic Republic of Pakistan*. Islamabad: Government of Pakistan.

Pakistan Bureau of Statistics. 2017. "National Health Accounts 2017–18." Government of Pakistan, Islamabad. https://www.pbs.gov.pk/sites/default/files/national_accounts /national_health_accounts/national_health_accounts_2017_18.pdf.

Pakistan, Ministry of Finance. 2021. "Pakistan Economic Survey 2021–22." Government of Pakistan, Islamabad. https://www.finance.gov.pk/survey_2022.html.

Planning Commission of Pakistan and UNDP (United Nations Development Programme). 2019. "Multi-Dimensional Poverty in Pakistan." Government of Pakistan and UNDP. https://www.undp.org/sites/g/files/zskgke326/files/migration/pk/MPI-4pager.pdf.

Rajan, Dheepa, Nanoot Mathurapote, Weerasak Putthasri, Tipicha Posayanonda, Poldej Pinprateep, Sana de Courcelles, Rozenn Bichon, et al. 2019. "Institutionalising Participatory Health Governance: Lessons from Nine Years of the National Health Assembly Model in Thailand." *BMJ Global Health* 4 (Suppl 7). https://doi.org/10.1136 /bmjgh-2019-001769.

Raza, Wajeeha, Wahaj Zulfiqar, Mashal Murad Shah, Maryam Huda, Syeda Shehirbano Akhtar, Urooj Aqeel, Saira Kanwal, et al. 2024. "Costing Interventions for Developing an Essential Package of Health Services: Application of a Rapid Method and Results from Pakistan." *International Journal of Health Policy and Management* 13 (8006). https://doi.org/10.34172/ijhpm.2023.8006.

Rodi, Paolo, Werner Obermeyer, Ariel Pablos-Mendez, Andrea Gori, and Mario C. Raviglione. 2022. "Political Rationale, Aims, and Outcomes of Health-Related High-Level Meetings and Special Sessions at the UN General Assembly: A Policy Research Observational Study." *PLoS Medicine* 19 (1). https://doi.org/10.1371/journal.pmed.1003873.

Tangcharoensathien, Viroj, Anne Mills, and Toomas Palu. 2015. "Accelerating Health Equity: The Key Role of Universal Health Coverage in the Sustainable Development Goals." *BMC Medicine* 13 (1). https://doi.org/10.1186/s12916-015-0342-3.

Torres-Rueda, Sergio, Anna Vassall, Raza Zaidi, Nichola Kitson, Muhammad Khalid, Wahaj Zulfiqar, Maarten Jansen, et al. 2024. "The Use of Evidence to Design an Essential Package of Health Services in Pakistan: A Review and Analysis of Prioritisation Decisions at Different Stages of the Appraisal Process." *International Journal of Health Policy and Management* 13 (8043). https://doi.org/10.34172/ijhpm.2024.8043.

UN (United Nations) General Assembly. 2019. "Political Declaration of the High-Level Meeting on Universal Health Coverage 'Universal Health Coverage: Moving Together to Build a Healthier World.'" https://www.un.org/pga/73/wp-content/uploads/sites/53/2019/07/FINAL-draft-UHC-Political-Declaration.pdf.

Vassall, Anna, Sedona Sweeney, Jim Kahn, Gabriela B. Gomez, Lori Bollinger, Elliot Marseille, Ben Herzel, et al. 2017. "Reference Case for Estimating the Costs of Global Health Services and Interventions." Global Health Cost Consortium. https://ghcosting.org/pages/standards/reference_case.

WHO (World Health Organization) and World Bank. 2017. *Tracking Universal Health Coverage: 2017 Global Monitoring Report*. Geneva: World Health Organization and Washington, DC: World Bank. https://iris.who.int/bitstream/handle/10665/259817/9789241513555-eng.pdf?sequence=1.

WHO (World Health Organization) and World Bank. 2021. *Global Monitoring Report on Financial Protection in Health 2021*. Geneva: World Health Organization and Washington, DC: World Bank. https://www.who.int/publications/i/item/9789240040953.

WHO (World Health Organization) and World Bank. 2023. *Tracking Universal Health Coverage: 2023 Global Monitoring Report*. Geneva: World Health Organization and Washington, DC: World Bank. https://www.who.int/publications/i/item/9789240080379.

World Bank. 2019. "High-Performance Health Financing for Universal Health Coverage: Driving Sustainable, Inclusive Growth in the 21st Century." World Bank, Washington, DC.

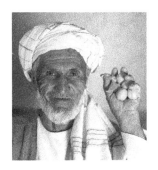

4

Lessons from the Development Process of the Afghanistan Integrated Package of Essential Health Services

Ataullah Saeedzai, Karl Blanchet, Safi Najibullah, Ahmad Salehi, Shafiq Mirzazada, Neha Singh, Gerard J. Abou Jaoude, Wahid Majrooh, Ahmad Jan, Jolene Skordis, Zulfiqar A. Bhutta, Hassan Haghparast-Bidgoli, Ala Alwan, Farhad Farewar, Bill Newbrander, Ritsuko Kakuma, Teri Reynolds, and Ferozuddin Feroz

ABSTRACT

In 2017, in the middle of the armed conflict with the Taliban, Afghanistan's Ministry of Public Health decided that the Afghan health system needed a well-defined priority package of health services that took into account the increasing burden of noncommunicable diseases and injuries and benefited from the latest evidence published in the third edition of *Disease Control Priorities* (Jamison, Gelband, et al. 2018). The resulting two-year process—involving data analysis, modeling, and national consultations—produced the country's integrated package of essential health services. Afghanistan's experience highlights the need to address not only the development of a more comprehensive benefit package but also its implementation and financing. This work, finalized just before the Taliban regime took over, has not been implemented.

INTRODUCTION

Despite an increasing number of armed conflict attacks since 2015, Afghanistan was on the path to universal health coverage (Lozano et al. 2020). Between September 2017 and August 2021 (before the arrival of the Taliban in power), the Ministry of Public Health (MoPH) set up context-specific health, disease, and intersectoral priorities. It carried out that work within the framework of Afghanistan's National

Health Policy 2015–2020 (Alkema et al. 2016), revising its basic and essential packages of health services using data from national surveys, reports, journal articles, and a costing study, and strengthening coordination and cooperation with key partners and line ministries.

The context for the development of a revised health package is one in which the Afghan government, since 2002, had achieved before the arrival of the Taliban substantial improvements in the health status of its population despite serious episodes of insecurity. For example, between 2000 and 2017, the maternal mortality ratio reduced from 1,100 to 638 deaths per 100,000 live births (Alkema et al. 2016) and under-five mortality decreased from 257 to 55 per 1,000 live births between 2000 and 2018 (You et al. 2015).

By 2020, there was clear evidence that the high level of insecurity in some provinces had negatively affected the delivery and coverage of health services, especially for maternal health and childhood vaccines (Akseer et al. 2019). Although all provinces in the country increased the coverage of maternal and child health services between 2005 and 2019 (Akseer et al. 2016; Akseer et al. 2018; World Bank 2018), significant differences remained between the poorest and the wealthiest populations, between rural and urban areas, and between provinces in terms of health outcomes and use and coverage of health services (Bartlett et al. 2017; Rahman et al. 2017). Direct out-of-pocket expenditure by households was high nationally, accounting for 76.5 percent of total health expenditure in 2018. Donors and the government accounted for 19.7 percent and 3.9 percent, respectively, of total health expenditure in 2018 (MoPH 2019).

Key weaknesses in population health observed in Afghanistan between 1990 and 2021 were the high burden of communicable diseases, poor status of maternal and newborn health, poor nutritional conditions, and largely neglected noncommunicable diseases (Shahraz et al. 2014). Among noncommunicable diseases, ischemic heart disease, congenital defects, and cerebrovascular disease all ranked among the leading causes of premature death (IHME 2016). The country had an additional high burden of mental health disorders (Kovess-Masfety et al. 2021; Shoib et al. 2022). According to the 2015 Afghanistan National Drug Use Survey, 2.5 million–2.9 million of Afghans (about 8 percent of the total population) used addictive drugs, and 1.9 million–2.3 million used opiates. The survey found drug use in 31 percent of all households. Nationally, 9 percent of Afghan children under the age of 14 tested positive for drugs, overwhelmingly opioids (APHI/MoPH et al. 2011).

In 2014, conflict-related injuries and road injuries ranked second and fifth, respectively, as causes of premature death (Shahraz et al. 2014). Furthermore, deaths from conflict and terror notably rose by almost 1,200 percent between 2005 and 2016 (IHME 2016). In 2017, Afghanistan recorded the highest number of civilian casualties from attacks in a single year since the United Nations mission in the country began systematic documentation of civilian casualties in 2009. Suicide and complex attacks accounted for 22 percent of all attacks that year, with 16 percent of the casualties taking place in Kabul. Just one attack in the city on May 31, 2017, killed over 200 people and injured nearly 600 (World Bank 2017).

PRIORITY HEALTH PACKAGES IN AFGHANISTAN

In 2001, after the end of the Taliban regime, MoPH had the challenging task of rebuilding the health system, including how best to address the key health challenges in the country—especially given that its maternal and child mortality rates represented the highest mortality rates in the world (UN IGME 2018). In 2002–03, MoPH designed a unique package of health services that helped bring coherence among health stakeholders in what was then a fragmented health system. Toward the end of 2003, MoPH, supported by its international partners, put in place the Basic Package of Health Services (BPHS) for the primary health care level throughout the country. The BPHS was followed in 2005 by the Essential Package of Health Services (EPHS) for hospitals up to the provincial level (Newbrander et al. 2014). The two packages of services have been provided in each province through either a contracting-in or a contracting-out mechanism—two different approaches that have produced similar benefits (World Bank 2018).

MoPH and health economists included in the Expert Committee advising MoPH estimated that the government and donors spent US$235 million on the BPHS and EPHS in 2018, equivalent to US$6.70 per capita. The BPHS accounted for 72 percent, or US$172 million, of that spending, whereas the EPHS accounted for about 28 percent, or US$63 million (Salehi and Blanchet 2021). Maternal and child health accounted for about 45 percent of total BPHS spending. Combined, government and donor spending on the BPHS and EPHS averted an estimated 1.04 million disability-adjusted life years (DALYs). Almost 60 percent (605,000) of DALYs averted by the BPHS and EPHS were related to maternal and child health interventions (Abou Jaoude, Haghparast-Bidgoli, and Skordis-Worrall 2019).

In 2017, MoPH decided that the BPHS and EPHS needed revising in light of the increasing burden of disease since 2006 related to noncommunicable diseases (2.5 percent increase annually) and injuries (4.4 percent increase annually), the international drive for universal health coverage (IHME 2017), and the recent publication of the third edition of *Disease Control Priorities*, or *DCP3* (Jamison, Alwan, et al. 2018). The BPHS had been only slightly revised in 2010, and the EPHS had never been reviewed for its relevance and usefulness since its creation in 2005. In August 2021, the new priority package, the Integrated Package of Essential Health Services (IPEHS), was finalized before the takeover by the Taliban (figure 4.1). Unfortunately, that takeover postponed the implementation of the IPEHS.

Figure 4.1 Timeline of the Development Process of the IPEHS in Afghanistan

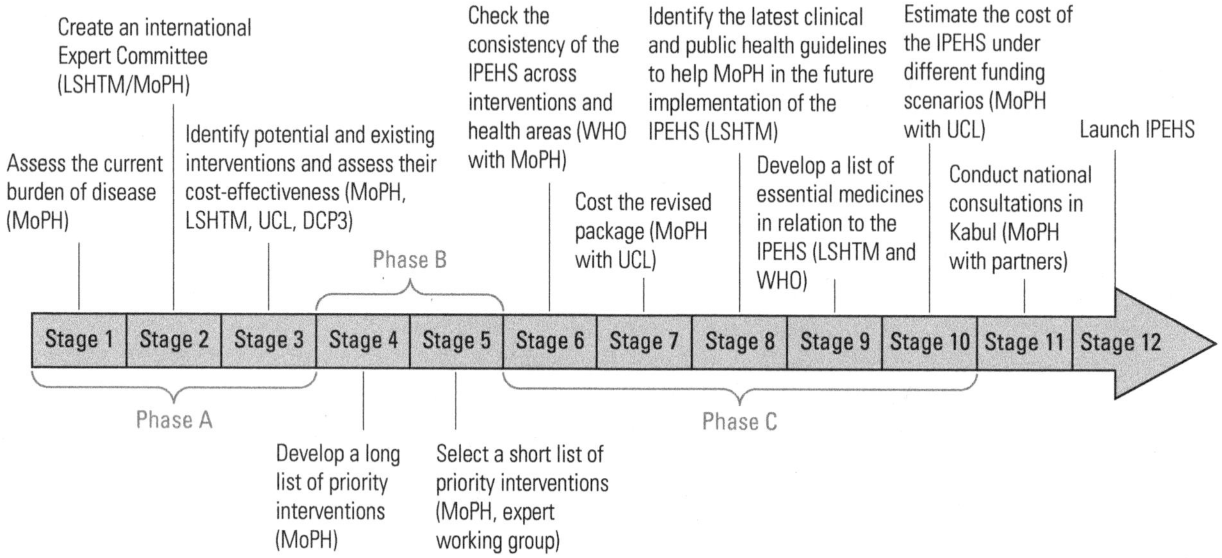

Stage	Time frame	Stage	Time frame
1	November 2017–February 2018	7	January–April 2019
2	December 2017–January 2018	8	January–April 2019
3	February–May 2018	9	January–April 2019
4	May–December 2018	10	January–May 2019
5	May–September 2018	11	February–May 2021
6	January–April 2019	12	August 2021

Source: Original figure created for this publication.

Note: DCP3 = *Disease Control Priorities,* third edition; IPEHS = Integrated Package of Essential Health Services; LSHTM = London School of Hygiene and Tropical Medicine; MoPH = Ministry of Public Health; UCL = University College London; WHO = World Health Organization.

PRIORITY-SETTING PROCESSES

Priority setting in public health and humanitarian contexts is a systematic process designed to allocate resources effectively to address the most critical health needs. It ensures that limited resources are used efficiently to achieve the greatest possible health impact. The priority-setting process involves multiple steps and considerations to ensure it is comprehensive, transparent, and equitable; however, several challenges and dilemmas are expected during the process.

The Various Trade-Offs

The difficult decisions made in Afghanistan when working on the IPEHS between 2018 and August 2021 reflected the need to respond to both the epidemiological transition and the level of violence generated by armed conflict while maintaining gains in maternal and child health, ensuring equitable access to interventions, and providing financial protection—all within a highly constrained government and donor budget envelope. Two key questions for MoPH guided the priority-setting process. First, which interventions in the exising BPHS and EPHS were no longer justified as top priorities and which additional health interventions were needed?

Second, how could the country ensure that the most underprivileged (that is, the poorest and populations living farthest from primary health care facilities) could access the new package of health services?

Priority setting in Afghanistan involved making trade-offs—not only between different health interventions from different disease groups but also between health services, public health interventions, and interventions tackling determinants of health. Those decisions carried with them value judgments and trade-offs between efficiency (cost-effectiveness) and equity. A priority-setting process usually takes place in an environment in which societal values are at stake and tensions exist between different perspectives and interests (González-Pier et al. 2016). Thus, the process requires legitimacy in order to gain any prospect of public and political acceptance. Consequently, the process in Afghanistan rigorously documented all decisions to make sure that every step grew from the previous ones (Lange et al. 2022).

In terms of governance, MoPH, led by the Minister of Public Health, drove the revision process. In its role of overseeing this activity, the MoPH core team created and managed nine in-country Working Groups and obtained and integrated expert opinion from members of the Ministry and the local stakeholder community including international organisations such as United Nations agencies. In Afghanistan, nine multi-stakeholder Working Groups were set up according to health domains (reproductive, maternal, child and adolescent health; mental health; surgery; cardiovascular health; infectious disease; surgery; cancer; palliative care; rehabilitation; and inter-sectoral policy) to provide expertise in reviewing the shortfalls in the BPHS and EPHS. An advisory mechanism in the form of an international Expert Committee was put in place to maximize the use of data and evidence, ensure the adequacy of the methodology, encourage creativity in data analysis, and provide accountability for use of the results by the Afghan government, as well as by national and global stakeholders (Lange et al. 2022, 3).

A Multicriteria Approach

MoPH adopted a multicriteria approach to enable a fair, transparent, and mutual process for setting priorities (Goetghebeur et al. 2017). The approach was based on the following principles: (1) use of the latest global and national evidence on burden of disease and cost-effectiveness of interventions, (2) well-defined selection criteria agreed by all key stakeholders, (3) transparent and documented process of selecting interventions, and (4) recognition that decisions made are reasonable, combining both analysis of evidence and expert discussions.

The selection criteria defined by the Expert Committee in May 2018 to guide decisions of MoPH and experts included the following:

- *Effectiveness*. What has been proven to work?
- *Local feasibility*. What local resources exist? Are staff in place? Are they trained? Does existing infrastructure support the intervention?

- *Affordability.* Are new drugs and equipment required? Is there a large setup cost?
- *Equity.* Will the intervention improve access to care? For whom?

The Expert Committee and MoPH also agreed on a set of priority conditions and risk factors to address the current burden of disease in Afghanistan. The priority conditions included reproductive, maternal, newborn, and child health; injuries (conflict and road traffic accidents); mental health (substance use, suicide, post-traumatic stress disorder); cardiovascular diseases (heart attack, stroke); undifferentiated emergency presentation (difficulty breathing, shock, meningitis, diarrheal disease, lower respiratory diseases); and diabetes. The priority risk factors identified included undernutrition, overnutrition, smoking, water sanitation and hygiene, air pollution, and hypertension.

MoPH designed a flexible process to examine the bigger picture that is internal and external to the setting of priorities by the institution. That process, which also reflected the connection and relationship between the different parts of the health system, involved the following steps:

1. MoPH research teams, with support from academic partners, conducted an analysis of the country's health needs and the health system's capacity.
2. An Expert Committee was established, chaired by the Minister of Public Health and composed of 12 national and international experts including from the DCP3 task force.
3. MoPH formed nine local working groups—one for each of the nine health volumes of DCP3 (Jamison, Gelband, et al. 2018)—to create an initial draft of priority interventions based on field experience.
4. Several opportunities were created for a wide range of stakeholders to help decide the priorities through consultative workshops and meetings with nongovernmental organizations, United Nations agencies, donors, and the president's office.
5. MoPH and the Expert Committee defined clear selection criteria for the setting of priority interventions and opportunities.
6. Academic partners costed the existing and new package of health services and identified relevant global cost-effective interventions.
7. Academic partners made projections of the fiscal space between 2018 and 2030 using different scenarios.
8. MoPH enhanced advocacy and negotiation to mobilize domestic revenue.
9. MoPH rigorously examined the short- and long-term implications of the new package of health services and developed relevant implementation approaches and systems including a tailored monitoring and information system.

At the same time, MoPH determined which of the DCP3 early intersectoral policy interventions was addressed as a priority using standardized and transparent criteria. It also worked on minimizing financial risks to people, especially the poor, in Afghanistan.

The priority-setting process was conducted within the available and projected fiscal space. According to the Ministry of Finance and the 2020 National Health Accounts, 52.0 percent of the national budget was funded by foreign aid, 44.8 percent by domestic revenue, and 3.2 percent by loans (MoPH 2019). From the total budget, MoPH was allocated 5 percent, of which about 79 percent was funded by donors covering the BPHS and EPHS. MoPH's budgetary prospect exercise developed three possible realistic scenarios for budget expansion in order to cover the potential expansion of services provided under the High Priority Programme for Afghanistan (MoPH 2020). The exercise estimated that—assuming stable support from international donors, stable economic growth, and a slight reduction in out-of-pocket spending—total per capita health expenditure would increase by 1 percent per year in a low variant projection, by 5 percent in a medium variant projection, and by 8 percent in a high variant projection (MoPH 2020).

ANALYSIS AND TOOLS

The development of the IPEHS in Afghanistan required not only extensive analyses of existing data sets at DCP3 and in Afghanistan but also some modeling to anticipate the effects of IPEHS on the Afghan population and health system.

Use of DCP3 Data

The third edition of *Disease Control Priorities*, published between 2015 and 2018 in nine volumes, provides a review of evidence on cost-effective interventions to address the burden of disease in low- and middle-income countries (Jamison, Alwan, et al. 2018). It does so by drawing on systematic reviews of economic evaluations, epidemiological data, and clinical effectiveness studies, and on the expertise and time of over 500 authors (Watkins et al. 2018).

DCP3 data, although generally considered thorough and to have been generated in a transparent manner, require considerable adaptation when applied at the country level, especially in those countries, like Afghanistan, where contextually adapted evidence was needed given the complexity brought about by sectarian violence and armed conflict. The DCP3 team advised national health officials that they should modify the DCP3 packages of interventions using local priorities, carry out country-specific analyses as to costs and impact, and consider the need for health system strengthening and implementation monitoring and evaluation.

To inform each health system building block, team members consulted additional sources, including the most recently available national health information systems data and results from the *Afghanistan Demographic and Heath Survey 2015* (CSO, MoPH, and ICF 2017), the mental health survey, and other national surveys (Mirzazada et al. 2020). To develop the list of interventions, working groups compared the DCP3 list of interventions with the existing BPHS and EPHS. MoPH decided that, instead of two distinct packages, one revised package of health services would cover the community level through the provincial level. That decision involved prioritizing the interventions in DCP3 and assigning them to the different categories of health system levels, categorized by health facility type. Contextual knowledge and specialist assessment as to which interventions would be possible given government and partner support at each level were critical for this task.

DALY-Driven Rationale

DALYs are a measure of the burden of disease accounting for the number of years lost because of ill health, disability, or early death. DALYs "measure the gap between a population's health and a hypothetical ideal for health achievement" (Gold, Stevenson, and Fryback 2002, 117–18) and are used in setting health research priorities, identifying disadvantaged groups, and targeting health interventions. Although estimates, projections, and modeling based on mortality—that is, how many deaths could be averted by offering a health service—are popular and compelling, unlike DALYs they do not capture morbidities such as chronic diseases, mental health, injuries, and disabilities that affect quality of life.

The Expert Committee made the decision to use DALYs through the Health Interventions Prioritization tool (HIPtool), a health resource categorized tool, using context-specific data on burden of disease and intervention cost-effectiveness to help stakeholders identify funding priorities and targets. Fraser-Hurt et al. (2021) provide full details on HIPtool, its methodology, and country applications. The reference point for that Expert Committee consultation, the essential universal health coverage package published by DCP3, was based on evidence of cost-effectiveness, presenting data in the form of "cost per DALY averted," an incremental cost-effectiveness ratio (Jamison, Alwan, et al. 2018). DALYs provided a single measure by which to compare interventions across the BPHS and the EPHS. Importantly, given the number of diseases and interventions considered, using a variety of inputs made interpretation of results less clear.

Summary of Analysis Findings

The first comprehensive list included 149 interventions for consideration. For the international Expert Committee meetings, HIPtool generated estimates of DALYs averted by (1) existing spending; (2) additional spending projections based on fiscal space assessments; (3) scaling up existing reproductive, maternal, newborn, and child health interventions in the package; and (4) categorizing spending on the basis of intervention cost-effectiveness and burden of disease. HIPtool categorized spending scenario–supported recommendations on the inclusion of emergency and trauma care as well as cost-effective mental health interventions in the IPEHS.

The IPEHS was organized by the seven levels of the health system: (1) community health posts, (2) mobile health teams, (3) sub health centers, (4) basic health centers, (5) comprehensive health centers, (6) first referral hospitals, and (7) second referral hospitals. To highlight the level of integration and the continuum between the various levels of the health system, the interventions were defined by level according to the resources and skills available at the level with an explicit link to the previous or next level of referral.

Nine domains were defined to help structure the interventions: (1) reproductive, maternal, and newborn health; (2) child and adolescent health and development; (3) infectious diseases; (4) chronic noncommunicable diseases; (5) mental, neurological, and substance use disorders; (6) emergency care; (7) surgical interventions; (8) palliative care; and (9) rehabilitation. These nine domains were complemented by 11 population-based interventions, such as a mass media campaign promoting healthy diet and physical exercise and a preparedness strategy in case of infectious disease outbreak.

Finally, the IPEHS included 15 intersectoral interventions, such as regulating emissions generated by transportation, industry, power, and households to reduce air pollution, and banning smoking in public places.

Cost of the IPEHS

Health care access, quality, and outcomes vary widely across geographies in Afghanistan. Variations in the financing and provision of health care services—along with population displacements, geographic remoteness, difficult terrain, sociocultural isolation, and health awareness—contribute to those differences. To address that challenge, the cost analysis included provinces from each region to achieve good geographic spread and sufficient representation: Daikundi, Faryab, Herat, Nangarhar, Paktya, Takhar, and Urzgan provided geographical representation from all regions of Afghanistan.

The BPHS cost analysis used the Cost Revenue Analysis Tool Plus for the health system levels of mobile health teams, sub health centers, basic health centers, comprehensive health centers, and district hospitals. The academic partners collected expenditure data in Afghanistan from 534 health facilities in seven selected provinces, and then converted expenses to US dollars using the 2020 exchange rate of Af 78.00 to US$1.00 (Salehi and Blanchet 2021). The studied health facilities covered 21 percent of the total population in 2020. The EPHS cost analysis looked at provincial hospitals and higher levels of the health system separately, using hospital data.

The difference between the combined costs of the BPHS and EPHS and the costs of the IPEHS was also assessed to understand the incremental costs of implementing the IPEHS. Health facilities were categorized into two groups: primary health care services and secondary health care services, including provincial hospitals. The total additional cost of the supplementary interventions was estimated at US$39,141,581. Compared to the BPHS at the primary health care level (community health posts, mobile health teams, sub health centers, basic health centers, comprehensive health centers, and district hospitals), the IPEHS would involve an additional cost of US$30,334,630; compared to the EPHS at the secondary health care level (provincial hospital and above), the IPEHS would cost US$8,808,951 more. In other words, primary health care accounts for 77.5 percent of the total required cost increase for the IPEHS, and secondary service accounts for 22.5 percent. The estimated overall average per capita cost of the IPEHS was US$6.90 (Salehi and Blanchet 2021).

METHODOLOGICAL LIMITATIONS

Because getting access to data presented a tremendous challenge for the working groups and the international Expert Committee, consensus panels were applied to capture expert opinion. That approach synthesizes expert opinion when other data are not available but is prone to various types of biases. Therefore, more studies on benefit-incidence analysis and cost-effectiveness will be necessary for future exercises in Afghanistan to better assess implications on equity and allocative efficiency.

Given the number of interventions, the project budget, and the time constraints to meet a policy reform window, this prioritization exercise did not conduct a cost-effectiveness study. HIPtool drew on national cost-analysis data, available by intervention, and cost-effectiveness data published by DCP3 to estimate existing and potential population health impacts for each intervention and for different health packages. HIPtool used the DCP3 volumes because they had just been released and provided up-to-date reviews of the effectiveness and cost-effectiveness of health interventions at the global level—with a focus on low- and lower-middle income countries. The international Expert Committee discussed the analysis of those reviews to verify the relevance of the DCP3 findings. Using existing evidence and HIPtool enabled the academic partners to carry out analyses to quantify the trade-offs between different decisions, in terms of population health, iteratively throughout the process and to inform three key discussions on IPEHS design.

The prioritization exercise mobilized many resources in and outside the country. It required more than two years to finalize the high-priority package and to ensure proper engagement of concerned parties (senior staff at MoPH, provincial authorities, and development partners). One possibility for reducing the transaction costs of the exercise would be to regularly update the priority package and review it every three years or in line with five-year national plans.

Because Afghanistan had conducted a similar exercise in 2012, this prioritization process greatly benefited from the experience of two successive ministers. With the arrival of the Taliban, many individuals with high-level expertise left the country. Future revision or conduct of such processes will require political willingness and rebuilding the country's expertise on health economics and public health, as well as the availability and modality of resource allocation.

LESSONS LEARNED

The prioritized package, the IPEHS, contained 144 health interventions and 14 intersectoral interventions that address the burden of communicable diseases; reproductive, maternal, newborn, and child health; chronic diseases; and injuries due to armed conflict. It included, for the first time, cost-effective services for chronic conditions, such as diabetes and hypertension, emergency trauma care, and palliative care, while maintaining a focus on addressing the country's high maternal and infant mortality rates. The package was finalized in August 2021, just before the Taliban took over the country.

Development of the IPEHS was supported by the Bill & Melinda Gates Foundation, as well as by United Nations agencies and Sehatmandi[1] donors (Canada, the European Union, the US Agency for International Development, and the World Bank). Despite high-level commitment at MoPH, the budgetary prospect was very limited and the implementation of the IPEHS was met with hesitancy from international donors. The emergence of a new package raised questions among donors on the government's financial capacity to increase financial commitment to cover the new interventions and ensure no increase in out-of-pocket payments. Earlier engagement of donors in the priority-setting process, from the outset of initial discussions and considerations of analysis methods, may have generated more support from donors.

The process of revising the health benefits package in Afghanistan identified a set of challenges and needs. The team faced difficulties in knowing how and when to start the process of revising the BPHS, citing lack of clear vision from the start regarding what the government thought was most needed in Afghanistan. Moreover, the political and health agendas clashed, creating increased pressure to deliver the revised package before the 2019 elections. The relative short timeline (18 months) to deliver a full revised package led to a shortened consultation process, seen by national stakeholders as a missed opportunity to create ownership. Although several government departments and provincial health directors participated in the process of revising the benefit package, information on the prioritized package did not cascade effectively down from top leadership across the health system. Two national consultations were organized in February and May 2021 to overcome that communication gap and receive feedback on the revised package. Consequently, the 2019 IPEHS was left aside after the departure of the minister. It was not until the end of 2020 that there was revived interest in the IPEHS by the president of Afghanistan. MoPH decided to finalize the IPEHS by emphasizing the national consultation process. The University of Geneva was called to provide guidance and help integrate feedback from national stakeholders into the IPEHS, which resulted in the 2021 IPEHS. Lange et al. (2022) offer a detailed account and review of the priority-setting process.

Change of MoPH leadership in the middle of the project in 2019 and from August 2021 impeded the finalization of costing the package, its implementation, and its sustainability. Inadequate commitment and engagement of the Ministry of Finance, low budget allocation, and overdependency on donor funding remain major challenges for universal health coverage in Afghanistan. Although the costing of the IPEHS was finalized in 2021, the arrival of the Taliban prevented MoPH and the University of Geneva from developing a realistic implementation plan.

With the Taliban's takeover in Afghanistan and the current political situation, implementation of the IPEHS is on hold. Afghanistan's experience in revising the IPEHS highlights the need to address not only the development of a more comprehensive benefit package but also its implementation, with careful deliberation on the prerequisites for implementing and financing the health benefits package and strengthening health systems. The IPEHS can be used as a foundation to define a new priority package—perhaps for primary care—under the Taliban rule.

NOTE

1   For more information about the Sehatmandi project, visit MoPH's project web page, https://moph.gov.af/en/sehatmandi-project.

REFERENCES

Abou Jaoude, G. J., H. Haghparast-Bidgoli, and J. Skordis-Worrall. 2019. "Optimisation of the National Budget in Afghanistan Using the HIP Tool." Unpublished manuscript. London.

APHI/MoPH (Afghan Public Health Institute, Ministry of Public Health), CSO (Afghanistan, Central Statistics Organization), ICF Macro, IIHMR (Indian Institute of Health Management Research), and WHO/EMRO (World Health Organization Regional Office for the Eastern Mediterranean). 2011. *Afghanistan Mortality Survey 2010*. Calverton, MD: APHI/MoPH, CSO, ICF Macro, IIHMR, and WHO/EMRO.

Akseer, N., A. Rizvi, Z. Bhatti, J. K. Das, K. Everett, A. Arur, M. Chopra, and Z. A. Bhutta. 2019. "Association of Exposure to Civil Conflict with Maternal Resilience and Maternal and Child Health and Health System Performance in Afghanistan." *JAMA Network Open* 2 (11): e1914819.

Akseer, N., Z. Bhatti, A. Rizvi, A. S. Salehi, T. Mashal, and Z. A. Bhutta. 2016. "Coverage and Inequalities in Maternal and Child Health Interventions in Afghanistan." *BMC Public Health* 16 (Suppl. 2): 797. https://doi.org/10.1186/s12889-016-3406-1.

Akseer, Nadia, Zaid Bhatti, Taufiq Mashal, Sajid Soofi, Rahim Moineddin, Robert E. Black, and Zulfiqar A. Bhutta. 2018. "Geospatial Inequalities and Determinants of Nutritional Status among Women and Children in Afghanistan: An Observational Study." *The Lancet Global Health* 6 (4): e447–59. https://doi.org/10.1016/S2214-109X(18)30025-1.

Alkema, L., D. Chou, D. Hogan, S. Zhang, A. B. Moller, A. Gemmill, D. M. Fat, et al. 2016. "Global, Regional, and National Levels and Trends in Maternal Mortality between 1990 and 2015, with Scenario-Based Projections to 2030: A Systematic Analysis by the UN Maternal Mortality Estimation Inter-Agency Group." *The Lancet* 387 (10017): 462–74. https://doi.org/10.1016/S0140-6736(15)00838-7.

Bartlett, L., A. LeFevre, L. Zimmerman, S. A. Saeedzai, S. Turkmani, W. Zabih, H. Tappis, et al. 2017. "Progress and Inequities in Maternal Mortality in Afghanistan (RAMOS-II): A Retrospective Observational Study." *The Lancet Global Health* 5 (5): e545–55. https://doi.org/10.1016/S2214-109X(17)30139-0.

CSO (Afghanistan, Central Statistics Organization), MoPH (Afghanistan, Ministry of Public Health), and ICF. 2017. *Afghanistan Demographic and Heath Survey 2015*. Kabul: CSO.

Fraser-Hurt, N., X. Hou, T. Wilkinson, D. Duran, G. J. Abou Jaoude, J. Skordis, A. Chukwuma, et al. 2021. "Using Allocative Efficiency Analysis to Inform Health Benefits Package Design for Progressing towards Universal Health Coverage: Proof-of-Concept Studies in Countries Seeking Decision Support." *PLOS ONE* 16 (11): e0260247. https://doi.org/10.1371/journal.pone.0260247.

Goetghebeur, M. M., H. Castro-Jaramillo, R. Baltbussen, and N. Daniels. 2017. "The Art of Medicine—the Art of Priority Setting." *The Lancet* 389: 2368–69.

Gold, M. R., D. Stevenson, and D. G. Fryback. 2002. "HALYs and QALYs and DALYs, Oh My." *Annual Review of Public Health* 23: 115–34.

González-Pier, E., C. Gutiérrez-Delgado, G. Stevens, M. Barraza-Lloréns, R. Porras-Condey, N. Carvalho, et al. 2016. "Priority Setting for Health Interventions in Mexico's System of Social Protection in Health." *The Lancet* 368 (9547): 1608–18.

IHME (Institute for Health Metrics and Evaluation). 2016. Afghanistan Health Data. IHME.

IHME (Institute for Health Metrics and Evaluation). 2017. Afghanistan Health Data. IHME.

Jamison, D. T., A. Alwan, C. N. Mock, R. Nugent, D. Watkins, O. Adeyi, S. Anand, et al. 2018. "Universal Health Coverage and Intersectoral Action for Health: Key Messages from *Disease Control Priorities*, 3rd Edition." *The Lancet* 391 (10125): 1108–20. https://doi.org/10.1016/S0140-6736(17)32906-9. https://doi.org/10.1016/S0140-6736(17)32906-9.

Jamison, D. T., H. Gelband, S. Horton, P. Jha, R. Laxminarayan, C. N. Mock, and Rachel Nugent, eds. 2018. *Disease Control Priorities* (third edition), Volume 9, *Disease Control Priorities: Improving Health and Reducing Poverty*. Washington, DC: World Bank. https://documents.worldbank.org/en/publication/documents-reports/documentdetail/527531512569346552/disease-control-priorities-improving-health-and-reducing-poverty.

Kovess-Masfety, V., K. Keyes, E. Karam, A. Sabawoon, and B. A. Sarwari. 2021. "A National Survey on Depressive and Anxiety Disorders in Afghanistan: A Highly Traumatized Population." *BMC Psychiatry* 21 (1): 314.

Lange, I. L., F. Feroz, A. J. Naeem, S. A. Saeedzai, F. Arifi, N. Singh, and K. Blanchet. 2022. "The Development of Afghanistan's Integrated Package of Essential Health Services: Evidence, Epertise and Ethics in a Priority Setting Process." *Social Science & Medicine* 305: 115010. https://doi.org/10.1016/j.socscimed.2022.115010.

Lozano, R., N. Fullman, J. E. Mumford, M. Knight, C. M. Barthelemy, C. Abbafati, H. Abbastabar, et al. 2020. "Measuring Universal Health Coverage Based on an Index of Effective Coverage of Health Services in 204 Countries and Territories, 1990–2019: A Systematic Analysis for the Global Burden of Disease Study 2019." *The Lancet* 396 (10258): 1250–84.

Mirzazada, S., Z. A. Padhani, S. Jabeen, M. Fatima, A. Rizvi, U. Ansari, J. K. Das, and Z. A. Bhutta. 2020. "Impact of Conflict on Maternal and Child Health Service Delivery: A Country Case Study of Afghanistan." *Conflict and Health* 14 (1): 1–13.

MoPH (Afghanistan, Ministry of Public Health). 2019. *National Health Accounts*. Kabul: Government of Afghanistan.

MoPH (Afghanistan, Ministry of Public Health). 2020. *Fiscal Space Analysis for Health 2020*. Kabul: Government of Afghanistan.

Newbrander, W., P. Ickx, F. Feroz, and H. Stanekzai. 2014. "Afghanistan's Basic Package of Health Services: Its Development and Effects on Rebuilding the Health System." *Global Public Health* 9 (1): S6–28.

Rahman, M., A. Karan, M. Rahman, A. Parsons, S. K. Abe, V. Bilano, R. Awan, et al. 2017. "Progress toward Universal Health Coverage: A Comparative Analysis in 5 South Asian Countries." *JAMA Internal Medicine* 177 (9): 1297–305. https://doi.org/10.1001/jamainternmed.2017.3133.

Salehi, A., and K. Blanchet. 2021. *Cost Analysis of the Integrated Package of Essential Health Services in Afghanistan*. Kabul: Afghanistan, Ministry of Public Health.

Shahraz, S., M. H. Forouzanfar, S. G. Sepanlou, D. Dicker, P. Naghavi, F. Pourmalek, A. Mokdad, et al. 2014. "Population Health and Burden of Disease Profile of Iran among 20 Countries in the Region: From Afghanistan to Qatar and Lebanon." *Archives of Iranian Medicine* 17 (5): 336–42. https://www.ncbi.nlm.nih.gov/pubmed/24784862.

Shoib, S., M Y. Essar, S. M. Saleem, Z. Legris, and M. Chandradasa. 2022. "The Children of Afghanistan Need Urgent Mental Health Support." *The Lancet* 399 (10329): 1045–46.

UN IGME (United Nations Inter-agency Group for Child Mortality Estimation). 2018. Child Mortality Estimates. UN IGME, New York, Geneva, and Washington, DC.

Watkins, D. A., D. T. Jamison, A. Mills, R. Atun, K. Danforth, A. Glassman, S. Horton, et al. 2018. "Universal Health Coverage and Essential Packages of Care." In *Disease Control Priorities* (third edition), Volume 9, *Disease Control Priorities: Improving Health and Reducing Poverty,* edited by D. T. Jamison, H. Gelband, S. Horton, P. Jha, R. Laxminarayan, C. N. Mock, and R. Nugent. Washington, DC: World Bank.

World Bank. 2017. "Strong Progress but Challenges Remain in Health Sector in Afghanistan." Press release, June 1, 2017. https://www.worldbank.org/en/news/press-release/2017/06/01/strong-progress-but-challenges-remain-in-health-sector-in-afghanistan.

World Bank. 2018. "Progress in the Face of Insecurity: Improving Health Outcomes in Afghanistan." Policy Brief, World Bank, Washington, DC. https://documents.worldbank.org/en/publication/documents-reports/documentdetail/330491520002103598/policy-brief.

You, D., L. Hug, S. Ejdemyr, P. Idele, D. Hogan, C. Mathers, P. Gerland, et al. 2015. "Global, Regional, and National Levels and Trends in Under-5 Mortality between 1990 and 2015, with Scenario-Based Projections to 2030: A Systematic Analysis by the UN Inter-agency Group for Child Mortality Estimation." *The Lancet* 386 (10010): 2275–86. https://www.ncbi.nlm.nih.gov/pubmed/26361942.

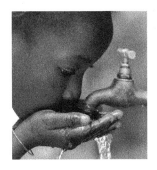

5

Economy Experiences with the Revision Process of the Zanzibar Essential Health Care Package

Omar Mwalim, Sanaa Said, Subira Suleiman, Fatma Bakar, Haji Khamis,
Dhameera Mohammed, Omar Mussa, Abdulmajid Jecha, Abdul-latif Haji,
Ole F. Norheim, Ingrid Miljeteig, Peter Hangoma, and Kjell Arne Johansson

ABSTRACT

Zanzibar, a semiautonomous region of Tanzanaia, undertook a revision of its essential
health care package in 2019–22 with the aim of providing a comprehensive,
inclusive, evidence-based, and fair package of health services. The revision gained
high-level political support and engaged many key stakeholders through a participatory
deliberative process. Several consensus-building workshops were held from the
community to the national level. Zanzibar's final health care package has a total of 302
interventions across 22 health program areas. Focusing on primary care, the package
will be scaled up over 10 years and is expected to cost US$198 per disability-adjusted
life year averted. With effective implementation, it is expected to save about 120,000
lives and increase life expectancy from 65 years to 71 years by 2032.

INTRODUCTION

Awareness and understanding of universal health coverage (UHC) have increased
both globally and in many specific settings such as Zanzibar (Hashimoto, Adrien,
and Rajkumar 2020; WHO 2020b). Key principles of UHC are to provide the
health services people need without exposing them to financial risk. In Zanzibar
and elsewhere, especially in low- and middle-income countries, resources are
scarce, and many competing priorities exist (Hanson et al. 2022; Kapiriri 2013).
An explicit national essential health care package (EHCP), or a list of high-priority
health services that the government promises to provide, is an important policy tool

for setting health priorities in achieving UHC fairly and efficiently (Verguet et al. 2021). Thus, transparent and fair priority setting is key in the development process of EHCPs (Barroy, Sparkes, and Dale 2016). It can replace conventional implicit priority-setting mechanisms like denial of services, dilution of quality of care, delay in providing services that patients have a right to, suboptimal standards of health facilities, and deterrence behavior of health workers due to an overwhelming number of tasks and responsibilities (Kapiriri and Martin 2007). An EHCP explicitly defines essential services that should be prioritized within a limited budget using specified criteria, describes how those services should be financed, and identifies who should receive them. Concretely, such an explicit list of high-priority services can serve as overarching policy guidance over a longer period to assure feasible health financing systems, like public health insurance, and investments in the most important services within a country. Further, it can guide future plans and policies on health personnel and essential medicines (Glassman, Giedion, and Smith 2017; Watkins et al. 2018).

Even though many countries have gone through an EHCP revision, implementation success will depend on the quality of the development process. Zanzibar has had two previous revisions of the EHCP, the latest one in 2018. Neither was comprehensive and both failed to be implemented with a consequence of low coverage of essential health services (Ministry of Health and Social Welfare 2017). Those revisions needed more comprehensive development processes rather than rapid expert-driven listing of essential health interventions. Selection of essential services and eligible populations into an EHCP requires a combination of robust methods and high-quality data as well as fair processes that include adequate institutionalization and legal frameworks (Baltussen et al. 2023). It also involves hard political choices, balancing the claims of various stakeholder groups engaged in the process (Gustavsson and Tinghög 2020; Mitton and Donaldson 2004).

Currently, many countries are developing and revising EHCPs (El-Jardali et al. 2019; Youngkong, Kapiriri, and Baltussen 2009). Ethiopia and Pakistan have recently conducted comprehensive revisions of their national EHCPs, and both countries are now in the implementation phase. Recent revisions of EHCPs have also taken place in countries like Somalia and Sudan, settings with fragile health systems. Further, many international expert guidance reports have been published in the last five years and they all emphasize the importance of having a fair and democratic process when making an EHCP (Jansen, Baltussen, and Bærøe 2018; Norheim 2018; WHO 2020a). A recent review of EHCP revisions in six countries presents a framework for decision-making processes, including both practical organizational and normative considerations in the revision of EHCPs (Baltussen et al. 2023). Countries that took part in that review appeared to follow the elements of that framework, although with organizational differences based on the specific context of each country.

Despite the importance of a democratic and transparent priority-setting process (Bhaumik et al. 2015), limited evidence exists from country experiences in conducting and applying democratic deliberative methods in priority setting of national EHCPs. Although the literature shows widespread application of sound technical and systematic processes in revising/developing EHCPs

(Bhaumik et al. 2015; Jansen, Baltussen, and Bærøe 2018; Nagpal et al. 2023; WHO 2020a), it offers limited clarity on whether priority decisions were made through democratic processes and how stakeholders were actually involved in the revision. We still need more evidence from actual decision-making on how substantial and complicated health economic analyses and equity impact assessments can be combined with input and participation of the people who will be affected by these decisions. Such evidence is needed in aiming for fairness, legitimacy, and impartiality in health priorities (Jansen, Baltussen, and Bærøe 2018; Razavi et al. 2019). Decision-making processes need to go beyond inclusion of only individuals in strategic positions who are trained in expressing their preferences and opinions (Allotey et al. 2019; Odugleh-Kolev and Parrish-Sprowl 2018; Warren et al. 2021). In the revision of its EHCP, Zanzibar has demonstrated a good practice of engaging community, and this chapter aims to describe the overall experience there.

Country Context

Zanzibar is a semiautonomous region of Tanzania. It consists of two islands (Pemba and Unguja) surrounded by smaller satellite islets in the Indian Ocean. Although part of Tanzania, Zanzibar addresses its health priorities independently because health remains among non-Union matters. It has a total per capita health expenditure of US$34 per year (Ministry of Health Zanzibar 2014), with 30 percent of that expenditure coming from donor funds and 16 percent from out of pocket.

The first EHCP in Zanzibar (ZEHCP), from 2007, was considered important as part of the strategy for improving population health, economic growth, and poverty reduction (Revolutionary Government of Zanzibar 2017). Evaluating the success of the first ZEHCP, and later revisions, presents difficulties because many of the specific priorities and health intervention targets were too broad to be evaluated (for example, "Conduct blood glucose screening"). The policies said little about the cost-effectiveness and actual resources needed for each intervention, or about finance mechanisms and which target coverage levels to aim for at various delivery platforms. Nevertheless, the fact that the Ministry of Health chose a national ZEHCP as one of the milestones for its overall health policy, the 2006–07 Plan of Action, reveals the importance that the national health authorities attached to the first edition of the EHCP.

Health Care System

The health care system in Zanzibar has for many years comprised four levels: (1) the primary level that includes Primary Health Care Units, Primary Health Care Units+, and Primary Health Care Centers; (2) the district level; (3) the regional level; and (4) the tertiary level. Because of the complicated categorization at the primary level, the Ministry of Health proposed in the 2019–22 ZEHCP revision to simplify the structure of health care delivery platforms and to map priorities to those platforms. Table 5.1 presents the revised delivery platforms, reflecting a current total of 167 public health care facilities through which the ZEHCP will be implemented (Ministry of Health Zanzibar 2018).

Table 5.1 Number of Health Facilities in Zanzibar, by District and Delivery Platform, 2022 and 2024

	Primary level		Secondary level		Tertiary level	
	Dispensary	Health center	District hospital	Regional hospital	Referral and specialty hospitals	Total
Pemba						
2022	52	15	2	1	0	70
2024	33	21	4	1	0	59
Unguja						
2022	73	19	2	0	3	97
2024	50	26	7	1	3	87
Total Zanzibar (2024)	83	47	11	2	3	146

Source: Ministry of Health Zanzibar 2024.

Note: The upper row for each district shows numbers of platforms in 2022, immediately after the revision of Zanzibar's essential health care package; the lower row shows numbers in January 2024, about one year after the revision.

Scope and Mandate

In 2019, Zanzibar's Minister of Health requested that the World Health Organization (WHO) and the Bergen Center for Ethics and Priority Setting (BCEPS) provide technical support in the revision of the EHCP. The revision process of the ZEHCP was locally driven; the first author of this chapter, who at the time was the head of the Noncommunicable Diseases Unit in Zanzibar's Ministry of Health and is currently a PhD candidate at BCEPS, led the core group in the entire process. That core group had a mandate to provide an explicit list of essential health services that address the most important health needs of Zanzibar's population across their life course, with special emphasis on services at the primary, secondary, and tertiary health care levels. The final ZEHCP report was intended to provide relevant guidance for future health policies and actual priority setting at all levels of Zanzibar's health system in the next 10 years, with subsequent regular reviews and updates. The revised ZEHCP forms part of the operationalization of the Zanzibar Health Sector Strategic Plan IV and Zanzibar's commitment to pursue the Sustainable Development Goals.

Description of methods and results is influenced by the authors' applied involvement in the process. The 2019 revision of the ZEHCP followed a participatory deliberative process involving many relevant stakeholders from the community level to the national level. Through various organized consensus-building workshops, the core team led the revision with support from Technical Working Groups. During the first six months, participants made decisions on which criteria to use for priority setting and which interventions to consider as candidates in the revised ZEHCP. The next 18 months focused on analytics and collection of evidence to use in the assessment of consequences of various priority decisions and information needed to set priorities. A budget space analysis was conducted and decision on the feasible size of the health budget increase up to 2032 was made, and final approval of the ZEHCP was made at the highest political level in Zanzibar. The final comprehensive

ZEHCP report, published in November 2022, included details about criteria for priority setting, interventions in the package, and financing scenarios (Ministry of Health Zanzibar 2022). The report also proposed implementation arrangements as well as a monitoring framework.

Priority-Setting Process

The revision of the ZEHCP began with a meticulous planning phase, with the core team following a 10-step revision process presented in detail elsewhere (Mwalim et al., forthcoming, a). The core team developed an initial comprehensive road map that underwent rigorous scrutiny and approval through workshops and consensus-building meetings, involving experts from various organizations, including WHO, as well as senior officials from the Ministry of Health and other stakeholders. Following input from diverse stakeholders, the Ministry of Health sanctioned the road map for operationalization.

Stakeholder engagement played a pivotal role in the process, involving participants from community to national levels, each representing distinct interests. The stakeholders actively contributed to defining criteria for intervention selection, acknowledging the crucial role of the ZEHCP in achieving UHC. Consultative meetings with civil society organizations, medical experts, and other key stakeholders resulted in agreement on six criteria—budget impact, disease burden, cost-effectiveness, financial risk protection, equity, and political/public acceptability—which formed the basis for intervention selection.

Subsequently, 11 extensive consultation meetings were conducted to review and accept 302 interventions spanning preventive, curative, rehabilitative, and intersectoral domains for inclusion in the EHCP. Controversial interventions, such as induced abortion, were excluded, considering feasibility, affordability, and positive gains during the selection process. Baseline and target coverages were assigned to each intervention.

Regarding financing, stakeholders recommended a budget increase for effective EHCP implementation, noting the inadequacy of the per capita expenditure, set at US$34 according to the National Health Accounts. They recommended doubling the health budget, prompting the government to introduce a health financing reform that included two enduring financing mechanisms—a new Universal Health Insurance scheme and a pro-poor Zanzibar Health Equity Fund—to support implementation of the ZEHCP.

Implementation considerations highlighted the crucial role of District Health Management Teams, especially in primary health care, where most interventions were concentrated. To ensure effective implementation, stakeholders agreed to assure proper resource allocation to facilities and to establish an efficient referral system, as well as robust links between health facilities and communities. Monitoring and evaluation was also considered, with responsibilities assigned to the Health Management Information System to ensure ongoing assessment of implementation progress. That collective effort aims to guide Zanzibar's health sector toward overarching goals, ultimately resulting in improved health outcomes for the population.

Analytics

The revision process of the ZEHCP included a comprehensive analysis using two analytical tools—the BCEPS FairChoices: DCP Analytics Tool and the WHO OneHealth Tool (OHT). The integration of FairChoices and OHT in the analytics of the ZEHCP revision facilitated a comprehensive assessment of costs, benefits, cost-effectiveness, and equity impact for various health interventions. Mwalim et al. (forthcoming, b) explains the details of the FairChoices methods in the Zanzibar revision. During the revision, a technical team prepared local parameters for both FairChoices and OHT, undertaking a thorough cost analysis that considered various scale-up scenarios for interventions within Zanzibar's health system over a 10-year period.

These tools employed distinct cost analysis approaches: OHT used an ingredient-based costing methodology, involving the summation of quantities and prices for all necessary components, whereas FairChoices employed a broader unit cost approach combined with population in need and baseline target coverage assumptions for each intervention. The unit cost approach encompassed aggregate cost to deliver health interventions per patient, including factors such as human resources, drugs, equipment, and other relevant elements. Local sources—including the Central Medical Store, Health Management Information System, published reports, and surveys—provided local data, which were further supplemented by information from published cost-effectiveness papers.

To align the policies of the ZEHCP and Health Sector Strategic Plan IV, the team undertook an intermediate cost analysis for the Health Sector Strategic Plan IV using OHT. Simultaneously, it employed FairChoices to estimate the health benefits and equity associated with the candidate interventions.

Cost-effectiveness played a pivotal role in ranking interventions by their potential to maximize population health. Whenever possible, the analysis used incremental cost-effectiveness ratio, representing the incremental cost and incremental effect of transitioning from the current baseline coverage of each intervention to a defined target coverage level. In that context, achieving coverage levels exceeding 90 percent was designated as the UHC endpoint. To ensure the robustness and validity of the incremental cost-effectiveness ratio values derived from FairChoices, the revision team conducted a thorough validation process. That process involved referencing peer-reviewed publications and the gray literature spanning the years 2010 to 2019.

RESULTS

The ZEHCP reflects the diverse health needs of Zanzibar's population. The package was carefully designed to address specific health challenges with the distribution of interventions hihghlighting strategic prioritization of resources. Primary health care facilities are central to the ZEHCP because they account for most interventions, costs, and health outcomes. The detailed and expansive nature of the ZEHCP underscores the commitment of the Ministry of Health to improving overall health outcomes and ensuring equitable access to essential health services across Zanzibar.

STRUCTURE OF THE ZEHCP

The ZEHCP encompasses a total of 302 interventions distributed across 22 health program areas (table 5.2). Each program area represents a distinct health domain, and the number of interventions allocated to each area highlights the comprehensive nature of the health care package. That comprehensive package strategically prioritizes a diverse array of health interventions, addressing a wide spectrum of health needs within Zanzibar's health care system.

Table 5.2 Overall Summary of Cost, Effect, and Health Outcomes of the ZEHCP, by Program Area, 2022–32

Program area	Cost-effectiveness (US$/HLY)	Cost (10 years, US$)	Healthy life years (10 years)	Life years (10 years)	Lives saved (10 years)
Surgery	2,348	15,402,854	6,560	4,303	35
Emergency care	25,956	11,498,754	443	493	4
Maternal and newborn health	52	18,583,478	359,765	411,720	6,171
Child and adolescent health	182	44,605,652	245,699	283,327	1,707
Reproductive health	—	—	—	—	—
HIV and sexually transmitted infections	86	6,413,687	74,443	89,743	1,202
Malaria	1,083	1,704,379	1,574	1,811	16
Tuberculosis	213	4,804,053	22,554	26,009	209
Neglected tropical diseases	904	321,263	355	119	1
Infections in general	720	11,596,866	16,104	17,912	173
Cancer	9	3,982,554	448,295	587,838	575
CVD and diabetes	4,748	58,976,782	12,422	14,899	347
Musculoskeletal disorders	21,612	651,210	30	18	1
Respiratory disorders	51,029	32,450,618	636	736	6
Mental and SUDs	5,864	21,833,853	3,723	3,461	35
Neurological disorders	117	629,111	5,386	2,493	20
Rehabilitation	—	—	—	—	—
Nutrition	414	3,841,319	9,271	7,604	72
Hearing and vision improvement	5,080	1,375,382	271	—	—
Interpersonal violence	—	—	—	—	—
Epidemic infections (including COVID-19)	—	—	—	—	—
Intersectoral interventions	—	—	—	—	—
Total	**198**	**238,671,814**	**1,207,531**	**1,452,485**	**10,572**

Source: Ministry of Health Zanzibar 2022.

Note: CVD = cardiovascular disease; HLY = healthy life year; SUD = substance use disorder; ZEHCP = Zanzibar essential health care package; — = not available.

The ZEHCP spreads interventions, expected costs, and health benefits (healthy life years) across various delivery platforms of the health care system. Primary health care facilities play a predominant role, constituting 68 percent of ZEHCP interventions, representing 65 percent of the associated costs, and contributing to 82 percent of the overall effects in terms of healthy life years. Secondary-level health care facilities follow, representing 22 percent of interventions and 31 percent of costs, and contributing to 16 percent of healthy life year impact. Referral hospitals, despite representing 10 percent of interventions, make up 3 percent of the overall cost and yield 1 percent of the total healthy life year impact.

Funding the ZEHCP

The revised ZEHCP anticipates an increase of US$39 per capita in annual health expenditure by 2032, necessitating a doubling of total health spending to US$73 per capita annually within the next decade. The team conducted a comprehensive 10-year fiscal space analysis in collaboration with the Ministries of Health and Finance and later presented and discussed it with policy makers, development partners, Ministry of Health program managers, and other stakeholders. That expert-driven analysis considered various factors such as economic growth expectations, population growth, government investment, donor funding, and the introduction of a social health insurance scheme.

The analysis projects an increase in the government's health care expenditure as a percentage of gross domestic product from the current 1.7 percent to 2.5 percent by 2032. Further, it proposed increasing government spending from 53 percent to 60 percent, reducing donor contributions from 29 percent to 15 percent, and decreasing out-of-pocket expenditure from 16 percent to 10 percent.

To fulfill commitments outlined in the updated 2022 ZEHCP, the government undertook significant financial reforms, including the introduction of Universal Health Insurance and the Zanzibar Health Equity Fund. Universal Health Insurance, initially targeting formal sector individuals, will later be extended to the informal sector, with the aim of improving health care accessibility and affordability. Meanwhile, the Equity Fund focuses on supporting vulnerable groups, particularly those below the poverty line. The reforms aim to ensure sustainable funding for ZEHCP implementation, highlighting the government's commitment to securing accessible and quality health care in Zanzibar.

However, when comparing the ambitious target of increasing per capita spending to US$73 with the reality on the ground, the team also considered and documented scenarios of increasing per capita spending by US$1 or US$2 per year.

Implementation Monitoring and Evaluation

The ZEHCP implementation plan is guided by strategic priorities aligned with Ministry of Health strategies. It focuses on enhancing the health care financing system, providing comprehensive health services, ensuring equitable distribution of the health workforce, improving the availability of drugs and equipment, strengthening health information systems and patient management, fostering community and stakeholder involvement, and reinforcing governance, leadership, and accountability within the health system.

In the realm of health care financing, the plan aims to progressively increase government health expenditure, provide health insurance to the entire population, introduce earmarked taxes on specific products, and establish trust funds to enhance mobilization of domestic resources. The provision of health services involves developing a clear referral system, updating treatment guidelines, and strengthening disease-specific registries. Additionally, the plan involves efforts to recruit qualified health workers, enhance training programs for equitable deployment, and improve the availability of drugs, supplies, and diagnostic equipment. The focus on health information systems and patient management includes strengthening national monitoring teams, enhancing digital medical record systems, increasing service access through partnerships, and aligning outcome metrics with ZEHCP objectives.

Responsibility for the continuous evaluation of the ZEHCP will lie with the planning unit through the Health Management and Information System and the Monitoring and Evaluation Division at the Ministry of Health, in collaboration with the Health Sector Reform Secretariat. In addition, heads of the departments and sections, and health care providers, shall ensure the smooth implementation of the health care package. The evaluation process will also engage the grassroots level, emphasizing the bottom-up approach to implementing the ZEHCP.

Lessons Learned

The design of benefit packages should reflect the priorities of respective countries. With that lesson in mind, it is highly recommended that countries manage the entire process themselves and ensure full participation of stakeholders at different levels. Additionally, the process requires the availability of sufficient and reliable evidence so that it can project costs and effects for the defined period. In its process, Zanzibar learned several lessons, discussed in the following paragraphs, that other countries could consider while doing similar work.

Ownership of the process. To carry out a benefit package development process efficiently, a country must lead the exercise. This aspect is crucial because local counterparts know who to involve and where to obtain the necessary information. Further, by leading the process, the country can build trust in what it has produced and can advocate for the resources needed.

Local capacity building. It has been common practice in many countries to employ foreign experts to undertake some assignments that local staff could do. Such was not the case in Zanzibar when it revised its benefit package. It recruited a core team, which was given basic health economic and priority-setting training organized by the Addis Center for Ethics and Priority Setting and BCEPS. The trainings, conducted in Ethiopia and Zanzibar, enabled the team to manage the entire exercise. The knowledge gained greatly helped in clarifying different issues that emerged during deliberative meetings.

Stakeholder engagement. The participatory process of designing a benefit package needs broad inclusion of different stakeholder groups (Heath 1997). During its revision process, Zanzibar held a total of 11 sessions that involved community-level stakeholders, development partners, health professionals, and various government leaders. The consultative meetings served as awareness-creation platforms for addressing several concerns. The biggest challenge for stakeholders was to understand the concepts of priority setting. Following detailed sessions, the stakeholders gave their opinions about the criteria to be used for selecting interventions, the list of interventions to include in the package, and the proposed increase in the health budget from the central government. The final package was approved by Zanzibar's highest decision-making bodies, including the Multisectoral Technical Committee—comprising all government principal secretaries—and the Minister's Cabinet, chaired by His Excellency the President of Zanzibar and the Chairman of the Revolutionary Council.

Advocacy for the package. During the evaluation of the previous package, it became apparent that most stakeholders were not aware of the benefit package, which had resulted from a more top-down expert-driven process. That lack of awareness was due to limited involvement during the earlier package's development and partly to the lack of its implementation. With proper advocacy, the package can be used as a tool to mobilize resources, which, if secured, will make its implementation successful. Zanzibar used the revision process as an opportunity to advocate for the package and explain the importance of setting priorities.

Aligning the package with existing financing mechanism(s). For efficient implementation of the package, the process must identify several sources of funding from which funds can be allocated to the prioritized interventions. Zanzibar has implemented a free health care policy for decades but recently decided to introduce public health insurance. The challenge that has emerged involves the lack of harmony between the insurance benefit package and the EHCP. Because neither was officially endorsed, the teams of experts are trying to align the two. Zanzibar's experience highlights the importance of ensuring proper intragovernment communication when developing policy documents to avoid inconvenience.

Prospects for future review. Other key lessons learned while revising the ZHECP relate to progress on achieving Sustainable Development Goal targets, efforts to address noncommunicable diseases, and the development of national strategies to combat emerging health conditions. Additionally, there is significant optimism regarding the potential availability of funds to support package implementation because of major financial reforms under way. These insights suggest that implementation of the package may evolve over time, indicating the possibility of reviewing this case study as its implementation progresses.

Legislation. Meanwhile, because the ZEHCP is not bound by law, its implementation may not be as effective as expected, which could hamper resource allocation. Following a conversation between the Ministry of Health, BCEPS, and Zanzibar's Attorney General, the Attorney General advised putting the ZEHCP's existence into law. Having a law in place will clearly identify a list of services that all Zanzibaris have the right to access and will necessitate resource allocation for ZEHCP implementation; however, it will also prevent introduction of health interventions that may have huge budget impact. Enacting such a law will require a process of gathering opinions at all levels, preparing a bill, and sending it to parliament for discussion and approval.

Limitations

The ZEHCP review team had major difficulties in collecting all the quantitative and qualitative data necessary to review the current service package; in some cases, it did not have reliable data readily available in the required format. For instance, inadequate data about service outputs (in terms of numbers of clients served) at the level of health institutions, about human resources, and about logistics had to be substantiated by data from the Health Management Information System, which lacked sufficient data at the time. Thus, the team used evidence from the Tanzania Demographic Health Survey 2010 and 2015/16 and OHT along with data from the Institute for Health Metrics and Evaluation's Global Burden of Disease study.

CONCLUSION

A national EHCP serves as an explicit mechanism for operationalizing entitlements to health. Ranking of services by priority should follow WHO recommendations, be evidence based, and align well with other social goals (WHO 2014). Competing priorities within the health sector and across other sectors need to be handled carefully using a fair process and rigorous and pragmatic methods. Successfully implementing UHC at the national level requires compromises on the parts of various stakeholders, including policy makers, providers, payers, insurance companies, product manufacturers, and patients. Local engagement is important when defining an EHCP at the country level. In Zanzibar, as elsewhere, multiple interests are involved, institutions are short of capacity, resources are extremely scarce, and the political setting is complex. The ZEHCP outlines key interventions that Zanzibar will make available to its population as it works to ensure high coverage with public financing, so it can assure population health and well-being.

ACKNOWLEDGMENTS

We extend our deepest gratitude to the Ministry of Health Zanzibar, along with all stakeholders and funders, for their invaluable support in making this study possible. Special thanks go to NORAD, the Trond Mohn Foundation, the Bill & Melinda Gates Foundation, and the World Health Organization for their generous funding.

REFERENCES

Allotey, P., D. T. Tan, T. Kirby, and L. H. Tan. 2019. "Community Engagement in Support of Moving toward Universal Health Coverage." *Health Systems & Reform* 5 (1): 66–77. https://doi.org/10.1080/23288604.2018.1541497.

Baltussen, R., O. Mwalim, K. Blanchet, M. Carballo, G. T. Eregata, A. Hailu, M. Huda, et al. 2023. "Decision-Making Processes for Essential Packages of Health Services: Experience from Six Countries." *BMJ Global Health* 8 (Suppl 1): e010704. https://doi.org/10.1136/bmjgh-2022-010704.

Barroy, H., S. Sparkes, and E. Dale. 2016. "Assessing Fiscal Space for Health Expansion in Low- and Middle-Income Countries: A Review of the Evidence." Health Financing Working Paper No. 3, World Health Organization, Geneva. https://iris.who.int/bitstream/handle/10665/251904/WHO-HIS-HGF-HFWorkingPaper-16.3-eng.pdf.

Bhaumik, S., S. Rana, C. Karimkhani, V. Welch. R. Armstrong, K. Pottie, R. Dellavalle, et al. 2015. "Ethics and Equity in Research Priority-Setting: Stakeholder Engagement and the Needs of Disadvantaged Groups." *Indian Journal of Medical Ethics*. 12 (2): 110–13. https://doi.org/10.20529/IJME.2015.030.

El-Jardali, F., R. Fadlallah, A. Daouk, R. Rizk, N. Hemadi, O. El Kebbi, A. Farha, and E. A. Akl. 2019. "Barriers and Facilitators to Implementation of Essential Health Benefits Package within Primary Health Care Settings in Low-Income and Middle-Income Countries: A Systematic Review." *International Journal of Health Planning and Management* 34 (1): 15–41. https://doi.org/10.1002/hpm.2625.

Glassman, A., U. Giedion, and P. C. Smith. 2017. *What's In, What's Out? Designing Benefits for Universal Health Coverage*. Washington, DC: Center for Global Development. https://www.cgdev.org/publication/whats-in-whats-out-designing-benefits-universal-health-coverage.

Gustavsson, E., and G. Tinghög. 2020. "Needs and Cost-Effectiveness in Health Care Priority Setting." *Health and Technology* 10 (3): 611–19. https://doi.org/10.1007/s12553-020-00424-7.

Hanson, K., N. Brikci, D. Erlangga, A. Alebachew, M. De Allegri, D. Balabanova, M. Blecher, et al. 2022 "The Lancet Global Health Commission on Financing Primary Health Care: Putting People at the Centre." *The Lancet Global Health* 10 (5): e715–72. https://doi.org/10.1016/S2214-109X(22)00005-5.

Hashimoto, K., L. Adrien, and S. Rajkumar. 2020. "Moving towards Universal Health Coverage in Haiti." *Health Systems & Reform* 6 (1). https://doi.org/10.1080/23288604.2020.1719339.

Heath, I. 1997. "Managing Scarcity: Priority Setting and Rationing in the National Health Service." *BMJ*. https://doi.org/10.1136/bmj.314.7076.313.

Jansen, M. P. M., R. Baltussen, and K. Bærøe. 2018. "Stakeholder Participation for Legitimate Priority Setting: A Checklist." *International Journal of Health Policy and Management* 7 (11): 973–76. https://doi.org/10.15171/IJHPM.2018.57.

Kapiriri, L. 2013. "How Effective Has the Essential Health Package Been in Improving Priority Setting in Low Income Countries?" *Social Science & Medicine* 85: 38–42. https://doi.org/10.1016/j.socscimed.2013.02.024.

Kapiriri, L., and D. K. Martin. 2007. "Bedside Rationing by Health Practitioners: A Case Study in a Ugandan Hospital." *Medical Decision Making* 27 (1): 44–52. https://doi.org/10.1177/0272989X06297397.

Ministry of Health and Social Welfare Zanzibar. 2017. "Mid-Term Review Report Zanzibar Health Sector Strategic Plan-III." Revolutionary Government of Zanzibar [not publicly available].

Ministry of Health Zanzibar. 2014. "National Health Account 2011–2012, 2012–2013." Revolutionary Government of Zanzibar [not publicly available].

Ministry of Health Zanzibar. 2018. "Zanzibar Annual Health Bulletin 2018." Revolutionary Government of Zanzibar [not publicly available].

Ministry of Health Zanzibar. 2022. *Zanzibar Essential Health Care Package Report.* Revolutionary Government of Zanzibar. https://mohz.go.tz/eng/zanzibar-essential-health -care-package-report/.

Mitton, C., and C. Donaldson. 2004. "Health Care Priority Setting: Principles, Practice and Challenges." *Cost Effectiveness and Resource Allocation* 2 (1): 2. https://doi.org/10.1186/1478 -7547-2-3.

Mwalim, Omar, Sanaa Said, Subira Suleiman, Fatma Bakar, Haji Khamis, Dhameera Mohammed, et al. Forthcoming, a. "A 10-Step Strategy for Fair Priority Setting Processes in Essential Health Care Package Revisions: A Qualitative Case Study from Zanzibar."

Mwalim, Omar, Sanaa Said, Subira Suleiman, Fatma Bakar, Haji Khamis, Dhameera Mohammed, Omar Mussa, et al. Forthcoming, b. "Enhancing Health Priorities in Zanzibar: Analysis of 302 Health Care Interventions for Cost Effectiveness, Equity, Budget Impact and Disease Burden Averted in the Essential Health Care Package."

Nagpal, S., N. Ahluwalia, L. O. Hashiguchi, K. McGee, and M. Lutalo. 2023. "Harnessing Country Experiences for Health Benefit Package Design: Evidence-Informed Deliberative Processes and Experiences from the Joint Learning Network: Comment on 'Evidence-Informed Deliberative Processes for Health Benefit Package Design—Part II: A.'" *International Journal of Health Policy and Management* 12 (1): 1–3. https://doi.org /10.34172/IJHPM.2023.7856.

Norheim, O. F. 2018. "Disease Control Priorities Third Edition Is Published: A Theory of Change Is Needed for Translating Evidence to Health Policy." *International Journal of Health Policy and Management* 7 (9): 771–77.

Odugleh-Kolev, A., and J. Parrish-Sprowl. 2018. "Universal Health Coverage and Community Engagement." *Bulletin of the World Health Organization* 96 (9): 660–61. https://doi.org /10.2471/BLT.17.202382.

Razavi, S. D., L. Kapiriri, J. Abelson, and M. Wilson. 2019. "Who Is In and Who Is Out? A Qualitative Analysis of Stakeholder Participation in Priority Setting for Health in Three Districts in Uganda." *Health Policy and Planning* 34 (5): 358–69. https://doi.org/10.1093 /heapol/czz049.

Revolutionary Government of Zanzibar. 2017. "The Zanzibar Strategy for Growth and Reduction of Poverty (ZSGRP)." https://www.sheriasmz.go.tz/docs/3FzvG7swbk_MKUZA _I_-_MKUZA_Final_Document_19_1_07_English.pdf.

Verguet, S., A. Hailu, G. T. Eregata, S. T. Memirie, K. A. Johansson, and O. F. Norheim. 2021. "Toward Universal Health Coverage in the Post-COVID-19 Era." *Nature Medicine* 27 (3): 380–87. https://doi.org/10.1038/s41591-021-01268-y.

Warren, C. E., B. Bellows, R. Marcus, J. Downey, S. Kennedy, and N. Kureshy. 2021. "Strength in Diversity: Integrating Community in Primary Health Care to Advance Universal Health Coverage." *Global Health: Science and Practice* (March): 1–5. https://doi.org/10.9745 /GHSP-D-21-00125.

Watkins, D. A., D. T. Jamison, A. Mills, R. Atun, K. Danforth, A. Glassman, S. Horton, et al. 2018. "Universal Health Coverage and Essential Packages of Care." In *Disease Control Priorities* (third edition), Volume 9, *Disease Contol Priorities: Improving Health and Reducing Poverty,* edited by D. T. Jamison, H. Gelband, S. Horton, P. Jha, R. Laxminarayan, and C. N. Mock. Washington, DC: World Bank.

WHO (World Health Organization). 2014. *Making Fair Choices on the Path to Universal Health Coverage: Final Report of the WHO Consultative Group on Equity and Universal Health Coverage.* Geneva: WHO. https://iris.who.int/bitstream/handle/10665/112671 /9789241507158_eng.pdf?sequence=1.

WHO (World Health Organization). 2020a. *Strengthening NCD Service Delivery through UHC Benefit Package.* Technical Meeting Report. Geneva: WHO. https://iris.who.int/bitstream /handle/10665/338690/9789240017528-eng.pdf?sequence=1.

WHO (World Health Organization). 2020b. *Universal Health Coverage Partnership Annual Report 2019. In Practice: Bridging Global Commitments with Country Action to Achieve Universal Health Coverage.* Geneva: WHO. https://iris.who.int/bitstream/handle/10665/341433/9789240012950-eng.pdf?sequence=1&isAllowed=y.

Youngkong, S., L. Kapiriri, and R. Baltussen. 2009. "Setting Priorities for Health Interventions in Developing Countries: A Review of Empirical Studies." *Tropical Medicine & International Health* 14 (8): 930–39. https://doi.org/10.1111/j.1365-3156.2009.02311.x.

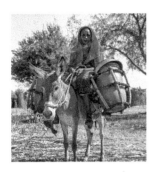

6

Developing Somalia's Essential Package of Health Services: An Integrated People-Centered Approach

Mohamed A. Jama, Abdullahi A. Ismail, Ibrahim M. Nur, Nur A. Mohamud, Teri Reynolds, Reza Majdzaheh, John Fogarty, Andre Griekspoor, Neil Thalagala, Marina Madeo, Sk Md Mamunur Rahman Malik, and Fawziya A. Nur

ABSTRACT

Somalia has a universal health service coverage index of 27 out of 100—significantly below the regional average of 57. Nonetheless, the country has committed to achieving progress toward universal health coverage targets by redesigning its essential package of health services (EPHS). The services package, tailored to address disparities in access to health services among communities including those in security-compromised areas, represents the minimum possible but has the capacity to respond to the most critical health challenges faced by the Somali people. Its integrated, people-centered approach is a key characteristic of this services package.

INTRODUCTION

Somalia has emerged from a long period of conflict that has rendered fragile the country's health system and continues to affect the delivery of health services. Over the past decade, the Federal Ministry of Health and Human Services (MoHHS) has embarked on a process of rebuilding and transforming the country's health system with the goal of improving access to essential health services for all and achieving universal health coverage (UHC) by 2030.[1]

Somalia is in the initial stages of a demographic and epidemiological transition, characterized by relatively declining maternal, infant, and child mortality and by life expectancy at birth that has reached 56.5 years (54.0 for men and 59.2 for women).[2] Despite a decline in the maternal mortality rate from an estimated 732 deaths per 100,000 live births in 2015 to 692 per 100,000 live births in 2020, the ratio remains alarmingly high (UN MMEIG 2020).[3] Similarly, the infant mortality rate fell from 86 deaths per 1,000 live births in 2014 to 75 deaths per 1,000 in 2019, yet it remains well above that of many neighboring countries.[4] Somalia lags behind its neighbors in coverage, as indicated by its low UHC service coverage index score of 27 out of 100, compared to the regional average of 57 (WHO and World Bank 2023).

The health sector in Somalia faces significant financial challenges, with public spending estimated at a mere 17 percent of total health expenditure. A combination of private spending and donor support accounts for most of the country's health expenditure, at 43 percent and 40 percent, respectively, of total health spending (GBD Health Financing Collaborator Network 2020). With per capita gross domestic product of US$445 in 2021, Somalia's economy relies heavily on remittances and international aid, with very limited domestic public financing options.

Added to those challenges is Somalia's growing population. Its population was estimated at 15.6 million in 2019, and its total fertility rate averaged 6.9 children per woman.[5] Individuals under 15 years of age make up nearly half of the population, and people under 30 make up three-quarters.[6] The high growth rate of 3 percent poses significant challenges for the health sector to keep up with the population.

Implementation from 2010 to 2019

The first EPHS, developed in 2009, was designed to address high rates of mortality and morbidity and to serve as the prime mechanism for an organized and standardized strategic service provision by directing available resources to EPHS implementation (UNICEF 2009). Uptake increased when complementary demand creation, household visiting, and outreach clinics initiatives were integrated into EPHS delivery. Those initiatives were accompanied by considerable innovations in the models of community care, with community health workers in primary health units and female health workers conducting household visits, and patient referrals, with creative use of mobile phone technology for data collection and for reporting.

Between 2010 and 2019, the EPHS covered an estimated 45 percent of the population in 47 out of 98 districts in the country (MoHHS 2020). Those substantial gains in service provision saved lives, notwithstanding the challenges encountered. Significant improvements in the capacity of regional and district health management teams were observed. The institutionalization of regular supervision using management tools such as score cards and checklists, quality assessment tools, procurement and supply chain management tools, and human resource management tools substantially enhanced the implementation of the services package. Even with those positive impacts, availability of the full package was limited by significant funding gaps, weak health system capacity, and lack of access to some areas due to security challenges. Furthermore, lack of resources meant that interventions in noncommunicable diseases, mental health, and trauma care remained unfunded despite the increasing disease burden.

Political Commitment as a Means for Achieving UHC

A change of government in February 2017 ushered in a renewed commitment to social and economic development as elaborated in Somalia's ninth National Development Plan (MoP 2020). Following the development of the Second Phase Health Sector Strategic Plan of 2017, which defined key priorities of the sector necessary for increasing access to health services, and the UHC road map of 2018, Somalia planned to revise the 2009 EPHS (MoHHS 2017, 2018)—figure 6.1. It made that decision on the basis of extensive review of experience, available evidence, the disease burden, the country context, and the lessons learned from the design and the fragmented and inefficient implementation of the 2009 EPHS. The decision was also informed by the improving political and security situation, and the reengagement with the World Bank, which opened new funding opportunities for the health sector.

Figure 6.1 Somalia's Road Map to Universal Health Coverage 2030

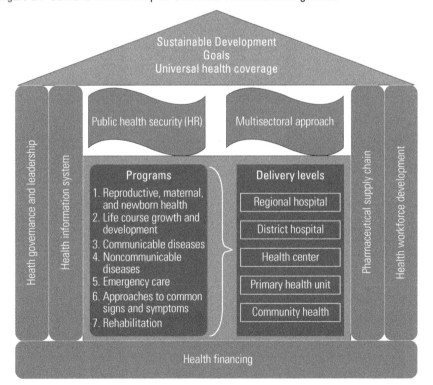

Source: Original figure created for this publication.

Despite that commitment, the EPHS revision process faced challenges because key stakeholders held different positions regarding the prioritization and financing of the package, the geographic scope and population coverage, and the delivery model. The situation necessitated an intensive policy dialogue to build consensus on the breadth of coverage and services in the package, which took 18 months to finalize.

THE EPHS REVISION PROCESS

As the first step of a more comprehensive plan for moving toward UHC, stakeholders made a collective decision to revise the services package in Somalia. A concept note was developed, and a multidisciplinary team constituted to lead the revision process (refer to figure 6.2 for the steps of the process).

Figure 6.2 Steps in Somalia's 2020 EPHS Revision Process

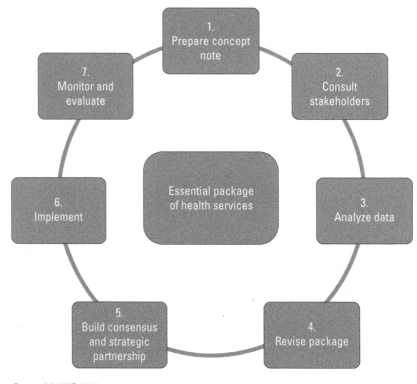

Source: MoHHS 2018.
Note: EPHS = essential package of health services.

Ownership and Governance

The decentralized management of Somalia's health care system necessitates the close collaboration and leadership of the subnational health management teams that play critical roles in planning, organizing, and implementing the EPHS at district and community levels. Somalia's revision process of the EPHS exemplified the power of building consensus and fostering collaboration among stakeholders. It entailed inclusive and in-depth discussions with all stakeholders, culminating in a harmonious agreement on the sequencing and scope of the package. That collective endeavor ensured the seamless and successful rollout of the revised EPHS, even amid resource constraints, significantly advancing the health care landscape in Somalia. Certain health services were thoughtfully prioritized for public accessibility, focusing on financing from available domestic and external resources. The dedication to equitable access extended to nomadic and security-compromised areas of the country, underscoring a solid commitment to enhancing health care accessibility and equity for all Somalis.

Somalia's heavy reliance on donor funding comes with disproportionate influence of development partners. That influence can potentially undermine country ownership and erode the principles agreed on in the 2005 Paris Declaration on Aid Effectiveness and the 2008 Accra Agenda for Action.[7] Nonetheless, development partners can play a pivotal role in shaping EPHS design and in strengthening the institutional capacity of the government in a way that strengthens the stewardship of the public sector and the delivery of homegrown solutions that are likely to succeed, instead of perpetuating past failed donor-driven solutions and approaches in many low-income countries (Noor 2022).

Stakeholder Consultation

Recognizing the need to address fragmented external aid, achieve synergy and alignment with national health priorities, and forge consensus on the prioritization and financing of highly cost-effective interventions that could address the leading causes of high mortality and morbidity in Somalia, MoHHS established an inclusive and participatory coordination structure and consultative process for the EPHS revision (Jama et al. 2023). The Federal MoHHS invited all key stakeholders to nominate representatives to a government-led task force, with members chosen for their technical expertise and knowledge of the health sector in Somalia. A concept note described the scope and purpose of the EPHS revision process, along with a timeline and the expected contribution to the different stages of the planning cycle, such as evidence generation (data collection and analysis), priority setting, implementation strategy, and monitoring and evaluation.

The resulting task force included representatives from MoHHS at the federal and state levels, the Ministry of Finance, civil society organizations, the private sector, academia, and development partners (the Canadian, German, Italian, and Swedish Embassies; Gavi, the Vaccine Alliance; the Global Financing Facility; the Global Fund; the UK Foreign, Commonwealth and Development Office; the United Nations Children's Fund and Population Fund; the World Bank; and the World Health Organization). The task force examined the adequacy of the components and scope of the 2009 EPHS against the burden of disease and the evolving health needs of the Somali people, actively soliciting, analyzing, and incorporating stakeholders' contributions and feedback early in the process.

Data Sources

The Global Burden of Disease database[8] and national data were used to prioritize services to address diseases with the highest burden of mortality and disability. Semistructured interviews conducted with public health experts helped develop a preliminary list of conditions of public health concern and hazards related to emergencies. Common symptomatic presentations at the primary care level were identified and shared with a broader group of managers, experts, and service providers for feedback through a web-based platform.

Somalia's Health and Demographic Survey of 2020 provided data on maternal and child health indicators, including use of services and vaccination coverages.[9] Because of the lack of information on baseline coverage for some noncommunicable diseases, the analysis used an assumption of 5 percent. A study reviewed service provision data and included interviews with implementers to find gaps in the 2009 EPHS. Information from the third edition of *Disease Control Priorities* and other materials highlighted cost-effective interventions and assisted with service prioritization (Glassman, Giedion, and Smith 2017; Hall et al. 2018; Jamison et al. 2018; Reich 2016; Tan-Torres Edejer et al. 2003).

Summary of Analysis Findings

Communicable diseases account for 48 percent of disability-adjusted life years in Somalia (figure 6.3), Tuberculosis, meningitis, acute hepatitis, measles, and other respiratory and infectious diseases make up nearly half of the communicable disease burden.[10] The order of the other causes of disability-adjusted life years is communicable diseases, noncommunicable diseases, maternal and neonatal disorders, malnutrition, and injuries.

Figure 6.3 Percentages of Causes of Disability-Adjusted Life Years in Somalia

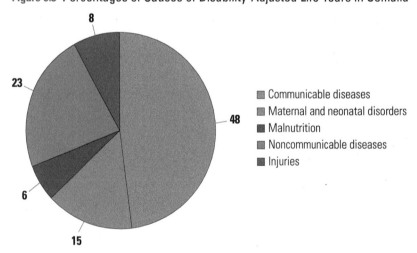

Source: Original figure based on data from Institute for Health Metrics and Evaluation, "Global Burden of Disease Study 2019 (GBD 2019) Data Resources," https://ghdx.healthdata.org/gbd-2019.

Priority-Setting Processes and Criteria Used

A deliberative process that accounted for people's health needs, economic realities, and societal preferences defined a set of evidence-informed, prioritized, individual, and population-based interventions including promotive, preventive, curative, rehabilitative, and palliative care and intersectoral actions. The guiding principles for the process highlighted consideration of (1) services that are likely to have the greatest impact on health outcomes, (2) services that are highly cost-effective and affordable within the available resources, and (3) services that can be scaled up and that give equal access to nomadic, rural, and urban populations.

Prioritization of the interventions took into account several important factors: (1) association with the high burden of disease; (2) cost-effectiveness information from the literature (Glassman et al. 2016; Glassman, Giedion, and Smith 2017; Tan-Torres Edejer et al. 2003; Waddington 2013) and from a generalized cost-effectiveness analysis for 106 proposed interventions given the limited data in the literature; and (3) the technical skills and infrastructure required for the interventions.

As a result of the priority-setting process, the 2020 EPHS is divided into a core package and an extended package. The core package constitutes a minimum service entitlement to be made available to most Somali people, whereas the extended package contains additional interventions to be progressively implemented when additional resources become available.

Scope and Content

The overarching goal of the revised EPHS was to achieve progressive expansion of and access to equitable, efficient, affordable, and quality essential health services, delivered as close to the communities they serve as possible—particularly nomadic, rural, and internally displaced populations. Certain elements of the EPHS design are specifically oriented to allow dynamic shifting of services to alternate delivery platforms and facilitate adaptation to different populations during implementation. The revision process was informed by several factors, including the evolving health needs of the Somali population, the gaps identified through a review of the 2009 EPHS, and the increasing strategic emphasis on progress toward UHC. Its overall objective was to develop an implementable package that responds to the priority health needs of the Somali people.

DESIGNING AN IMPLEMENTABLE PACKAGE

Development of the revised EPHS progressed from data to dialogue to decision-making underpinned by principles such as country values, inclusiveness, equity, effective collaboration, and partnership. Recognizing that it is the actual implementation of a package that results in effectiveness, key package design elements to support service delivery implementation included entries expressed as services rather than diseases, which supported translation to the delivery context, including monitoring and mapping of health worker competencies.

The task force used normative guidance from the third edition of *Disease Control Priorities* (Jamison et al. 2018) and the World Health Organization's UHC Compendium.[11] The task force adopted an integrated service delivery approach covering complementary elements including the response of the health system to people's demands, the continuum of care across delivery platforms, and a package design that supported implementation.

The task force adopted a rationalized architecture of interventions with consistent and nested levels of granularity for different needs. It formulated services with adequate detail and organized them to support mapping of relevant human and material resources required for implementation. This activity guided decisions about the appropriateness of the total list of services assigned to a given platform.

The structures of the package allowed for visual representation of the relationship of services across platforms (that is, related interventions were aligned across rows, and interdependent interventions were reviewed and prioritized together). The structure also supported mapping to integrated channels of service delivery.

A visual mechanism to indicate links to burden of disease was used and included a color coding system for services that addressed the top causes of death and disability. The mechanism allowed for ongoing consideration of that criterion as others were discussed. Arrows indicated progressive goals for implementation—both for the initial delivery platform and for the intended shift to the optimal delivery platform once health capacity is strengthened and funding becomes available. Figure 6.4 illustrates Somalia's health services pyramid.

Figure 6.4 The Five Delivery Platforms of Somalia's Health Care System

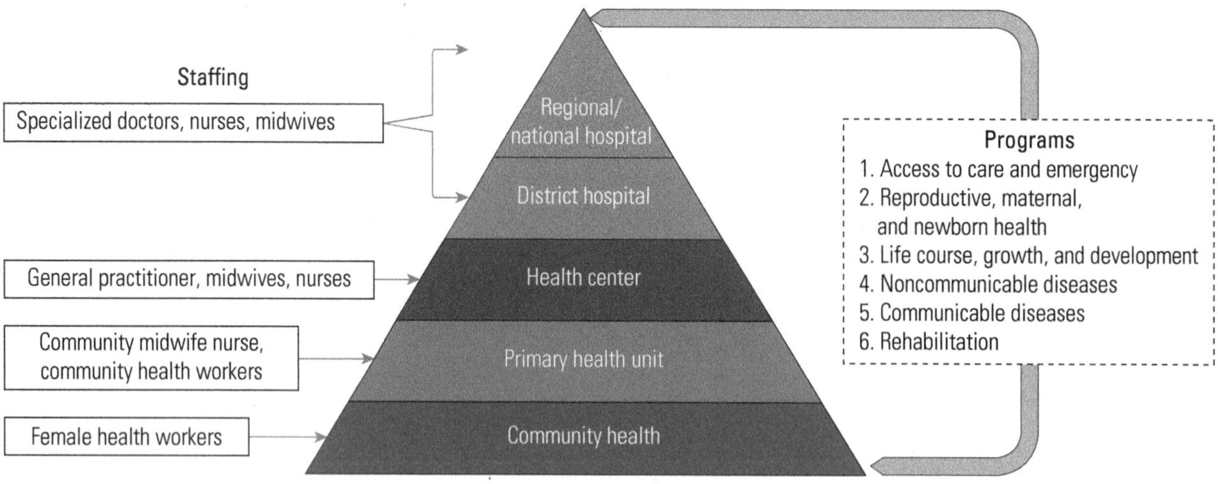

Staffing
- Specialized doctors, nurses, midwives
- General practitioner, midwives, nurses
- Community midwife nurse, community health workers
- Female health workers

Regional/national hospital
District hospital
Health center
Primary health unit
Community health

Programs
1. Access to care and emergency
2. Reproductive, maternal, and newborn health
3. Life course, growth, and development
4. Noncommunicable diseases
5. Communicable diseases
6. Rehabilitation

Source: Original figure based on MoHHS 2021a.

Emphasizing Integrated People-Centered Health Services

Somalia's EPHS 2020 was built on the notion that frontline health workers deliver care across a range of conditions based on the demands of people. People routinely seek care for symptoms (for example, cough or fever) rather than for diseases (for example, pneumonia or tuberculosis), and many of those symptoms and syndromes are managed and even resolved without a specific diagnosis. The task force therefore highlighted the importance of including demand-driven services for common symptoms and syndromes to avoid distortion of services delivery based only on diseases and to ensure a package responsive to people's demands.

All interventions proposed were highly cost-effective and considered as a minimum set of services. The package was deemed affordable based on costing analysis, and none of the selected services was excluded from the list. During the implementation plan, however, a core list of services was selected for initial implementation; an expanded list of interventions will be added to ensure progressive realization of services.

Costing and Impact Analysis

Somalia's 2020 EPHS contains 412 interventions aggregated into six program areas:

- Emergency care and approaches to common signs and symptoms
- Reproductive, maternal, and newborn health
- Life course, growth, and development
- Noncommunicable diseases
- Communicable diseases
- Rehabilitation and palliative care.

The cost of the interventions was estimated using the OneHealth Tool (OHT).[12] The costing exercise determined the impact of some interventions for which OHT impact data were available. The scope of cost estimates included the (1) cost of drugs and other supplies, (2) capital and recurrent costs of health institutions, (3) cost of remunerating health staff participating in EPHS implementation, (4) logistics costs, and (5) program costs.

OHT uses a three-step process to estimate drug and supply costs. First, it estimates potential numbers of patients/recipients of interventions based on user-defined target populations and intervention coverages. Second, it estimates the average cost of supplying drugs and other supplies of an intervention based on the user-defined treatment inputs, management protocols, and unit prices of drugs and other supply items. Third, it multiplies the number of patients/recipients of intervention by the average cost of managing a patient to produce the drugs and supply estimates of the intervention. That procedure was repeated for all interventions in the package throughout the costing period to obtain annual costs.

The proposed cost scenario did not envisage new construction of health facilities. Annualized capital costs of existing health facilities and the medical equipment and furniture attached to them were estimated as rehabilitation cost requirements. Estimates of the running costs of the facilities—electricity, water, and so on—were based on current reported expenditures. Relevant baseline and target numbers of infrastructures and respective cost parameters were obtained from MoHHS sources and entered into OHT for analysis.

Human resource costs were estimated using salary rates provided by MoHHS. Because the number of health workers would increase over time to fill staffing gaps and meet facility-based standards, the costing analysis factored that increase into the human resource costs over the projection period. Because of data constraints, logistics costs were calculated as a percentage (25 percent) of drug and supply costs. However, human resource and infrastructure costs related to the regional drug supply stores were estimated using the actual parameters.

The analysis considered that creating an enabling environment would require certain types of activities. Consequently, it calculated (using the "quantity × price" approach) the cost of program activities related to (1) the adaptation of guidelines to suit the revised EPHS package; (2) in-service training related to the EPHS; (3) supervision of the EPHS implementation; (4) monitoring and evaluation, including the adaptation of the information system; and (5) health promotion and community mobilization. It enumerated the resource requirements of each activity according to the nature of the activity and past program experiences in Somalia for similar activities, obtaining that information and various unit costs from implementation partners.

The impact analysis of EPHS scale-up in Somalia used OHT impact modules and was based on scaling up the interventions from baseline population coverage of 45 percent to 80 percent coverage in 2030. Looking at the key resources required, the cost analysis suggested a gradual scale-up of the implementation of the 2020 EPHS interventions across the five delivery platforms. At the baseline (2020) with existing coverage, EPHS implementation would cost US$105 million. That cost would gradually increase to an estimated US$626 million in 2030 at universal coverage (table 6.1). The 2030 figure reflects an estimated per capita expenditure of US$33, with the largest portion of the cost increase attributed to the expansion of priority intervention coverage for people currently not covered and to account for projected population growth.

Table 6.1 Costs of Implementing Somalia's EPHS 2020, by Cost Item, 2020–30
US dollars, million

Cost item	2020	2021	2022	2023	2024	2025	2026	2027	2028	2029	2030	Total
Total human resources	48.2	54.1	60.2	66.6	73.2	80.0	87.2	94.6	102.3	110.3	118.6	895.3
Total infrastructure, all facilities	10.5	10.7	11.0	11.2	11.4	11.7	12.0	12.2	12.5	12.8	13.0	128.9
Infrastructure rehabilitation	4.4	4.5	4.6	4.7	4.8	4.9	5.0	5.1	5.2	5.3	5.4	53.6
Maintenance and operations, all existing facilities	6.1	6.3	6.4	6.5	6.7	6.8	7.0	7.1	7.3	7.5	7.6	75.3
Total medicines and supplies	36.0	43.3	54.3	68.2	85.7	107.8	136.7	174.4	223.9	288.9	375.1	1,594.3
Total logistics	9.6	11.7	14.8	18.9	24.1	30.7	39.6	51.5	67.4	88.6	117.3	474.2
Warehouse	0.1	0.1	0.1	0.1	0.1	0.1	0.1	0.1	0.1	0.1	0.1	1.1
Logistics workers	0.5	0.5	0.6	0.6	0.6	0.6	0.6	0.6	0.6	0.6	0.7	6.5
Drug transportation	9.0	11.1	14.2	18.2	23.4	30.1	38.9	50.8	66.6	87.9	116.6	466.6
Total program	0.2	1.5	1.1	1.3	1.2	1.3	1.3	1.3	1.3	1.4	1.5	13.3
Grand total	104.6	121.3	141.5	166.1	195.6	231.6	276.7	334.1	407.3	501.9	625.5	3,106.0

Source: Adapted from table 6 in MoHHS 2021a.

Note: EPHS = Essential Package of Health Services.

The largest share of the EPHS implementation cost is attributed to human resources at 46 percent, followed by medicines and other supplies at 34 percent (figure 6.5). Infrastructure and logistics costs account for 10 percent and 9 percent, respectively. The distribution of those resources is similar to results identified in a 2014 costing study of the EPHS in Somalia (Blaakman 2014). Analysis of EPHS implementation costs by facility type shows that community, primary health unit, and health center levels of care would consume nearly 80 percent of EPHS implementation costs (figure 6.6).

Figure 6.5 Percent of Estimated Baseline Cost of EPHS, by Cost Component, 2020

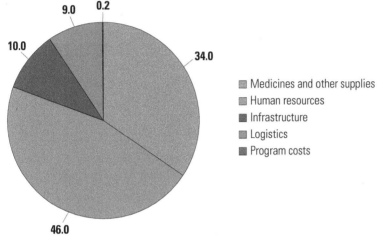

Source: Adapted from figure 3 in MoHHS 2021a.
Note: EPHS = essential package of health services.

Figure 6.6 Total Cost of EPHS Implementation, by Type of Facility, Somalia, 2020–2030

Cost of EPHS implementation (unit, US$, million)

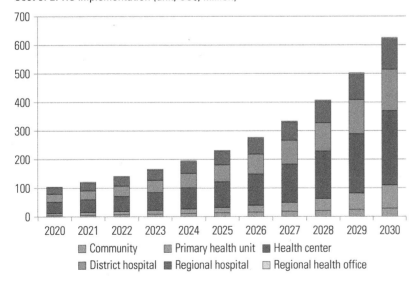

Source: Adapted from figure 7 in MoHHS 2021a.
Note: EPHS = Essential package of health services.

The revised EPHS was designed to be flexible and adaptable to resource constraints, with core and extended scenarios to support progressive realization and future expansion of the services package. The design allows for the need to ramp up capacity and for flexible operationalization for different contexts that may have distinct platforms or constraints, including geographical or security constraints affecting access.

Linking with Monitoring and Evaluation

MoHHS adopted a right-to-health approach with an emphasis on ensuring access for the most vulnerable. The EPHS sets the direction for the development of an implementation plan that progressively adds more services of increased quality made available to more people.

At the time of the EPHS design, the country did not yet have a unified and standardized national Health Information Management System, or a harmonized list of indicators. The EPHS implementation plan sets measurable objectives that can be monitored with a well-established information system. It gives special attention to sex-disaggregated data and data on vulnerable populations. It also includes mechanisms designed to enhance access to EPHS services, including an integrated disease surveillance system and complaint mechanisms.

The EPHS design process was used as the entry point to define the purpose and scope of the system. It supports an area-based, district health management approach with supportive supervision as a cornerstone for implementing the package and improving overall accountability. Users of the information include facility managers who oversee quality improvement processes, health management teams that manage EPHS implementation and plan services based on population health needs, and national authorities who report achievements, increase accountability, and design incentives.

Routine data collection systems, complemented by surveys and community-based surveillance systems and mechanisms to collect qualitative information, constitute the basis of an integrated health information system (table 6.2). District Health Information System 2 (DHIS2),[13] already introduced in Somalia, is used to calculate a range of key performance indicators that monitor trends in outputs, use, and coverage such as the number of outpatient department visits (per person per year), proportion of births attended by skilled health personnel, or immunization coverage levels.

The Integrated Disease Surveillance and Response system complements the Routine Health Information System collected through DHIS2 to manage alerts, investigations, and response to potential epidemics. The system has defined indicators, including timeliness and completeness of the reporting, and investigations done within 48 hours build on the experience of the countries in the region (Fall et al. 2019).

A national list and mapping of all public and private health facilities obtained from Somalia's 2016 Service Availability and Readiness Assessment Survey and the Health Resources and Services Availability Monitoring System allow regular updating of facilities' functionality to support the humanitarian program (MoHHS 2016).[14] A standard list of key indicators was developed to monitor the number of health facilities offering specific services per 10,000 population and meeting minimum service standards based on tracer criteria for specific services, the percentage of the population living within a 5-kilometer radius or one hour's travel to a health facility, and the total number of beds per 10,000 population.[15]

Table 6.2 Overview of Data Sources Used to Improve Data Completeness and Quality for Somalia's 2020 EPHS

| M&E domain | Facility-based routine information and data | | | Household surveys | |
	RHIS	IDSR	Facility mapping	SHDS	Expenditure, health-seeking behavior, and barriers
Availability of package	✓		✓	✓	✓
Provider performance	✓				
Quality of services					
Use and barriers				✓	✓
Preparedness		✓			
Patient satisfaction				✓	
Service coverage	✓		✓	✓	✓
Financial protection					✓
Burden of disease	✓			✓	

Source: Original table developed for this publication.

Note: EPHS = essential package of health services; IDSR = Integrated Disease Surveillance and Response; M&E = monitoring and evaluation; RHIS = Routine Health Information System; SHDS = Somalia Health and Demographic Survey.

The data sources and indicators generated through those systems are integrated in comprehensive district and regional dashboards. Dashboards include indicators on service availability, their effective use, unmet needs, service quality, and outcome measures necessary for monitoring and evaluating the EPHS and quality of services and their impact. For accountability, the implementation strategy includes independent monitoring and evaluation by a third-party monitoring agency and a complaint resolution mechanism so that people can receive support in reaching a solution to problems.

Linking to Other Health System Functions

The EPHS translates the Second Phase Health Sector Strategic Plan of 2017 and the road map to UHC into an implementable package to address the significant gaps in service delivery (MoHHS 2017, 2018). The EPHS also serves as the foundation for improving the overall effectiveness of the health system's performance. The policy options elaborated in the revised Health Sector Strategic Plan of 2022 guide the health system strengthening strategy (MoHHS 2022).

Implementation of the EPHS has revealed a critical shortage and the unequal distribution of health workers, particularly in rural and nomadic communities. Those problems have led to a review of human resources for health, which identified priority areas for action related to production and deployment of critical midlevel health workers, including, but not limited to, midwives, nurses, and community health workers (MoHHS 2021b). Other reforms carried out by the government to ensure the delivery of quality health services to the Somali population include improving oversight and regulatory functions, and strengthening procurement and supply chain management, health financing, and public health management.

Strengthening Subnational Governance

Because regional and district health offices are key to ensuring successful implementation of the 2020 EPHS, regional and district health authorities have been tasked with ensuring that services are available and delivered effectively. Being close to the field, regional and district health offices are well positioned to hold providers accountable and to collect feedback on service delivery from users. They play a key role in informing policy makers on the need for package adjustments and delivery modalities, as well as in providing input on resource allocations in their districts.

District management teams serve as an interface with the community to generate demand and provide crucial oversight of resources to optimize service delivery, increase equity and efficiency, and improve how patients access and move through the health system. Those roles are defined in the revised EPHS (MoHHS 2021a).

Adapting the Package to Different Contexts to Foster the Humanitarian-Development Nexus

The design of the EPHS allows for a quick ramp-up of capacity as well as for flexible operationalization for different contexts that may have distinct platforms or constraints. Nevertheless, the package is intended to be delivered through a district primary health care approach that includes standards on the number of delivery platforms per district to serve the population in the district. The package includes additional adaptations for nomadic populations to facilitate referral pathways and support transportation. Special considerations are applied for outreach and mobile facilities in insecure/limited accessibility areas.

Table 6.3 illustrates possible adaptations for district health and service delivery platforms in different operational contexts. Although some general benchmarks are proposed, they are adapted to local conditions. Adaptations are led by district health management teams responsible for assessing and managing the accessibility and functionality of the health facilities in their areas.

Table 6.3 Adapting Package Operationalization in Different Contexts, Somalia's 2020 EPHS

Context characteristics	Rural districts	Urban districts	Nomadic populations	Insecure and/or inaccessible areas
Operational context and local conditions	Lower population per district, with lower population density	Larger population per district, with higher population density	Populations that move across administrative boundaries of districts	Boundaries based on accessibility and security; areas served through humanitarian hubs
Assumption for adaptation	Local differences in population density need to be considered when planning locations for the facilities for upgrading the health network to progressively increase coverage of service availability based on 5 km distance and/or 1 hour travel time	More efficient to increase the capacity of one health center or district hospital to serve the catchment population within 5 km/1 hour travel, rather than rigidly adhering to the standards for rural contexts	For smaller nomadic populations, it is more efficient to invest in first aid and stabilization capacities of the community health worker, and transportation for referral	Referral pathways defined for each hub, whereby it may be desirable to upgrade a health center to district hospital or district hospital to regional hospital. Special consideration is given to support transportation to referral facilities
Community services	1 community health worker per 600–1,000 population	Same	Same	Same in accessible areas
Primary health unit	1 primary health unit per 7,500–10,000 population	Same	Same	Same in accessible areas
Health centers	1 health center per 20,000–30 000 population	1 health center per 30,000 to 50,0,000 population, with capacity adapted to catchment population within 5 km or 1 hour	Mobile clinic that follows the population, or flexible referral pathways to nearest health center with investment in transportation capacities within nomadic population	Mobile health and nutrition teams to provide services
District hospitals	1 district hospital per 120,000–150,000 population	1 district hospital per 150,000–300,000 population, with capacity adapted to catchment population within 5 km/1 hour	Flexible referral pathways to nearest district hospital, with investment in transportation capacities within nomadic population	District hospital in a town that serves as the humanitarian hub for a geographical area or upgrade to district hospital in the accessible area
Regional/ national hospital	Existing national, regional, or specialized hospitals			
Surge capacity or specialized treatment centers linked to acute or chronic emergencies	Temporary treatment centers in the event of epidemics, drought, or floods; nutrition rehabilitation units in the event of increased food insecurity. Additional temporary staff recruited for the duration of the increased health needs; in other cases, existing staff repurposed to temporary treatment centers. This adaptation inevitably affects the capacity to maintain services outlined in EPHS, requiring anticipation of further reprioritization in contingency plans to suspend temporarily noncritical services.			

Source: Original table based on MoHHS 2016.

Note: EPHS = essential package of health services; km = kilometers.

Linking to Service Delivery Reforms

The revised EPHS aims to address all high-burden conditions through simple, low-cost, high-impact interventions; establish demand-driven services to facilitate more accurate costing and integrated service delivery; link services to level of care; allow operationalization of the package in variable contexts with distinct delivery platforms; provide a foundation for service planning, workforce mapping, and training competencies; support progressive realization and account for the need to increase service delivery capacity over time; and support expansion to additional services when additional resources become available.

Although the private sector plays a critical role in Somalia's health sector, it is largely concentrated in urban centers and focuses predominantly on clinical and surgical care. Somalia's private sector delivers an estimated 60 percent of health services and supplies 70 percent of medicines (Buckley, O'Neill, and Aden 2015). To realize the full potential of the private sector, the government is strengthening its regulatory bodies with the objective of ensuring the quality and safety of pharmaceuticals and medical devices (MoHHS 2021b).

Linking to Financing Mechanisms

During the EPHS revision process, Somalia encountered several challenges related to financial affordability, limited implementation capacity, and weak governance. Those challenges were compounded by the COVID-19 pandemic, which pressured the already-stretched service delivery capacity of the available resources to ensure the feasibility and success of the revised EPHS. Somalia has developed an investment case for the health sector as the main instrument to support transformation and financial reforms that can unlock and accelerate efforts to secure predictable financing for the delivery of the EPHS (MoHHS 2021c). Despite expectations for sustainable public financing in the long term, the short-term implementation of the EPHS will depend on a combination of domestic resources and sustainable and predictable foreign aid and private financing that can reduce the country's high out-of-pocket payments and their devastating impact on household income.

LIMITATIONS

Weak health system capacity, inconstant quality of care, data gaps and lack of financial information, limited analytical skills in economic evaluation and fiscal space analysis, and ensuring community consultation and institutionalization were some of the key challenges the EPHS revision process encountered. Although the Somalia Health and Demographic Survey of 2020 and the Global Burden of Disease database filled some of the data gaps, the absence of some critical data required the use of expert opinion, complemented by data extracted from other reports. In addition, to overcome the data gaps and fragmentation, the government developed an integrated Health Information Management System that uses a single digital platform—provided by DHIS2—for data collection, validation, and analysis. It has also deployed digital mobile solutions for data collection and reporting in remote areas.

LESSONS LEARNED

Achieving consensus on a prioritized, highly cost-effective package of health services that responds to the health needs of the people requires country preparation and the establishment of a deliberative approach through structured coordination and an inclusive consultation process involving all stakeholders. Ensuring government ownership of EPHS design and implementation, and mapping potential financial resources available for EPHS service delivery, was an integral part of the EPHS development process and provided a clear road map for implementation.

National governments need to ensure that decision-making processes on package development are inclusive and participatory. Similarly, countries should also endeavor to achieve the target Abuja Declaration of 2001 by allocating sufficient domestic resources to the health sector and demonstrate value for money by improving transparency and accountability for results.

Implementation models must continue to prioritize the capacity of Regional and District Health Management Teams with supervision and integrated action planning and tracking at all levels. Similarly, expenditure tracking and strategic rationalization decisions need to be made annually by region and district to improve coverage (breadth) and to determine package size (depth).

The establishment of clear criteria supported by locally generated evidence on the prioritization of EPHS interventions is essential. Similarly, development of the package requires local capacity building for skills on burden of disease analysis, economic evaluation, and costing of the services packages.

The inclusion of implementation considerations and the ability to adapt the package to various local conditions as part of the design and organization of the EPHS facilitated the planning process of the district management teams. Similarly, the implementation of public administration reforms, including public financial management and establishment of functioning supply chain management, were deemed critical for the implementation of the package.

The establishment of a monitoring and evaluation mechanism, which includes the generation of evidence such as the UHC service index, was considered central for garnering the support of decision-makers and stakeholders.

Expanding the EPHS will require engagement of the private sector to enhance access to quality primary health care services. Similarly, the engagement of other sectors in the design of the package and the promotion of a multisectoral approach are necessary for tackling the social determinants of health.

ACKNOWLEDGMENTS

The authors express their gratitude to the Ministry of Health and Human Services of Somalia and the World Health Organization (WHO) for their invaluable assistance in improving the quality and completeness of the data used in this chapter. We also extend our thanks to the World Bank; the United Nations Children's Fund; and the Foreign, Commonwealth, and Development Office of the United Kingdom and Northern Ireland for their support and cooperation.

We are deeply grateful for the substantial contributions and suggestions from our colleagues in the Ministry of Health and Human Services at both the federal and state levels, as well as from colleagues at WHO and the World Bank country office.

In particular, we acknowledge our late friend and colleague, Dr. Peter Salama, executive director of WHO's Division for Universal Health Coverage – Life Course. Dr. Salama was a champion for global health equity, and his vision and unwavering commitment to delivering an effective, implementable package of health services in fragile and conflict settings, such as Somalia, were truly inspirational. Driven by his conviction and passion to serve populations in challenging circumstances, Dr. Salama, in collaboration with the Ministry of Health and Human Services of Somalia, brought together a team from WHO, the United Nations Children's Fund and Population Fund, the World Bank, bilateral donors, and civil society organizations in January 2020. That team initiated the design and implementation of a highly cost-effective package of health services in Somalia, which continues to save lives today. Dr. Salama was a great public health leader of our time. May his soul rest in eternal peace.

NOTES

1. One of the United Nations' Sustainable Development Goals; for more information, refer to United Nations, "The 17 Goals," https://sdgs.un.org/goals.
2. World Health Organization, "Global Health Observatory data repository," https://apps.who.int/gho/data/node.main.688?lang=en.
3. Also refer to the Somali National Data Archive, "Somali Health and Demographic and Survey 2020," https://apps.who.int/gho/data/node.main.688?lang=en (accessed July 10, 2022).
4. United Nations Children's Fund, "Country Profiles: Somalia," https://data.unicef.org/country/som/ (accessed December 22, 2021).
5. United Nations Population Fund, "World Population Dashboard: Somalia," https://www.unfpa.org/data/world-population/SO (accessed December 28, 2021).
6. Somali National Data Archive, "Somali Health and Demographic and Survey 2020."
7. Organisation for Economic Co-operation and Development, "Paris Declaration and Accra Agenda for Action," https://web-archive.oecd.org/temp/2021-08-02/73869-parisdeclarationandaccraagendaforaction.htm.
8. Institute for Health Metrics and Evaluation, "Global Burden of Disease Study 2019 (GBD 2019) Data Resources," https://ghdx.healthdata.org/gbd-2019.
9. Somali National Data Archive, "Somali Health and Demographic Survey 2020," https://microdata.nbs.gov.so/index.php/catalog/50.
10. Institute for Health Metrics and Evaluation, "Global Burden of Disease Study 2019."
11. World Health Organization, "UHC Compendium" (database), https://www.who.int/universal-health-coverage/compendium (accessed July 20, 2022).
12. Avenir Health, "OneHealth Tool," https://www.avenirhealth.org/software-onehealth.
13. For more information about DHIS2, refer to the University of Oslo's DHIS2 web page, https://dhis2.org.
14. World Health Organization, "Health Resources and Services Availability Monitoring System (HeRAMS)," https://www.who.int/initiatives/herams.
15. WHO, "AccessMod 5: Supporting Universal Health Coverage by Modelling Physical Accessibility to Health Care," https://www.accessmod.org.

REFERENCES

Blaakman A. 2014. "Cost Analysis of the Essential Package of Health Services (EPHS) in Somalia." HEART (Health & Education Advice & Resource Team), Oxford. https://assets.publishing.service.gov.uk/media/57a089e8e5274a27b2000305/Somalia-cost-analysis-of-the-essential-package-of-health-services-.pdf.

Buckley, J., L. O'Neill, and A. M. Aden. 2015. "Assessment of the Private Health Sector in Somaliland, Puntland and South Central." HEART (Health & Education Advice & Resource Team), Oxford. https://assets.publishing.service.gov.uk/media/57a0899bed915d622c0002e3/Assessment-of-the-Private-Health-Sector-in-Somaliland-Puntland-and-South-Central.pdf.

Fall, I. S., S. Rajatonirina, A. A. Yahaya, Y. Zabulon, P. Nsubuga, M. Nanyunja, J. Wamala, et al. 2019. "Integrated Disease Surveillance and Response (IDSR) Strategy: Current Status, Challenges and Perspectives for the Future in Africa." *BMJ Global Health* 4 (4): e001427. https://gh.bmj.com/content/4/4/e001427.

GBD (Global Burden of Disease) Health Financing Collaborator Network. 2020. "Health Sector Spending and Spending on HIV/AIDS, Tuberculosis, and Malaria, and Development Assistance for Health: Progress towards Sustainable Development Goal 3 (2020)." *The Lancet* 396 (10252): 693–724. https://doi.org/10.1016/S0140-6736(20)30608-5.

Glassman, A., U. Giedion, Y. Sakuma, and P. C. Smith. 2016. "Defining a Health Benefit Package: What Are the Necessary Processes?" *Health Systems & Reform* 2 (1): 39–50. https://doi.org/10.1080/23288604.2016.1124171.

Glassman, A., U. Giedion, and P. C. Smith. 2017. *What's In, What's Out? Designing Benefits for Universal Health Coverage.* Washington, DC: Center for Global Development. https://www.cgdev.org/publication/whats-in-whats-out-designing-benefits-universal-health-coverage.

Hall, W., I. Williams, N. Smith, M. Gold, J. Coast, L. Kapiriri, M. Danis, and C. Mitton. 2018. "Past, Present and Future Challenges in Health Care Priority Setting: Findings from an International Expert Survey." *Journal of Health Organization and Management* 32 (3): 444–62. https://doi.org/10.1108/JHOM-01-2018-0005.

Jama, M. A., R. Majdzadeh, T. Reynolds, I. M. Nur, A. A. Ismail, N. A. Mohamud, A. Griekspoor, et al. 2023. "Revising the Essential Package of Health Services through Stakeholder Alignment, Somalia." *Bulletin of the World Health Organization* 101 (11): 738–42. http://dx.doi.org/10.2471/BLT.23.289733.

Jamison, D. T., H. Gelband, S. Horton, P. Jha, R. Laxminarayan, C. N. Mock, and Rachel Nugent, eds. 2018. *Disease Control Priorities* (third edition), Volume 9, *Disease Control Priorities: Improving Health and Reducing Poverty.* Washington, DC: World Bank. https://documents.worldbank.org/en/publication/documents-reports/documentdetail/527531512569346552/disease-control-priorities-improving-health-and-reducing-poverty.

MoHHS (Somalia, Ministry of Health and Human Services). 2016. "Service Availability and Readiness Assessment (SARA) of Somalia, 2016." Federal Government of Somalia, Mogadishu. https://moh.gov.so/so/pdfs/somalia-sara-report-2016/.

MoHHS (Somalia, Ministry of Health and Human Services). 2017. *Second Phase Health Sector Strategic Plan 2017–2021.* Mogadishu: Federal Government Somalia. https://www.somalimedicalarchives.org/media/attachments/2021/09/18/fgs-hssp-ii-2017-2021---final.pdf.

MoHHS (Somalia, Ministry of Health and Human Services). 2018. "Roadmap towards Universal Health Coverage in Somalia, 2019–23." Federal Government of Somalia, Mogadishu. https://extranet.who.int/countryplanningcycles/sites/default/files/country_docs/Somalia/final_draft_somali_roadmap_towards_uhc_2019-23-2.pdf.

MoHHS (Somalia, Ministry of Health and Human Services). 2020. "Implementation of the Somali EPHS 2008–2019." Report, Federal Government of Somalia, Mogadishu. https://moh.gov.so/so/wp-content/uploads/2024/08/Implementation-of-Somali-EPHS-2009-2019.-9-March-2020.pdf.

MoHHS (Somalia, Ministry of Health and Human Services of Somalia). 2021a. *Essential Package of Health Services (EPHS) Somalia, 2020*. Mogadishu: Federal Government of Somalia. https://reliefweb.int/report/somalia/essential-package-health-services-ephs-somalia-2020.

MoHHS (Somalia, Ministry of Health and Human Services). 2021b. "HRH Regulatory Landscape Mission Report September 30, 2021." Federal Government of Somalia, Mogadishu. https://moh.gov.so/so/pdfs/hrh-regulatory-landscape-mission-report_september-30-2021/.

MoHHS (Somalia, Ministry of Health and Human Services). 2021c. "Investment Case for the Somalia Health Sector, 2022–2027." Federal Government of Somalia, Mogadishu. https://moh.gov.so/en/wp-content/uploads/2022/11/Investment-Case-for-the-Somali-Helath-Sector.pdf.

MoHHS (Somalia, Ministry of Health and Human Services). 2022. *Somalia Health Sector Strategic Plan 2022–2026*. Mogadishu: Government of Somalia. https://moh.gov.so/so/wp-content/uploads/2022/11/Health-Sector-Strategy-Plan-III.pdf.

MoP (Somalia, Ministry of Planning, Investment and Economic Development). 2020. *Somalia National Development Plan 2020–2024*. Mogadishu: Federal Government of Somalia. https://mop.gov.so/national-development-plan/.

Noor, A. M. 2022. "Country Ownership in Global Health." *PLoS Global Public Health* 2 (2): e0000113. https://doi.org/10.1371/journal.pgph.0000113.

Reich, M. R. 2016. "Introduction to the PMAC 2016 Special Issue: 'Priority Setting for Universal Health Coverage.'" *Health Systems & Reform* 2 (1): 1–4. https://doi.org/10.1080/23288604.2016.1125258.

Tan-Torres Edejer, T., R. Baltussen, T. Adam, R. Hutubessy, A. Acharya, D. B. Evans, and C. J. L. Murray, eds. 2003. *Making Choices in Health: WHO Guide to Cost-Effectiveness Analysis*. Geneva: World Health Organization. https://iris.who.int/bitstream/handle/10665/42699/9241546018.pdf?sequence=1&isAllowed=y.

UNICEF (United Nations Children's Fund). 2009. "Essential Package of Health Services: Somalia 2009." Report 2, UNICEF. https://moh.gov.so/en/wp-content/uploads/2020/07/Essential-Package-of-Health-Services-2009.pdf.

UN MMEIG (United Nations Maternal Mortality Estimation Inter-Agency Group). 2020. *Trends in Maternal Mortality 2000 to 2017: Estimates by WHO, UNICEF, UNFPA, World Bank Group and the United Nations Population Division*. Geneva: World Health Organization. https://www.who.int/publications-detail-redirect/9789241516488.

Waddington C. 2013. "Essential Health Packages: What Are They For? What Do They Change?" HLSP Institute, London. https://www.mottmac.com/download/file/6125?cultureId=127.

WHO (World Health Organization) and World Bank. 2023. *Tracking Universal Health Coverage: 2023 Global Monitoring Report*. Conference edition. Geneva: WHO and Washington, DC: World Bank. https://iris.who.int/bitstream/handle/10665/374059/9789240080379-eng.pdf?sequence=1.

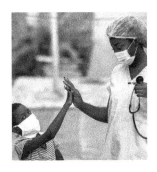

7

Malawi's Universal Health Coverage Country Translation Process

Pakwanja Desiree Twea, Paul Revill, Sakshi Mohan, Gerald Manthalu, Dominic Nkhoma, Collins Owen Francisco Zamawe, and Collins Chansa

ABSTRACT

Malawi has developed and implemented Essential Health Packages (EHPs) since 2001. EHPs in Malawi have focused on addressing the burden of disease and equity challenges in health care, with the multistakeholder EHP Technical Working Group leading the EHP development and review process. This chapter documents the health sector prioritization process for the development of Malawi's EHPs with a focus on its third EHP (2017–22). Key criteria for that EHP were health maximization, equity, the continuum of care, and complementarities. The EHP review team used local costing data, and effectiveness data came from the second edition of *Disease Control Priorities* (Jamison et al. 2006), the World Health Organization Choosing Interventions That Are Cost-Effective (WHO-Choice), and the Tufts Global Health Registry.[1] The final EHP had a cost-effectiveness threshold of US$61 per disability-adjusted life year averted with 97 health interventions.

INTRODUCTION

The government of Malawi is committed to meeting its domestic and international commitments to health service delivery. Those commitments are enshrined in the National Health Policy 2018–30 (MoH 2018) and medium-term strategic frameworks such as the five-year Health Sector Strategic Plan (HSSP) III (MoH 2023). Domestically, the law mandates that the government provide adequate health care to the population in accordance with the health needs of the population and international standards of care (Government of Malawi 1994). To deliver on the universality mandate, government policy is to reduce health care access barriers by providing a health benefits package (known in Malawi as the Essential Health Package or EHP) that residents can access for free at the point of consumption.

Like most countries, Malawi has inadequate financial, human, and material resources available to provide free and quality health care. For instance, its per capita total health expenditure of US$39.60 (MoH 2020b) is insufficient to provide quality essential health services universally (figure 7.1). With fiscal space challenges worsening because of the advent of the COVID-19 pandemic (World Bank 2020), Malawi's aspiration of adequate quality public health care services at the point of access and attainment of universal health coverage by 2030 remains improbable. Access to health care continues to present a challenge, with about 53 percent of women facing financial and geographical barriers (NSO and ICF 2017). The first EHP developed by the government sought to address those and other access barriers by providing a framework for targeting available resources to a prioritized package of health services. In that way, available resources could be rationalized and provided at scale to more people and to increase financial protection.

Figure 7.1 Total Health Expenditure Trends, Malawi, 2002/03–17/18

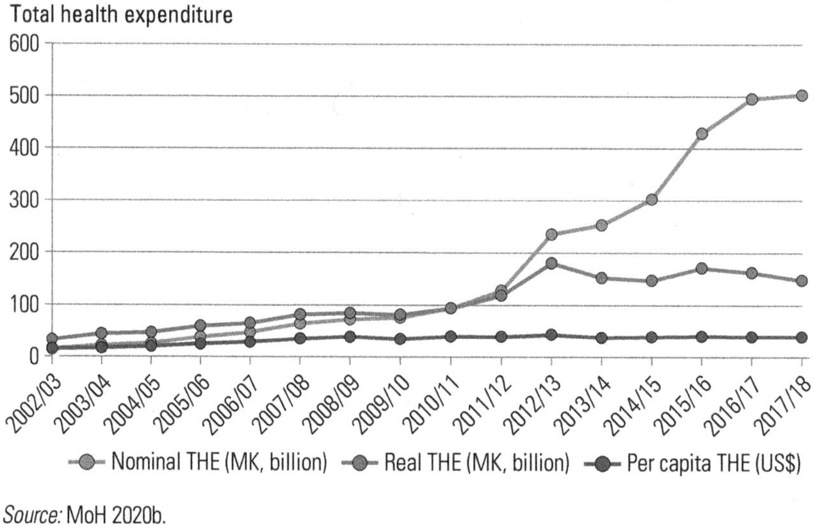

Total health expenditure

Source: MoH 2020b.

Note: MK = Malawian kwacha; THE = total health expenditure.

This chapter documents the priority-setting process in Malawi's health sector as it relates to the development, implementation, and review of EHPs over the years. It also discusses the content and lessons learned from implementing the third EHP (2017–22) and future directions. By documenting the implementation process and lessons learned, the chapter can help inform future design and implementation of health benefits packages in Malawi and other developing countries.

EVOLUTION OF THE EHP IN MALAWI

The concept of an EHP for Malawi was first envisaged in the fourth National Health Plan (MoH 1999). However, an EHP was not formally adopted until the successor plan, the Joint Programme of Work, the medium-term health strategy covering the period 2004–10 (MoH 2004). Apart from addressing health access barriers, the first EHP also aimed to contribute to poverty reduction in line with recommendations of the *World Development Report 1993* (World Bank 1993). At the core of the introduction of the EHP in the Joint Programme of Work was the use of burden of disease data to identify diseases and conditions that contributed the most to mortality and morbidity, and to prioritize the interventions that could cost-effectively address those diseases. The objectives of that EHP were "to improve technical and allocative efficiency in the delivery of health care; to ensure universal coverage of health services, and to provide cost-effective interventions that can control the main causes of disease burden in Malawi" (MoH 2004, 17). Limitations of that EHP included not explicitly accounting for equity and resource availability in its design, as evidenced by higher access among the nonpoor than among the poor.

The EHP was first revised in 2011 as part of informing the first HSSP, and the revision maintained the same criteria of disease burden and cost-effectiveness of interventions (MoH 2011). For the burden of disease criterion, The EHP included interventions for diseases/conditions contributing to at least 10,000 disability-adjusted life years (DALYs) per year across Malawi's population and excluded interventions for diseases/conditions that imposed fewer than 10,000 DALYs. It considered cost-effective any interventions with an incremental cost-effectiveness ratio below US$150 per DALY averted per year. Interventions with an incremental cost-effectiveness ratio higher than US$1,050 were automatically excluded as cost-ineffective because they represented more than three times the country's gross domestic product at the time (Phoya et al., n.d.). Unlike its predecessor, the second EHP was designed to be more equitable by including more interventions targeting vulnerable population groups.

The Ministry of Health then developed the third EHP to inform the second HSSP for the period 2017–22. With previous EHPs, a recurrent challenge was that the cost of implementation exceeded the available resources. In the third EHP, the cost-effectiveness threshold (US$61 per DALY averted) takes into account the resource constraints at implementation (MoH 2017). Thus, the third EHP had lower financing gaps compared to its predecessors because it included fewer interventions than if it had used World Health Organization thresholds based on gross domestic product per capita. However, without reforming service delivery, resource allocation, provider payment, and provider organization, among others, the Ministry of Health found it challenging to enforce the package because public health facilities continued to deliver a broader range of services than those included in the EHP.

Figure 7.2 shows the cost and affordability[2] trends of EHPs in Malawi. Notably, except for 2005 07 and 2017, the cost of EHP delivery has exceeded available resources (MoH 2016a, 2020b) as characterized by per capita total health expenditure—especially for the second EHP, which covered the period 2011–16. Although the first EHP covered the years 2004–10, costs escalated because more and more interventions were added between 2008 and 2010. EHP cost per capita again rose with the introduction of the second EHP in 2011. Costs reduced to within the level of total health expenditure resources only with the introduction of the third EHP in 2017.

Figure 7.2 EHP Cost Trend, Malawi, 2004–17

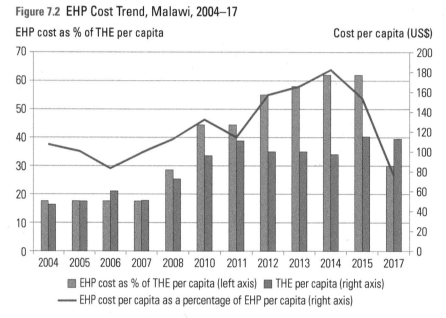

Sources: Adapted and updated from MoH 2004, 2011, 2017; THE (total health expenditure) per capita data are from MoH 2016a, 2020b.

EHP PRIORITY-SETTING PROCESS

The Ministry of Health leads and coordinates the health sector priority-setting process at the national level. It coordinates the EHP development and review processes and acts as the secretariat to the EHP Technical Working Group (EHP-TWG), which leads those processes. As the secretariat to the EHP-TWG, the Ministry of Health is responsible for developing the EHP road map, terms of reference, and any other required guidance documents. The EHP-TWG is multidisciplinary in its composition and has the leadership role in making the EHP review process as inclusive and transparent as possible.

Among its responsibilities, the EHP-TWG collects and assesses the evidence on health care interventions and provides objective recommendations that inform inclusion and exclusion decisions. Specifically, it provides technical input to inform policy decisions on EHP provision, ensures that the EHP reflects the latest evidence, regularly updates the EHP Cost-Effectiveness Tool, monitors EHP implementation and suggests policies for improvement, and provides evidence to decision-makers to inform EHP decisions (MoH 2016b). Ministry of Health Senior Management makes the final decisions on the list of interventions to include in the EHP, which is then reviewed and disseminated among key stakeholders for consensus building before approval. Upon finalization and approval, the HSSP and the EHP are then shared with key national- and subnational-level stakeholders.

The composition of the EHP-TWG is based primarily on inclusiveness and on the competencies and expertise of members. The focus on inclusiveness ensures representation of all important stakeholders, including the Ministry of Health at the headquarters and district levels, academia, civil society, private nonprofit health providers, development partners, and nongovernmental organizations. EHP-TWG members are chosen also for their competency and expertise in areas including economic evaluation of health care interventions, evidence synthesis, health economic modeling, and clinical and economic evidence interpretation. Figure 7.3 outlines the stakeholders involved in each stage of the EHP development and implementation process.

Figure 7.3 EHP Review Process Stakeholders

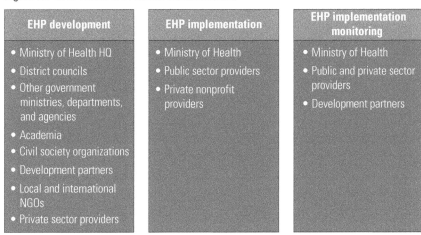

Source: MoH 2016b.

Note: EHP = Essential Health Package; HQ = headquarters; NGOs = nongovernmental organizations.

For the third EHP, the review process consisted of three main phases: setting goals and criteria, operationalizing criteria and defining the appraisal methods, and undertaking appraisal and budget impact analysis. The first phase included review of the previous EHP and identification of implementation challenges. Data collection and development of analytical tools took place during the second phase, along with appraisal of collected data. Finally, the data were analyzed and validated using the agreed-upon criteria.

Criteria Used to Guide the Design of the Third EHP

Several criteria were used to inform the inclusion of interventions in the third EHP. The first criterion was health maximization, considered in the context of cost-effectiveness. The revision process used the EHP Tool, a specially designed

Excel tool for EHP development. The Ministry of Health collected information on the costs and effectiveness of the health interventions considered for EHP inclusion. Because the country had not commissioned any new cost-effectiveness studies to inform the process, most of the data used in the tool were based on cost-effectiveness evidence from other countries, converted to Malawi cost equivalent, and applied to the Malawi context.

A cost-effectiveness threshold of US$61 was applied to determine whether an intervention was cost-effective. That threshold was derived from previous studies by Ochalek, Lomas, and Claxton (2015) and Woods et al. (2016), which estimated Malawi's cost-effectiveness threshold to range from US$24 to US$37 and from US$3 to US$116, respectively. The final threshold of US$61 was calculated as a midpoint of the two estimates converted to 2016 US dollars (Ochalek et al. 2018). Results were presented using a net health benefit measure, calculated as total health gains less health opportunity costs (costs divided by the cost-effectiveness threshold), multiplied by the size of the population in need of each intervention, to show the magnitude of total population health gains expected from implementing an intervention. That measure was also used to show the population health losses as a result of systems weaknesses leading to less than full implementation of most interventions (Ochalek et al. 2018).

The second criterion for the benefits package was equity. Equity considerations were based on geographic area, age, gender, and socioeconomic status. Equity was effectively implemented by reviewing the target populations for each intervention and placing greater weight on the interventions targeting marginalized demographic groups, in this case women and children under five years of age (MoH 2017). Greater weight was also given to cost-effective community-level interventions targeting rural communities with disproportionate barriers to health access. The equity implications of the EHP were subsequently evaluated on the basis of an assessment of which population groups most benefited from EHP implementation using the approach of distributional cost-effectiveness analysis (Arnold, Nkhoma, and Griffin 2020). Table 7.1 presents an example of the evaluation of equity implications of rotavirus vaccines.

A third criterion, the continuum of care, was also used to facilitate links between interventions. For instance, where feasible, considerations were made to include all treatments along a continuum to ensure continuity of services. Considerations were also made to include interventions fully financed by development partners. That approach was designed to optimize the costs of additional interventions and allow the population to access "bundled services" more effectively, thus improving financial risk protection (MoH 2017).

The fourth criterion was complementarities between interventions in line with the organization of services at all levels of service delivery. For instance, in the case of pregnant women, considerations were made for all the services that need to be delivered as part of antenatal care. The fourth criterion accounts for horizontal complementarities in the delivery of health care interventions.

Table 7.1 Sample EHP Equity Calculations with Rotavirus Vaccines, Malawi

Rotavirus vaccination for children under 1

Total population (A)	521,300
Incremental health benefit (B)	0.14
Incremental cost (C)	$0.69
Total cost (A × C)	$359,697

	Poorest	Poorer	Middle	Richer	Richest	Total
% survey reported cases of rotavirus (D)	36	16	23	13	12	100
DALYs averted if everyone vaccinated (A × B × D)	26,274	11,677	16,786	9,488	8,758	72,982
Uptake of vaccination (%) (E)	48	39	46	49	43	45
1. DALYs averted at current uptake (A × B × D × E)	12,611	4,554	7,721	4,649	3,766	32,842
Proportion of direct health benefit by subgroup	0.38	0.14	0.23	0.14	0.11	1
Cost by subgroup (A × 0.2 × C × E)	$34,531	$28,056	$33,092	$35,250	$30,934	$161,864
Proportion of opportunity cost by subgroup (F)	0.23	0.22	0.2	0.19	0.16	1
2. Health opportunity cost by subgroup [F × (A × C/61)]	1,356	1,297	1,179	1,120	943	5,897
3. Net health benefit by subgroup (1−2)	11,255	3,257	6,542	3,529	2,822	26,945
Proportion of net health benefit by subgroup	0.42	0.12	0.24	0.13	0.10	

Source: Arnold, Nkhoma, and Griffin 2020, revised 2024.

Note: DALY = disability-adjusted life year; EHP = Essential Health Package.

Analyses and Tools

Implementation of the priority-setting process for the third EHP took place in two parts. The first part consisted of reviewing available evidence on cost-effectiveness and selecting the interventions considered cost-effective in the Malawian setting. The second part applied the criteria described earlier and used a consultative process to finalize the interventions that would become part of the EHP. The second step of the process relied on expert opinion and occurred through consensus building with experts from district health offices and tertiary hospitals. The consultative process included consultations for interventions with and without cost-effectiveness evidence.

For the cost-effectiveness analysis part, the process used an Excel-based tool developed specifically for the EHP design process (Ochalek et al. 2018). With that tool, the team aggregated available information on the costs and effectiveness of interventions. The tool allowed the secretariat to collate and analyze the data in a convenient format for the analyses planned and to extend the analysis beyond what was feasible in previously existing tools. The analysis used other tools, such as the OneHealth Tool,[3] for health system cost analysis and the EHP Tool to analyze the available information on cost-effectiveness and for health service planning and costing. The costing considered the current and targeted levels of service delivery as well as the implementation levels considered more realistic given the health system's capacity. It conducted additional simulations to ascertain the level of health system expansion required to accommodate higher service delivery levels. Resource Mapping[4] data were used to inform medium-term resource availability and to compare the available resources to the cost of implementing the interventions in the EHP.

Data on per-patient costs and health benefits of interventions came primarily from the Tufts Global Health Cost Effectiveness Analysis Registry—Center for the Evaluation of Value and Risk in Health (CEVR) at Tufts Medical Center—and from *Disease Control Priorities*, second edition;[5] WHO-CHOICE papers; and systematic reviews. Per-unit costs of medicines, vaccines, and commodities for delivering interventions came from the Central Government Procurement Agency and other procurement agencies in the health sector. Because of limited evidence, the first analysis phase did not include cost-effectiveness data for some health interventions, particularly multisectoral interventions. Such interventions were assessed for inclusion during the second consultative phase. The OneHealth Tool was used to ascertain coverage rates in terms of what would be realistic based on the capacity of the health system (Ochalek et al. 2018).

SUMMARY OF INTERVENTIONS, COST-EFFECTIVENESS, AND COST OF THE THIRD EHP

The total number of potential interventions was 258, but complete data were available for only 71 of those interventions. Based on the cost-effectiveness threshold, only 52 EHP interventions were sufficiently cost-effective to be included in the Malawi EHP. However, in the second consultative phase, which considered the criteria outlined in the previous section and broader policy needs, the list of interventions included in the package increased to 97 (refer to table 7A.1 in the annex).

The EHP costing considered four scenarios. The first (total demand) scenario included all interventions that could be delivered, including those eventually excluded from the EHP. In addition to including all interventions, the assumption of complete coverage of the services made the first scenario unaffordable and unattainable within the implementation time frame. The second scenario, 100 percent coverage of all the interventions included in the EHP, was also unattainable because of significant coverage gaps at baseline that could not realistically be addressed during the five-year implementation period. The third (scale-up) scenario allowed for a gradual increase in the coverage rates during the five-year period of implementing the HSSP and had more realistic costs. The third scenario was, therefore, used as a basis for planning. For the fourth (status quo) scenario, costs were calculated using current coverage rates for the duration of the HSSP II. The revised EHP cost 31 percent less than its predecessor package and had a greater potential to generate population health impact (DALYs averted). Implementing the previous package (the second EHP) would have cost

US$7.91 per DALY averted, whereas the third EHP cost US$5.97 per DALY averted (MoH 2017). Figure 7.4 shows the costs of each of these scenarios across the implementation period.

Figure 7.4 Summary of Estimated EHP Costs, Malawi, 2017/18–2020/21

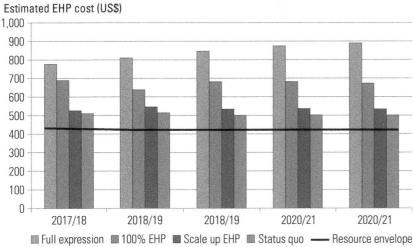

Estimated EHP cost (US$)

Source: Reprinted from Barker 2018. Used with permission; further permission required for reuse.
Note: EHP = Essential Health Package.

The cost assumptions were based on data collected during the resource mapping exercises. Resource mapping is based on self-reported data on financing projections and informs the collective projections for the health sector. Further assumptions on fiscal space were based on a previous World Bank study that indicated limited possibilities for expanding the fiscal space in the medium term (World Bank Group 2017).

PRACTICAL APPLICATION AND EFFECT OF THE EHP

Implementation of the EHP occurs at the service delivery level, where providers are expected to prioritize the delivery of its interventions. In practice, because Malawi has a policy of free health care at the point of access, providers have found it difficult to restrict access to non-EHP interventions when intervention inputs were centrally procured and, in some cases, fungible across EHP and non-EHP interventions. That practical implementation challenge, among others, prompted subsequent analyses exploring how public financial management mechanisms could better align with EHP prioritization. The following paragraphs highlight some of the EHP analytical and practical applications.

Development of the geographical Resource Allocation Formula (RAF). The health sector geographical RAF was instituted as the primary resource allocation mechanism for drug and recurrent expenditures at the subnational level. Development of the first geographical RAF dates to 2002, just before development of the first EHP. The Ministry of Health updated the RAF in 2008. Following review and approval of the updated RAF, it was implemented for a few years before the government reverted to the incremental historically based allocation pattern. In 2017, the Ministry of Health started revising the RAF to improve efficiency, equity, and accountability in resource allocation (McGuire et al. 2020; Twea, Manthalu, and Mohan 2020). The updated RAF is based on the estimated cost of EHP implementation for each district and allocates available resources proportional to need. The cost-of-service delivery is calculated using the unit cost of providing the intervention and the expected number of cases based on incidence, prevalence, and utilization rates. That RAF design allowed for an alignment between resource allocation and the expected level of service delivery.

Use of the EHP in national and subnational planning. During the implementation period of the third EHP, the Ministry of Health sought to align national and subnational level planning with the EHP. The district health planning guidelines (2018–22) recommended budget prioritization through the lens of EHP service delivery. More specifically, a bottleneck analysis approach was used to identify health systems gaps for low-performing (in terms of coverage and quality) EHP interventions (Kiwanuka Henriksson et al. 2017). The process was designed to align health planning, resource allocation, implementation, and monitoring and evaluation with EHP delivery. Not only did the process bring about a greater focus on performance in planning and continuous improvement, but it also allowed district managers greater visibility across the spectrum from planning to evaluation and EHP prioritization activities, which would result in improved EHP delivery.

Alignment of resource tracking efforts with the EHP. The Ministry of Health has conducted resource mapping exercises since 2011 as part of its resource tracking efforts. Resource mapping is one way of augmenting other financial tracking instruments used by the Ministry. A key requirement for the Ministry of Health was to track resource availability and expenditure according to the EHP. The reporting of data in this manner allowed for the estimation of health financing gaps and provided evidence for resource allocation at the domestic and international levels.

EHP distribution impact. One of the health sector objectives, as stated in the HSSP II, was to ensure equitable implementation of the EHP. A study by Arnold, Nkhoma, and Griffin (2020) used distributional cost-effectiveness analysis to evaluate Malawi's EHP interventions on the basis of two objectives: increasing population health and reducing health inequality. The study assessed equity by geographical location (urban versus rural residence) and wealth, using the International Wealth Index. Overall, the authors found that incorporating the impact on health inequality alongside impact on overall population health would result in prioritization of a similar set of interventions. When comparing EHP impact by socioeconomic group, the findings showed that use of EHP interventions was higher among the poorest. Such analysis can render support to the usefulness of the EHP design and its implementation as a health policy instrument toward achieving the universal health coverage objectives underlying the EHP.

LIMITATIONS AND FUTURE DIRECTIONS

One of the limitations is that EHP financing gaps still exist, perhaps because of the mismatch between planned budgets and actual expenditures by development partners and the government. As such, the interventions in the EHP have limited linkage to financing and results. Other EHP implementation challenges highlighted in the medium-term implementation strategies include limited awareness of the EHP among stakeholders, lack of policy enforcement, lack of clarity about excluded but otherwise cost-effective interventions, vertical organization of program management, and input-based expenditure tracking under the Integrated Financial Management Information System. Fully implementing the EHP will require aligning the entire policy and implementation machinery with it, including but not limited to consumables and equipment purchase, donor guidance, health systems investments, budgeting, and service delivery and purchasing mechanisms. At present, Malawi has adopted a light-touch approach to prioritizing EHP services across the country; however, it might adopt a firmer approach through a more comprehensive revision of purchasing processes.

Despite those challenges, and as highlighted earlier in the chapter, the EHP has been used adequately at various levels of the health system to guide policy, planning, and budgeting in Malawi's health sector. Further, the monitoring and evaluation system has continued to improve during the EHP implementation period for public health services with reporting links for community health care workers. The revision of the third EHP considered those challenges and best practices.

ANNEX 7A

Table 7A.1 List of EHP Interventions, Malawi

Category	Intervention package	Intervention	Level of care
RMNCH	ANC package	Tetanus toxoid (pregnant women)	Community/Primary/Secondary
		Deworming (pregnant women)	Community/Primary/Secondary
		Daily iron and folic acid supplementation (pregnant women)	Community/Primary/Secondary
		Syphilis detection and treatment (pregnant women)	Community/Primary/Secondary
		IPT (pregnant women)	Community/Primary/Secondary
		ITN distribution to pregnant women	Community/Primary/Secondary
		Urinalysis (four per pregnant woman)	Primary/Secondary
	Modern family planning	Injectable	Community/Primary/Secondary
		IUD	Primary/Secondary
		Implant	Primary/Secondary
		Pill	Community/Primary/Secondary
		Female sterilization	Secondary
		Male condom	Community/Primary/Secondary

table continues next page

Table 7A.1 List of EHP Interventions, Malawi (continued)

Category	Intervention package	Intervention	Level of care
RMNCH	Delivery package	Clean practices and immediate essential newborn care (in facility)	Primary/Secondary
		Active management of the third stage of labor	Primary/Secondary
		Management of eclampsia/preeclampsia (magnesium sulfate, methyldopa, nifedipine, hydralazine)	Primary/Secondary
		Neonatal resuscitation (institutional)	Primary/Secondary
		Caesarean section with indication	Secondary
		Caesarean section with indication (with complication)	Secondary
		Vaginal delivery, skilled attendance (including complications)	Primary/Secondary
		Management of obstructed labor	Primary/Secondary
		Newborn sepsis—full supportive care	Primary/Secondary
		Newborn sepsis—injectable antibiotics	Primary/Secondary
		Antenatal corticosteroids for preterm labor	Primary/Secondary
		Maternal sepsis case management	Primary/Secondary
		Cord care using chlorhexidine	Primary/Secondary
		Hysterectomy	Primary/Secondary
		Post-abortion case management	Secondary
		Treatment of antepartum hemorrhage	Primary/Secondary
		Treatment of postpartum hemorrhage	Secondary
		Antibiotics for pPRoM	Primary/Secondary
Vaccine-preventable diseases	Essential vaccines package	Rotavirus vaccine	Community/Primary/Secondary
		Measles rubella vaccine	Community/Primary/Secondary
		Pneumococcal vaccine	Community/Primary/Secondary
		BCG vaccine	Community/Primary/Secondary
		Polio vaccine	Community/Primary/Secondary
		DPT-Heb-Hib / Pentavalent vaccine	Community/Primary/Secondary
		HPV vaccine	Community/Primary/Secondary
Malaria	First line uncomplicated malaria treatment	Uncomplicated (adult, <36 kg)	Community/Primary/Secondary
		Uncomplicated (adult, >36 kg)	Community/Primary/Secondary
		Uncomplicated (children, <15 kg)	Community/Primary/Secondary
		Uncomplicated (children, >15 kg)	Community/Primary/Secondary
	Complicated malaria treatment	Complicated (adults, injectable artesunate)	Primary/Secondary
		Complicated (children, injectable artesunate)	Primary/Secondary
	Malaria diagnosis	RDTs	Community/Primary/Secondary
		Microscopy for malaria	Primary/Secondary
Integrated management of childhood illnesses	ARIs	Pneumonia treatment (children)	Community/Primary/Secondary
		Treatment of severe pneumonia (oxygen)	Primary/Secondary
	Diarrheal disease	ORS	Community/Primary/Secondary
		Zinc	Community/Primary/Secondary
		Treatment of severe diarrhea (intravenous fluids)	Primary/Secondary

table continues next page

Table 7A.1 List of EHP Interventions, Malawi (continued)

Category	Intervention package	Intervention	Level of care
	Nutrition	Community management of nutrition in under-5—Plumpy Peanut	Community/Primary
		Community management of nutrition in under-5—micronutrient powder	Community/Primary
		Community management of nutrition in under-5—vitamin A	Community/Primary
	Malaria diagnosis	RDTs for under-5	Community/Primary
Community health	Community health package	Growth monitoring	Community/Primary
		Vermin and vector control and promotion	Community/Primary
		Disease surveillance	Community/Primary
		Community health promotion and engagement	Community/Primary
		Village inspections	Community/Primary
		Promotion of hygiene (handwashing with soap)	Community/Primary
		Promotion of sanitation (latrine refuse, drop hole covers, solid waste disposal, hygienic disposal of children's stools)	Community/Primary
		Occupational health promotion	Community/Primary
		Household water quality testing and treatment	Community/Primary
		Home-based care of chronically ill patients	Community/Primary
		Child protection	Community/Primary
NTDs	Treatment and MDA	Schistosomiasis mass drug administration	Community/Primary
		Case finding and treatment of trypanosomiasis	Primary
		Trachoma mass drug administration	Community/Primary
HIV/AIDS	HIV Prevention	Cotrimoxazole for children	Community/Primary/Secondary
		PMTCT	Community/Primary/Secondary
	HIV testing	HIV testing services	Community/Primary/Secondary
	HIV treatment	HIV treatment for all ages—ART and viral load	Community/Primary/Secondary
Nutrition		Vitamin A supplementation in pregnant women	Community/Primary/Secondary
		Management of severe malnutrition (children)	Community/Primary/Secondary
		Deworming (children)	Community/Primary/Secondary
		Vitamin A supplementation in infants and children 6–59 months	Community/Primary/Secondary
Tuberculosis (TB)		Isoniazid preventive therapy for children in contact with TB patients	Primary/Secondary
		First-line treatment for new TB cases for adults	Primary/Secondary
		First-line treatment for retreatment TB cases for adults	Primary/Secondary
		First-line treatment for new TB cases for children	Community/Primary/Secondary
		First-line treatment for retreatment TB cases for children	Community/Primary/Secondary
		Case management of MDR cases	Primary/Secondary
	TB testing	LED test	Primary/Secondary
		Xpert test	Primary/Secondary
		MGIT test	Primary/Secondary
		LJ test	Primary/Secondary

table continues next page

Table 7A.1 List of EHP Interventions, Malawi *(continued)*

Category	Intervention package	Intervention	Level of care
Noncommunicable diseases		Treatment of injuries	Primary/Secondary
	Mental health treatment	Basic psychosocial support, advice, and follow-up	Community/Primary/Secondary
		Anti-epileptic medication	Community/Primary/Secondary
		Treatment of depression (first line)	Community/Primary/Secondary
		Testing of precancerous cells (vinegar)	Primary/Secondary
	Diabetes treatment	Diabetes type I	Primary/Secondary
		Diabetes type II	Primary/Secondary
		Hypertension	Primary/Secondary
Oral health	Tooth pain treatment	Management of severe tooth pain, tooth extraction	Primary/Secondary
		Management of mild tooth pain, tooth filling	Primary/Secondary

Source: MoH 2011.

Note: ANC = antenatal care; ARIs = acute respiratory infections; ART = antiretroviral therapy; BCG = Bacillus Calmette-Guerin; DPT-Heb-Hib = diphtheria, tetanus, pertussis, polio, hepatitis B, and Haemophilus influenzae type b; EHP = Essential Health Package; IPT = intermittent preventive treatment; ITN = insecticide-treated nets; kg = kilogram; LED = fluorescent light-emitting diode; LJ = Löwenstein-Jensen; MDA = mass drug administration; MDR = multidrug resistance; MGIT = Mycobacteria Growth Indicator Tube; NTD = neglected tropical diseases; ORS = oral rehydration salts; PMTCT = prevention of mother to child transmission; pPRoM = preterm premature rupture of membranes; RDTs = rapid diagnostic tests; RMNCH = reproductive, maternal, newborn, and child health.

NOTES

1. For more on WHO-CHOICE, refer to the World Health Organization's WHO-CHOICE web page, https://www.who.int/news-room/questions-and-answers/item/who-choice-frequently-asked-questions; for more on the Tufts Global Health Registry (now the Global Health Cost Effectiveness Analysis Registry), refer to Tufts Medical Center, Center for the Evaluation of Value and Risk in Health, "GH CEA Registry," https://cevr.tuftsmedicalcenter.org/databases/gh-cea-registry.
2. Affordability refers to the cost of the EHP relative to total health expenditure—that is, the package is considered affordable if the cost of implementation is lower than the EHP.
3. Avenir Health, "OneHealth Tool," https://www.avenirhealth.org/software-onehealth.
4. "Resource Mapping (RM) tracks forward-looking budget data for all organisations in the Malawian health sector, including relevant government ministries, departments, and agencies (MDAs), the Christian Health Association of Malawi (CHAM), bilateral and multilateral partners, as well as nongovernmental organisations (NGOs), though private health facilities are not included" (MoH 2020a, 10).
5. Because of the timing of the EHP development process, it did not consider DCP3 evidence because it was finalized only after the completion of the EHP review process.

REFERENCES

Arnold, Matthias, Dominic Nkhoma, and Susan Griffin. 2020. "Distributional Impact of the Malawian Essential Health Package." *Health Policy and Planning* 35 (6): 646–56. https://doi.org/10.1093/heapol/czaa015.

Barker, Catherine. 2018. *Costing of Malawi's Second Health Sector Strategic Plan Using the OneHealth Tool.* Washington, DC: Palladium, Health Policy Plus.

Government of Malawi. 1994. *Constitution of the Republic of Malawi*. Lilongwe: Government of Malawi. https://www.malawi.gov.mw/index.php/resources/documents/constitution-of -the-republic-of-malawi.

Jamison, Dean T., Joel G. Breman, Anthony R. Measham, George Alleye, Mariam Claeson, David B. Evans, Prabhat Jha, et al. 2006. *Disease Control Priorities in Developing Countries* (second edition). Washington, DC: World Bank and Oxford University Press. https://www .dcp-3.org/sites/default/files/dcp2/DCPFM.pdf.

Kiwanuka Henriksson, Dorcus, Mio Fredriksson, Peter Waiswa, Katarina Selling, and Stefan Swartling Peterson. 2017. "Bottleneck Analysis at District Level to Illustrate Gaps within the District Health System in Uganda." *Global Health Action* 10 (1): 1327256. https://doi .org/10.1080/16549716.2017.1327256.

McGuire, Finn, Paul Revill, Pakwanja Twea, Sakshi Mohan, Gerald Manthalu, and Peter C. Smith. 2020. "Allocating Resources to Support Universal Health Coverage: Development of a Geographical Funding Formula in Malawi." *BMJ Global Health* 5 (9): e002763. https://doi.org/10.1136/bmjgh-2020-002763.

MoH (Malawi, Ministry of Health). 1999. *Malawi Fourth National Health Plan 1999–2004*. Lilongwe, Government of Malawi.

MoH (Malawi, Ministry of Health). 2004. *A Joint Programme of Work for a Health Sector Wide Approach (SWAp) (2004–2010)*. Lilongwe: Government of Malawi.

MoH (Malawi, Ministry of Health). 2011. *Malawi Health Sector Strategic Plan 2011–2016*. Lilongwe: Government of Malawi.

MoH (Malawi, Ministry of Health). 2016a. *The Malawi National Heath Accounts Report for Fiscal Years 2012/2013–2014/2015*. Lilongwe: Government of Malawi. https://p4h.world /app/uploads/2023/02/The20Malawi20National20Health20Accounts20Report202012_201 3E280932014_2015.x23411.pdf.

MoH (Malawi, Ministry of Health). 2016b. "Terms of Reference for the EHP Technical Working Group." Government of Malawi, Lilongwe [not publicly available].

MoH (Malawi, Ministry of Health). 2017. *Health Sector Strategic Plan II 2017–2022*. Lilongwe: Government of Malawi. https://extranet.who.int/countryplanningcycles/sites/default/files /public_file_rep/MAL_Malawi_HSSP_II_2017-2022.pdf.

MoH (Malawi, Ministry of Health). 2018. *National Health Policy*. Lilongwe: Government of Malawi. https://www.health.gov.mw/download/national-health-policy-2/?wpdmdl=3850&r efresh=669fce88513eb1721749128.

MoH (Malawi, Ministry of Health). 2020a. "Health Sector Resource Mapping Round 6." Government of Malawi, Lilongwe [not publicly available].

MoH (Malawi, Ministry of Health). 2020b. *Malawi National Health Accounts Report for Fiscal Years 2015/16–2017/18*. Lilongwe: Government of Malawi.

MoH (Malawi, Ministry of Health). 2023. *Malawi Health Sector Strategic Plan III 2023–2030*. Lilongwe: Government of Malawi. https://www.health.gov.mw/download/hssp-iii/?wpdmd l=4458&refresh=669fd0980f6001721749656.

NSO (Malawi, National Statistical Office) and ICF. 2017. *Malawi Demographic and Health Survey 2015–16*. Zomba, Malawi, and Rockville, MD: NSO and ICF. http://dhsprogram .com/pubs/pdf/FR319/FR319.pdf.

Ochalek, Jessica Marie, James Lomas, and Karl Philip Claxton. 2015. "Cost per DALY Averted Thresholds for Low- and Middle-Income Countries: Evidence from Cross Country Data." CHE Research Paper No. 122, Centre for Health Economics, University of York.

Ochalek, Jessica, Paul Revill, Gerald Manthalu, Finn McGuire, Dominic Nkhoma, Alexandra Rollinger, Mark Sculpher, and Karl Claxton. 2018. "Supporting the Development of a Health Benefits Package in Malawi." *BMJ Global Health* 3 (2): e000607. https://doi .org/10.1136/bmjgh-2017-000607.

Phoya, Ann, Trish Araru, Rabson Kachala, John Chizonga, and Cameron Bowie. No date. "Setting Strategic Health Sector Priorities in Malawi." Disease Control Priorities in Developing Countries, 3rd Edition Working Paper #9, DCP3 Secretariat. https://www.dcp-3.org/sites/default/files/resources/DCP%20Working%20Paper%209_Malawi%20Case%20Study_0.pdf.

Twea, Pakwanja, Gerald Manthalu, and Sakshi Mohan. 2020. "Allocating Resources to Support Universal Health Coverage: Policy Processes and Implementation in Malawi." *BMJ Global Health* 5 (8): e002766. https://doi.org/10.1136/bmjgh-2020-002766.

Woods, Beth, Paul Revill, Mark Sculpher, and Karl Claxton. 2016. "Country-Level Cost-Effectiveness Thresholds: Initial Estimates and the Need for Further Research." *Value in Health* 19 (8): 929–35.

World Bank. 1993. *World Development Report 1993: Investing in Health*. Washington, DC: World Bank. https://documents.worldbank.org/en/publication/documents-reports/documentdetail/468831468340807129/world-development-report-1993-investing-in-health.

World Bank. 2020. "Malawi Public Expenditure Review 2020: Strengthening Expenditure for Human Capital." World Bank, Washington, DC. https://openknowledge.worldbank.org/handle/10986/35855.

World Bank Group. 2017. "Fiscal Space for Health in Malawi and Revenue Potential of 'Innovative Financing.'" World Bank Group, Washington, DC. https://openknowledge.worldbank.org/handle/10986/28404.

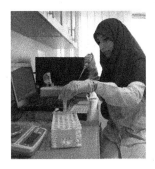

8

Health Services Packages in the Islamic Republic of Iran: The Need for Comprehensive and Effective Institutionalization

Reza Majdzadeh, Haniye Sadat Sajadi, Hamidreza Safikhani,
Alireza Olyaeemanesh, and Mohsen Aarabi

ABSTRACT

The Islamic Republic of Iran has expanded its primary health care network, yielding notable enhancements in health indicators. The core health services portfolio now encompasses primary health care, diagnostic and specialty treatment services, and inpatient care. Challenges posed by economic sanctions and the COVID-19 pandemic have imposed strains on the country's health care system. In response, the Islamic Republic of Iran has undertaken revisions to its service package, aiming for enhanced efficiency and equity and substantial investments in augmenting its human resources capacity. Nevertheless, despite recent efforts to systematically embed service package prioritization within the health system, achieving sustainability remains a challenge. To establish a lasting institutional foundation for its service packages, the Islamic Republic of Iran must continue dismantling institutional obstacles and creating robust stakeholder engagement platforms. However, the success of those initiatives will require ongoing work and time to see whether they yield the desired outcomes. Such measures will facilitate the prioritization of services, fostering improved efficiency within the health system.

INTRODUCTION

The Islamic Republic of Iran has a per capita gross national income of 13,338 international dollars (2020) at purchasing power parity (Hamadeh, Van Rompaey, and Metreau 2021). It has been under sanctions since 1979, and the United Nations has imposed sanctions since 2011 over nuclear development activities. Economic sanctions were lifted in 2015 through the Joint Comprehensive Plan of Action; however, economic sanctions were reimposed in 2018 with severe restrictions (Danaei, Harirchi, et al. 2019; Sajadi, Gloyd, and Majdzadeh 2021).

The country has implemented remarkable initiatives to strengthen the health system and provide accessible health care to all citizens (Doshmangir et al. 2019; Sajadi, Ehsani-Chimeh, and Majdzadeh 2019). Those outstanding initiatives began in the early 1980s with the expansion of the primary health care (PHC) network. For example, life expectancy before the Islamic Revolution in 1976 was 55.7 years and reached 78.7 years in the 2019 census. Changes in life expectancy in the country primarily reflect the reduction in child mortality, a reduction that has accelerated with the development of PHC throughout the country and the rural development after the revolution (Danaei, Farzadfar, et al. 2019). Table 8.1 provides selected health system indicators related to package definition and revision.

Table 8.1 Selected Health System Indicators, Islamic Republic of Iran

Indicator	Estimate	Year
UHC service coverage index	77/100	2019
Incidence of catastrophic expenditure (>25%) (NIHR 2023)	1.04	2022
Total health expenditure from gross domestic product (%) (WHO 2020a)	8.7	2018
Domestic general government health expenditure as a percentage of general government expenditure	21.4	2019
Out-of-pocket expenditure as a percentage of current health expenditure (WHO 2020a)	41.2	2018
Percentage of primary health care expenditure from domestic general government health expenditure (WHO 2020a)	30.0	2018
Medical doctors per 10,000 population	15.8	2018
Nursing and midwifery personnel per 10,000 population	20.8	2018

Sources: As shown in table; data with no reference come from World Health Organization, Global Health Observatory, https://www.who.int/data/gho (accessed March 7, 2023).

Note: UHC = universal health coverage.

The COVID-19 pandemic affected the Islamic Republic of Iran more than other countries in the Eastern Mediterranean Region (Takian, Raoofi, and Kazempour-Ardebili 2020). According to official statistics, more than 137,000 people in the country had died from COVID-19 as of March 1, 2022.[1] The pandemic has also had an extensive economic impact: government revenue from April to December 2020 was only 55 percent of the approved budget for the fiscal year, whereas health and social assistance costs increased to 28 percent because of the pandemic (World Bank 2022). Consequently, the combination of economic sanctions and the social and economic consequences of COVID-19 have deepened financial constraints on the country's health system. During these many years, cumulative financial constraints have eroded the health infrastructure (equipment and buildings) and limited the provision of health resources (Sajadi and Majdzadeh 2019).

The Universal Insurance Law 1994 sought to cover nearly 60 percent of uninsured Iranians, leading to the creation in October 1994 of the Medical Services Insurance Organization, later renamed the Iran Health Insurance Organization. The organization was established to cover all people within five years, including government employees and community individuals of various socioeconomic levels who were not eligible for coverage by other health insurance organizations.

Most health insurance schemes have faced numerous challenges during the last two decades. For example, they failed to meet the Universal Insurance Law's target of covering all Iranians by 1999. They underperformed in their primary functions, such as strategic purchasing and cost containment, which led to a considerable increase in out-of-pocket (OOP) health expenditures. A new Ministry of Welfare and Social Security was established to overcome the challenges, with mandates including the integration of all basic health insurance organizations under one structure. Because the merger of insurance funds did not materialize, however, the pooling function is still fragmented (Doshmangir et al. 2021; Mohammadi et al. 2014).

Since 2014, the General Health Policies (GHPs) have defined a road map for the future direction of the Islamic Republic of Iran's health system. The content analysis of the GHPs shows two fundamental goals of the system: equity in access to services and financial protection against health expenditures (Sajadi, Gholamreza Kashi, and Majdzadeh 2020). Clause 9 of the GHPs aims for a quantitative and qualitative development of health insurance and states:

> Determining the package of comprehensive health services at the level of basic and supplementary insurance by the Ministry of Health and Medical Education (MoHME), purchasing by the insurance system, and adequate supervision over the accurate implementation of packages by eliminating unnecessary measures and unnecessary costs.

In the same year, health sector reform in the country began under the Health Transformation Plan (HTP). The estimated incidence of catastrophic health expenditures (that is, OOP payments for health that represent more than 10 percent of household income) increased from 11.3 percent in 2005 to 16.0 percent until the HTP in 2014 (Hsu et al. 2021). Evidence shows that OOP spending had no stability or decrease before that. Through HTP, a basic insurance scheme covered 9 million people to complete population coverage in the country. The share of people's direct payment for health services in the public sector decreased significantly, and many public hospitals and primary health care centers were renovated. The HTP increased MoHME's budget by over one-third and health insurance organizations by two-thirds to finance the plan. In addition, it allocated 1 percent of value added tax to the health system (Harirchi et al. 2020). Although initiated as a comprehensive health system reform, the HTP faced instability of resources because of the economic constraints of sanctions and the COVID-19 pandemic. Consequently, financial resources after HTP were not sustainable, and government spending on health at a constant price shows a decline from 2016 (Aminlou 2022).

The Islamic Republic of Iran's service package is provided through three service platform levels. The first level of the public sector includes mostly promotive and PHC services provided at no charge to individuals. Private offices are the main provider of first-level care, however, particularly in urban areas and populated cities where basic insurance schemes cover their services and because of the lack of a Family Physician Program (FPP) in urban areas with populations greater than 20,000. In those private offices, insurance covers 70 percent of the public or government doctor's tariff and patients must pay the difference. Community health workers in comprehensive public health centers in cities with a population of more than 20,000 actively provide health service packages to almost the entire population, with one community health worker for every 3,000 people. They receive funding from the public sector through MoHME.

The second level consists of specialists and subspecialists services in outpatient offices and district hospitals, and the third level of care is provincial hospital services. Basic health insurance organizations purchase the second and third levels of care by paying 90 percent of public/government tariffs. Because the private sector is a significant secondary and tertiary care provider, basic health insurance organizations cover only 70 percent and 90 percent of public tariffs for outpatient and inpatient services, respectively. Complementary, noncompulsory, or commercial insurances cover co-payment of those services based on the private tariffs, partially paid by the basic insurance and additional health care services. Additional support comes from the public fund that directly subsidizes most of the costly services.

Because basic health insurance does not provide adequate coverage for outpatient services, especially para-clinic services in the private sector, complementary health insurance has been expanded in recent years. Complementary health insurance covers not only those services not covered by the basic service package (such as advanced dental services and some medications) but also partial costs of diagnosis and treatment services partly covered by basic insurance. Despite the legal framework, basic health insurance obligations have not been clearly defined, so a few differences exist between basic and complementary health insurance services.

The decision to divide services between basic and complementary insurance is not systematic and is based on criteria such as willingness to pay, public health importance, and financial protection. Consequently, some essential services may be left out of public insurance schemes (Akbari et al. 2022; Keshavarzian and Mofidian 2015). In addition, because of the lack of strategic purchasing, insurance funds operate passively, with the service provider determining what services should be purchased. Currently, the difference between the price of services in the public and private sectors is due to the difference in the technical component of the tariff, which includes depreciation rates and capital gains. As noted earlier, basic insurance pays 70 percent of the government tariff for outpatient services and 90 percent of the inpatient tariff for the second and third levels of basic services. The existence of tariffs higher than the approved ones has led to widespread informal payments (Doshmangir et al. 2020; Sajadi et al. 2022).

Of the more than 1,054 hospitals providing inpatient services, almost 80 percent are public (NIHR 2023). Private hospitals have a dramatically higher tariff than public hospitals, although both private and public tariffs are approved by the Supreme Council of Health Insurance (SCHI). Individuals insured by complementary insurance benefits pay 10 percent to 20 percent of inpatient service expenses in private hospitals (Keshavarzian and Mofidian 2015).

A significant amount of induced demand exists, as evidenced by the nonadherence of clinical practice with service standards (Akbari et al. 2022). Induced demand has not been comprehensively investigated in the country; however, the results of existing studies indicate that the payment mechanism is based on the fee-for-service method, many physicians are shareholders of hospitals and medical laboratories, and there is poor adherence to clinical practice guidelines (Mounesan et al. 2013). The development of those guidelines in the Islamic Republic of Iran dates back more than two decades. A department in the MoHME supports various research centers in developing the clinical practice guidelines, but no drastic measure has been adopted for encouraging or supervising their application (Baradaran-Seyed and Majdzadeh 2012) and adherence is not enforced.

APPROACH

This chapter does not follow the conventional methodology of detailing the various stages of designing a service package, such as assessing the cost-effectiveness of interventions or the budget impact. Instead, this chapter partly represents the outcome of a study whose detailed methodology and results were previously published elsewhere (Sajadi et al. 2024). It adopts the framework presented in the World Health Organization's *Institutionalizing Health Technology Assessment Mechanisms: A How To Guide* (Bertram, Dhaene, and Tan-Torres Edejer 2021). That guidance introduces a conceptual framework encompassing the establishment of a mandate, a legal framework, institutional arrangements, and procedural aspects required for initiating an evidence-informed decision-making system. However, the process requires inputs further augmented by human and financial resources (Bertram, Dhaene, and Tan-Torres Edejer 2021).

Following that framework, the significance of institutionalization for formulating a service package is proposed as a vital element of fair decision-making in the priority-setting process (Sajadi, Jama, and Majdzadeh 2023). Having already described the context of the Islamic Republic of Iran's health system, the chapter will provide an overview of the evolution of priority setting for health service packages in the country and the current challenges. It will subsequently employ this framework to provide recommendations for institutionalizing the priority-setting decision-making process for the service package.

EVOLUTION OF PRIORITY SETTING FOR HEALTH SERVICES PACKAGES

The Islamic Republic of Iran's basic health services package consists of two main categories: essential PHC services ("A" in the descriptions provided in the following paragraphs) and more advanced diagnostic and treatment services ("B"), provided in both the secondary and tertiary levels of care. Figure 8.1 shows the actions the country has taken to define or revise each of the two categories.

A: Preventive and PHC services. The first level of care provides the services. The package includes mostly promotive and preventive services, with a small number of surgical, pharmaceutical, and diagnostic services. The government funds this package of services, and the country's entire population has access to the services for free.

A1: Pilot of PHC package. The design and use of PHC service packages in the country date back to the 1970s and the Urmia project carried out by the Institute of Public Health Research at Tehran University in West Azerbaijan. Thirty health houses in rural areas were set up as an intervention compared with a similar area without health houses. In that initial design, the package included services needed by mothers and children. It then defined environmental health and infectious diseases services to be delivered by community health workers (Pileroudi, Shadpour, and Vakil 1981). The target diseases were identified by studying reasons for admission to service delivery points and causes of mortality. The content was defined according to World Health Organization and United Nations Children's Fund recommendations.

A2: Revision and scale-up of PHC package. Since the early 1980s, PHC has been deployed across the country. This round involved completing the package and reviewing the technical details of the planned package for nationwide implementation, and defining services related to family and school health, infectious diseases, noncommunicable diseases (NCDs), oral health, environmental health, and health education. The critical point in this round was considering the human resources needed and defining the link between different health system levels for continuity of care (referral system).

A3: Addition of the FPP. In 2005, the package implemented the FPP, established a referral system, and established the rural health insurance system. The family physician or health team package provides PHC services in rural, nomadic areas and in cities with less than 20,000 people. Since 2012, the FPP has expanded to cities with higher populations and has been fully implemented as a pilot program in two provinces of Fars and Mazandaran.

Figure 8.1 Timeline of Significant Events Related to Determining Health Interventions, Islamic Republic of Iran

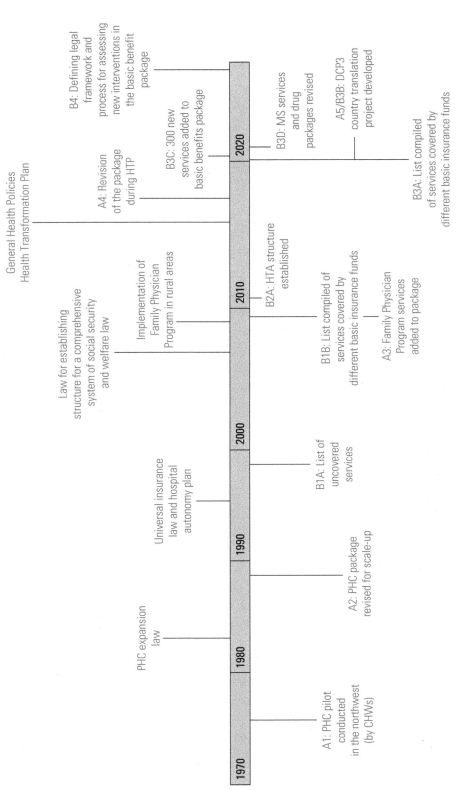

Source: Original figure developed for this publication.

Note: Blue = the preventive and PHC services package; red = the diagnostic and therapeutic services package. A = PHC services; B = diagnostic and therapeutic services; CHW = community health worker; DCP3 = *Disease Control Priorities*, third edition; HTA = Health Technology Assessment; HTP = Health Transformation Plan; MS = multiple sclerosis; NCD = noncommunicable disease; PHC = primary health care.

A4: Revision of the package during the HTP. In 2015, during the HTP, the preventive and PHC services packages were reviewed. The approach to package definition changed to the care of population groups (children, adolescents and young people, the middle-aged and elderly, and pregnant mothers). The review included NCDs; nutrition; and mental, infectious, environmental, and occupational health service packages at the primary level. The revised services were implemented, and funds for these services came from the government without any payment from people at the first level of services.

B: Diagnostic and therapeutic services. This category comprises diagnostic and paraclinical services, clinical interventions, medicines, medical equipment and supplies, and specialized medical care, delivered mainly through general and specialized hospitals and ambulatory care centers. The actions taken fall into three categories: passive purchasing (B1), Health Technology Assessment, or HTA (B2), and moving toward strategic purchasing of the service package (B3).

B1: List of uncovered services. The need for defining a package arose in 1995 after the approval and implementation of the country's Universal Insurance Law and hospital self-governance policy. With its formation, the SCHI took on the responsibilities of policy making, planning, coordination, and supervision of insurance organizations. Previously, each insurance organization prepared and implemented its package according to the population covered and the available resources. One of the SCHI's first decisions was to publish a negative list of noncovered services. Examples of noncovered services included cosmetic procedures, organ transplantation, and infertility services (B1A). After approval in 2004 of the comprehensive welfare and social security system law, some services (for example, rehabilitation devices and oral health) were removed from the package to reduce the financial burden on insurance funds. In 2007, a comprehensive list of all services covered by different insurance funds was compiled (B1B).

B2: Establishment of HTA structure. Strategic purchase through HTA began in 2007 as a national program. Since 2010, an office in MoHME has been assigned to HTA. The first cohort of students has been admitted to the HTA master's program. So far, more than 150 HTA projects in medicine, medical equipment, and treatment procedures have been conducted, making the Islamic Republic of Iran one of the leading countries in the Eastern Mediterranean Region in HTA (B2A). However, a study of 23 completed HTA projects finds that HTA evidence is unsatisfactory and that the lack of institutionalization prevents HTA from providing evidence for decision-making (Mohtasham et al. 2016).

B3: Strategic purchasing. The implementation of the HTP made evident that inefficiency is one of the main problems of the country's health system. Encompassing challenges include constrained allocation to PHC, fragmentation among insurance funds, weak strategic purchasing, catastrophic costs, and inadequate financial protection (Danaei, Farzadfar, et al. 2019). Attempts to address those challenges included a workshop on strategic purchasing (B3A) and review of the package using the reference list from the third edition of *Disease Control Priorities* (DCP3). This initiative started with maternal care, HIV/AIDS, and NCDs services, but did not continue (A5/B3B). With the mobilization of resources through HTP, basic insurance covered 300 new services (B3C). Finally, in 2018, the service package review began with the evidence-informed deliberative process approach. The SCHI reviewed the service package and medicines related to multiple sclerosis (MS) and diabetes (Mataria et al. 2023) and endorsed the package in 2021 for implementation (B3D).

With the shift in disease burden, the initial package containing services such as those related to communicable diseases and maternal and child health has changed to include NCDs, their risk factors, and mental health. A study on the NCD interventions to determine how the Iranian intervention package complies with World Health Organization recommendations identifies five criteria for prioritization: number of people affected by the intervention, cost-effectiveness, attributable burden, hospitalization, and variations among income levels (Bakhtiari et al. 2020). According to multiple-criteria decision analysis used for prioritization, the only best buy for NCDs is the papillomavirus vaccination, which is not available in the country. Another study demonstrates that evidence-informed decision-making in the Islamic Republic of Iran remains a challenge when defining health programs within the PHC context of public facilities (Majdzadeh et al. 2022). Fundamentally, because the services at this level encompass essential health care provisions (such as maternal and neonatal health), they attract the attention of United Nations agencies. Also, the MoHME maintains robust connections with those agencies.

To assess the eligibility of benefits, the SCHI Secretariat has used specific criteria, including effectiveness, safety, and financial burden. Disease burden was included after the first study in the country in 1999. Later, the financial burden on vulnerable groups was added as a criterion. Decisions were made by consensus or voting, and criteria were not scored. Until 2001, the purchase of services was passive, with services reviewed at the request of service providers, scientific groups, or companies. The development of managed care began at that time. In 2004, 42 managed care guidelines were published in the country outlining activities to address specific health issues, such as monitoring children's health or pain control in cancer patients. This initiative can be considered a move toward strategic purchasing.

In 2008, MoHME endorsed a procedural guide for HTA. At that time, HTA was applied to capital equipment entering the country for the first time. A domestic HTA model has existed in the country since 2011 (Arab-Zozani et al. 2020) with a decision support system that specifies what to do for each outcome (Yazdani and Jadidfard 2017). Research projects have studied fundamental methodological aspects of package development, determining, for example, the willingness to pay for each quality-adjusted life year (Moradi et al. 2019) and for social health insurance (Nosratnejad et al. 2014). A study on public opinion regarding private and social time preference for health outcomes finds that the discounting rate for distant health outcomes should include lower values than global standards (Mahboub-Ahari et al. 2019). In prioritization methodologies, the Technique for Order of Preference by Similarity to Ideal Solution approach was applied to three technologies: adenosine, tissue plasminogen activator, and mechanical thrombectomy (Mobinizadeh et al. 2021). Another study used expert opinion to identify nine criteria: efficiency/effectiveness, safety, population size, vulnerable population size, availability of alternative technologies, cost-effectiveness in other countries, budget impact, financial protection, and quality of evidence (Mobinizadeh et al. 2016). A study assessing the public perspective regarding prioritization criteria recognizes disease severity, age, daily care needs, number of alternative interventions, individuals' economic status, and diseases with absence from work (Darvishi et al. 2022).

Despite the methodological advancements pursued in the Islamic Republic of Iran over the years, most approaches remained exemplar-based at the level of individual research projects, and an evidence-informed decision-making system for prioritization was not fully institutionalized. The primary evidence stems from a qualitative study on the basic insurance package between 2014 and 2016. That study reveals that political and financial factors heavily influenced package design, with limited incorporation of evidence-informed methodology. Additionally, conflicts of interest played a role, necessitating proactive measures to mitigate potential negative consequences (Mohamadi, Takian, et al. 2020).

In 2018, a comprehensive study was conducted on the country translation of DCP3. Its initial assessment indicates that DCP3 has limited added value in the Islamic Republic of Iran as a lower-middle-income country (at the time of the study). DCP3's list of services is suitable for countries with constrained resources and few services in the package but needs more information for countries with more financial resources or extended service packages. For example, a review of maternal health services in the Islamic Republic of Iran shows that all DCP3 services already exist in the country, highlighting the need for more information about benefits (such as surgeries) at the second and third levels of service delivery. Nevertheless, DCP3's approach can play a crucial role as a model package capable of establishing a unified approach to prioritization, steering the national health system toward a prioritization system, and shaping the necessary governance in the country (Alwan et al. 2023). For example, countries' experiences demonstrate how having a model package has significantly contributed to multiple funding agencies' convergence of pooling functions (Soucat, Tandon, and Gonzales Pier 2023).

After May 2019, another effort to implement the evidence-informed deliberative process involved reviewing previous studies that address the criteria for prioritizing the basic services package. It identified and used three pillars: quality of care (effectiveness and safety), necessity (OOP and alternative availability), and sustainability (budget impact) (Nouhi et al. 2022). The project fostered deliberation among technical experts, medical professionals, patients, scientists, and insurance company representatives to select services. World Bank (2023) cites it as an example illustrating how well a fair and democratic process can work. This initiative demonstrated two additional advantages. First, stricter coverage conditions at lower prices were implemented for specific interventions, which could be considered a type of disinvestment (Gheorghe and Baker 2024). Second, a model for monitoring and evaluating the decision-making process for the package's priority-setting process was developed, which requires an assessment to validate its performance. In addition to the pilot on MS, the methodology developed in this work has been applied to cases of diabetes, breast and colorectal cancers, schizophrenia, hypertension, and dementia. The resulting structure and process have provided input for the resolution of the SCHI, which is introduced subsequently.

The review of important events in service prioritization shows that the Islamic Republic of Iran has been developing and implementing service packages for decades. In all those years, expert opinion highly influenced the process, first implicitly and then explicitly from 15 years ago, before the evolution of the priority-setting process and the adoption of criteria used in other countries (Baltussen et al. 2023). The country has also engaged in adequate capacity building of skilled human resources. However, the need to revise many more services, which has yet to be addressed, has caused the country's health system to suffer from inefficiency (Mohamadi, Manesh, et al. 2020; Sajadi et al. 2020). Therefore, the financial protection provided to the people against health expenditure is less than the capacity of the country's health system (Abdi et al. 2020; Hsu et al. 2021).

B4: Establishing a legal framework and process for assessing new interventions in the basic benefits package. Fundamental steps have been taken to use evidence in the health service package. Notably, insurance funds are mandated to conduct HTA for new interventions in the five-year plan scheduled for implementation starting in 2024. Should the HTA be realized, a legal framework for this level of services will be established (Iran's Islamic Consultative Assembly 2024).

Since early 2020, the SCHI has approved the structure and decision-making process for prioritizing services that define the obligations of basic insurance funds concerning specialized health services. The process involves technical groups, patient advocacy, ethical development, and benefit management, all of which are expected to assess interventions on the basis of predefined criteria (as outlined in the pilot program detailed in section B3D). The criteria for determining voting rights, ensuring confidentiality during reviews, and avoiding conflicts of interest among these individuals have been defined. Additionally, the decision-making method, the weight assigned to each criterion, and the appeal process have been anticipated (MoHME 2020). In terms of resource allocation, the SCHI has approved the allocation of up to 1 percent of the growth in revenue from service tariffs to cover new services; additionally, 0.01 percent of the resources from the major basic insurance funds is to be dedicated to conducting cost-effectiveness and budget impact studies. Time is needed to observe how well this process and structure are implemented and to evaluate their impact on the health service package.

CURRENT CHALLENGES

Applying the framework introduced earlier in the chapter, figure 8.2 summarizes current challenges and the way forward for the Islamic Republic of Iran's health system in terms of service package development. The lack of institutionalization of evidence use to prioritize health interventions is the fundamental challenge of service package development in the country.

Institutionalization refers to how a collection of actions becomes a sustainable part of a system (Sajadi, Jama, and Majdzadeh 2023). Health care organizations' complex individualized, organizational, and system relations and contextual factors make it difficult to institutionalize the use of evidence to set priorities (Bertram, Dhaene, and Tan-Torres Edejer 2021; Kuchenmüller et al. 2022). Removing barriers and moving toward evidence-informed priority setting will require identifying requisites and health system readiness (Alwan et al. 2023). The following paragraphs explain the most critical challenges of institutionalization according to the Islamic Republic of Iran's experience in developing and revising its service package.

Figure 8.2 Challenges and Way Forward for the Islamic Republic of Iran's Health System

Challenges	The Way Forward
Lack of institutionalization of evidence use to prioritize health interventions	Remove barriers related to institutional factors and conflict of interest management
The necessity of revising the health package as a mandate to achieve UHC, particularly at the second and third level of care	Remove barriers related to institutional factors and conflict of interest management
Need for a legal framework to support evidence in prioritizing services	Strengthen transparency and accountability
Lack of a structure and processes for deliberative evidence-informed prioritization	Consolidate the process to clearly define the participation of stakeholders and the public
Challenges in stakeholder engagement and conflict of interest management	Implement the structure and processes for evidence-informed prioritization

Source: Original figure developed for this publication.

Note: UHC = universal health coverage.

First, the need to revise the health package, particularly at the second and third levels of care, is not considered part of the health system's mandate to achieve UHC. Upstream laws and policies include revision of the health package through an evidence-informed approach (Sajadi, Gholamreza Kashi, and Majdzadeh 2020); however, that change in approach has not led to sustainable practice in the health system because it is considered a separate initiative, not part of achieving UHC. Consequently, packages of different levels of care (intersectoral interventions, PHC, and secondary and tertiary care) are considered separately rather than as part of a comprehensive package for achieving health and equity for the whole society. The service packages are not designed to implement the GHPs (in line with UHC) and are not developed or revised in a systematic and integrated way. Some services overlap with others, and their structure is unclear. Without an integrated scientific system to prioritize health interventions, vulnerable groups' access to essential, cost-effective services is threatened. That situation, along with high OOP payments, jeopardizes their financial protection.

Second, the country needs more than its current legal framework to support evidence in prioritizing services. Revising the health package—as endorsed in the country's development plans and GHPs—will require adequate enforcement and regulatory support as well as a more robust accountability mechanism (Doshmangir, Moshiri, and Farzadfar 2020; Sajadi, Gholamreza Kashi, and Majdzadeh 2020).

Third, the country must expand a structure and processes for deliberative, evidence-informed prioritization and ensure robust implementation of it for a basic benefits package. The institutional arrangement has some weaknesses despite the formation and operation of the Secretariat of the SCHI (to decide on basic insurance packages and government support), the PHC Network Development Center (for the first level of public services), and the HTA office (for data work). For example, the organizational position of the SCHI in playing its stewardship role has been established and needs to be implemented.

Although the 2010 formation of the HTA office in the MoHME marked a significant turning point, separate offices for HTA have recently been set up in different departments of the MoHME and insurance organizations. As those different offices have undertaken evaluation work, it has created a dispersion in the production and implementation of HTA. The lack of harmonization in the prioritization process has resulted in the use of various technical methods by the diverse centers.

Part of this challenge involves lack of stakeholder participation and conflicts of interest. The outcome of the service package definition and revision process affects the interests of various groups, and a significant challenge persists in ensuring that the process is evidence-informed and that it properly manages the participation and interests of all stakeholders, including patients. This issue has been anticipated in the new process for the insurance funds and must be implemented.

HTA offices' outsourcing of evidence production to the private sector (suppliers or importers of drugs) increases the likelihood of conflicts of interest. Given the private sector's role in the provision of health services, the interplay between the private and public sectors for dual-practice professionals can exacerbate conflicts of interest and substitute the use of power for evidence in the prioritization process.

Another challenge in managing interests is people's preferences. Over the years, specialization has dramatically dominated the service-seeking culture. People have an extreme desire to go directly to specialist and subspecialist physicians and to have unconditional access to expensive diagnostic and treatment services.

The diversity and inconsistency between licensing bodies for health technologies is another concern, making it difficult to apply the results of studies (Yazdizadeh et al. 2016). A study examining the feasibility of setting up a hospital HTA in the country finds limited use of evidence for prioritization not only at the macro level but also at the hospital level (Mohtasham, Majdzadeh, and Jamshidi 2017).

THE WAY FORWARD

As shown in figure 8.2, the Islamic Republic of Iran needs to remove barriers related to institutional factors and conflict of interest management. It needs to redefine the structure and processes associated with the evidence-informed approach to prioritization and develop the necessary platforms for stakeholder participation. Institutionalizing the use of evidence in prioritization will require changing the attitude of policy makers to recognize the need for a scientific approach to reviewing the service package. Otherwise, the country cannot solve the health system's current problems, especially those related to financing and service delivery, and they will become more acute over time. Revising the health package should include a comprehensive definition of UHC of services from promotional to palliative. Given the vital role of social factors affecting health, establishing a relationship between the health system and the social services system can accelerate the promotion of people's physical, mental, and social health. Doing so will require strengthening the intersectoral sections of the service package.

Regardless of the need to align package definition and revision with a comprehensive approach to health and UHC, the country needs to implement three primary strategies: (1) enforce the legal framework of prioritization, (2) strengthen transparency and accountability, and (3) consolidate the process to clearly define stakeholder and public participation (Sajadi, Jama, and Majdzadeh 2023).

The experience of the Universal Insurance Law 1994 shows the possibility of full enforcement with the support of the legal framework. That framework should consider revising the package as part of achieving UHC. It should create commitment and motivation of policy makers and ministries and convince them that using evidence to define health interventions for public funding is part of ensuring health for all. To institutionalize the process, decisions to add or remove services from the health package at all levels of service delivery (from promotional to palliative care) must meet specific requirements.

Recent pilots conducted for MS and other diseases show the possibility of optimizing resources allocated for each disease. Although the changes did not achieve the advantage of increasing the health system's efficiency because of their lack of generalization, it is promising that the SCHI has approved the pilots' recommendations. As a strategy for progressing the work, focusing independently on each disease and program removes initial sensitivities and allows for optimization between the diseases and the programs. For example, when services are optimized in the MS package, MS's public resources no longer move to other programs, and entitlements of MS patients or related service providers do not change to create challenges. However, until the health package is comprehensively revised to achieve UHC, it cannot lead to positive changes in increasing health system efficiency.

Transparency and accountability processes also need to be established or strengthened. A salient feature of the recent SCHI resolution is transparency, which is essential for service package review work and has been a challenge in recent HTA in the country. A recent comprehensive study in the Islamic Republic of Iran clearly shows the need to establish accountability mechanisms to persuade policy makers to make informed decisions (Majdzadeh et al. 2022). Without establishing mechanisms to monitor what individuals do in response to decisions and, consequently, what rewards or penalties to impose on them, one cannot expect the results of using evidence for prioritization. Other measures to increase transparency and accountability include establishing policies and decisions related to the basic health insurance package based on studies and expert opinions, and reducing political decisions, especially for expensive technologies and medicines.

One of the critical elements for fairness in the decision-making process for priority setting—and a principle for preparing health care services packages— is the participation of the public, including vulnerable groups (Kapilashrami, Razavi, and Majdzadeh 2023; WHO 2020b). Despite the legal capacities for public participation in Iranian policy making, which could be employed in priority setting, those capacities have not been effectively used yet (Rahbari Bonab, Majdzadeh, and Rajabi 2023). Irananian public participation structures take two forms—the health participation house (for brokering between people and managers) and the health assembly (public participation in policy making)—which can be used to institutionalize their capacity or similar structures in the evidence-informed deliberative prioritization process of the service package.

ACKNOWLEDGMENTS

The authors are grateful for the significant contributions of Dr. Mohammad-Hassan Abolhassani and Dr. Effat Mohammadi, whose insights into historical perspectives and recent advancements have significantly enriched this work.

NOTE

1. World Health Organization, Eastern Mediterranean Region, "COVID-19 Situation Reports," https://www.emro.who.int/health-topics/corona-virus/situation-reports.html (accessed August 20, 2024).

REFERENCES

Abdi, Zhaleh, Justine Hsu, Elham Ahmadnezhad, Reza Majdzadeh, and Iraj Harirchi. 2020. "An Analysis of Financial Protection Before and After the Iranian Health Transformation Plan." *Eastern Mediterranean Health Journal* 26 (9): 1025–33.

Akbari, Mohammad, Abbas Assari Arani, Mohammad Esmaeil Akbari, Bahram Sahabi, Alireza Olyaeemanesh, and Sajad Noorian. 2022. "Unnecessary Ultrasonography as Supplier-Induced Demand in Diagnosis of Primary Breast Cancer in Iran: A Cross-Sectional Study." *International Journal of Health Planning and Management* 37 (2): 873–85.

Alwan, Ala, Reza Majdzadeh, Gavin Yamey, Karl Blanchet, Alemayehu Hailu, Mohamed Jama, Kjell Arne Johansson, et al. 2023. "Country Readiness and Prerequisites for Successful Design and Transition to Implementation of Essential Packages of Health Services: Experience from Six Countries." *BMJ Global Health* 8 (Suppl 1): e010720.

Aminlou, Hassan. 2022. *Health Expenditure in Iran (2016–2021)*. Tehran: Ministry of Health and Medical Education.

Arab-Zozani, Morteza, Mobin Sokhanvar, Edris Kakemam, Tahereh Didehban, and Soheil Hassanipour. 2020. "History of Health Technology Assessment in Iran." *International Journal of Technology Assessment in Health Care* 36 (1): 34–39.

Bakhtiari, Ahad, Amirhossein Takian, Reza Majdzadeh, and Ali Akbar Haghdoost. 2020. "Assessment and Prioritization of the WHO 'Best Buys' and Other Recommended Interventions for the Prevention and Control of Non-communicable Diseases in Iran." *BMC Public Health* 20 (1): 1–16.

Baltussen, Rob, Omar Mwalim, Karl Blanchet, Manuel Carballo, Getachew Teshome Eregata, Alemayehu Hailu, Maryam Huda, et al. 2023. "Decision-Making Processes for Essential Packages of Health Services: Experience from Six Countries." *BMJ Global Health* 8 (Suppl 1): e010704.

Baradaran-Seyed, Z., and R. Majdzadeh. 2012. "Evidence-Based Health Care, Past Deeds at a Glance, Challenges and the Future Prospects in Iran." *Iranian Journal of Public Health* 41 (12): 1.

Bertram, Melanie, Gwenaël Dhaene, and Tessa Tan-Torres Edejer. 2021. *Institutionalizing Health Technology Assessment Mechanisms: A How To Guide*. Geneva: World Health Organization. https://iris.who.int/bitstream/handle/10665/340722/9789240020665-eng.pdf?sequence=1.

Danaei, Goodarz, Farshad Farzadfar, Roya Kelishadi, Arash Rashidian, Omid M. Rouhani, Shirin Ahmadnia, Alireza Ahmadvand, et al. 2019. "Iran in Transition." *The Lancet* 393 (10184): 1984–2005.

Danaei, Goodarz, Iraj Harirchi, Haniye Sadat Sajadi, Faeze Yahyaei, and Reza Majdzadeh. 2019. "The Harsh Effects of Sanctions on Iranian Health." *The Lancet* 394 (10197): 468–69.

Darvishi, Ali, Rajabali Daroudi, Mehdi Yaseri, and Ali Akbari Sari. 2022. "Public Preferences Regarding the Priority Setting Criteria of Health Interventions for Budget Allocation: Results of a Survey of Iranian Adults." *BMC Public Health* 22 (1): 1–16.

Doshmangir, Leila, Mohammad Bazyar, Reza Majdzadeh, and Amirhossein Takian. 2019. "So Near, So Far: Four Decades of Health Policy Reforms in Iran, Achievements and Challenges." *Archives of Iranian Medicine* 22 (10): 592.

Doshmangir, Leila, Mohammad Bazyar, Arash Rashidian, and Vladimir Sergeevich Gordeev. 2021. "Iran Health Insurance System in Transition: Equity Concerns and Steps to Achieve Universal Health Coverage." *International Journal for Equity in Health* 20 (1): 1–14.

Doshmangir, Leila, Esmaeil Moshiri, and Farshad Farzadfar. 2020. "Seven Decades of Primary Healthcare during Various Development Plans in Iran: A Historical Review." *Archives of Iranian Medicine (AIM)* 23 (5).

Doshmangir, Leila, Haniye Sadat Sajadi, Maryam Ghiasipour, Ali Aboutorabi, and Vladimir Sergeevich Gordeev. 2020. "Informal Payments for Inpatient Health Care in Post-Health Transformation Plan Period: Evidence from Iran." *BMC Public Health* 20 (1): 1–14.

Gheorghe, Adrian, and Peter Baker. 2024. "Disinvesting From Low-Value Health Technologies in Low- and Middle-Income Countries: Between a Solution to the Current Fiscal Crises and a Costly Mirage." CGD Policy Paper 327. Washington, DC: Center for Global Development. https://www.cgdev.org/publication/disinvesting-low-value-health -technologies-low-and-middle-income-countries-between.

Hamadeh, Nada, Catherine Van Rompaey, and Eric Metreau. 2021. "New World Bank Country Classifications by Income Level: 2021–2022." *World Bank Data Blog*, July 21, 2021. https://blogs.worldbank.org/opendata/new-world-bank-country -classifications-income-level-2021-2022.

Harirchi, Iraj, Mohammad Hajiaghajani, Aliakbar Sayari, Rassoul Dinarvand, Haniye Sadat Sajadi, Mahdi Mahdavi, Elham Ahmadnezhad, et al. 2020. "How Health Transformation Plan Was Designed and Implemented in the Islamic Republic of Iran?" *International Journal of Preventive Medicine* 11: 121.

Hsu, Justine, Reza Majdzadeh, Anne Mills, and Kara Hanson. 2021. "A Dominance Approach to Analyze the Incidence of Catastrophic Health Expenditures in Iran." *Social Science & Medicine* 285: 114022.

Iran's Islamic Consultative Assembly. 2024. *Seventh Five-Year Cultural, Economic, and Social Development Plan of the Islamic Republic of Iran*, Article 70(c). http://shenasname.ir.

Kapilashrami, Anuj, Donya Razavi, and Reza Majdzadeh. 2023. "Enhancing Priority-Setting Decision-Making Process Through Use of Intersectionality for Public Participation." *International Journal of Health Policy and Management* 12: 8095.

Keshavarzian, Maryam, and Sharareh Mofidian. 2015. "An Overview on Iran Health Care Financing System: Challenges and Solutions." *Journal of Health Policy and Sustainable Health* 1 (4).

Kuchenmüller, Tanja, Laura Boeira, Sandy Oliver, Kaelan Moat, Fadi El-Jardali, Jorge Barreto, and John Lavis. 2022. "Domains and Processes for Institutionalizing Evidence-Informed Health Policymaking: A Critical Interpretive Synthesis." *Health Research Policy and Systems* 20 (1): 1–18.

Mahboub-Ahari, Alireza, Abolghasem Pourreza, Ali Akbari Sari, Trevor A. Sheldon, and Maryam Moeeni. 2019. "Private and Social Time Preference for Health Outcomes: A General Population Survey in Iran." *PloS One* 14 (2): e0211545.

Majdzadeh, Reza, Haniye Sadat Sajadi, Bahareh Yazdizadeh, Leila Doshmangir, Elham Ehsani-Chimeh, Mahdi Mahdavi, Neda Mehrdad, et al. 2022. "Policy Options for Strengthening Evidence-Informed Health Policymaking in Iran: Overall SASHA Project Findings." *Health Research Policy and Systems* 20 (1): 1–13.

Mataria, Awad, Reza Majdzadeh, Deena Al Asfoor, Hassan Salah, and Zafar Mirza. 2023. "Translating Political Commitments into Actions by Designing and Implementing Packages for Priority Services for Universal Health Coverage in the Eastern Mediterranean Region." *Eastern Mediterranian Health Journal* 29 (12): 980–86.

Mobinizadeh, Mohammadreza, Efat Mohamadi, Hosein Arman, AmirAshkan Nasiripour, Alireza Olyaeemanesh, and Sara Mohamadi. 2021. "Topic Selection for Health Technology Assessment: An Approach Combining Multiple Attribute Decision Making and Decision Rules." *Medical Journal of the Islamic Republic of Iran* 35: 40.

Mobinizadeh, Mohammadreza, Pouran Raeissi, Amir Ashkan Nasiripour, Alireza Olyaeemanesh, and Seyed Jamaleddin Tabibi. 2016. "A Model for Priority Setting of Health Technology Assessment: The Experience of AHP-TOPSIS Combination Approach." *DARU Journal of Pharmaceutical Sciences* 24 (1): 1–12.

Mohamadi, Efat, Alireza Olyaee Manesh, Amirhossein Takian, Reza Majdzadeh, Farhad Hosseinzadeh Lotfi, Hamid Sharafi, Matthew Jowett, et al. 2020. "Technical Efficiency in Health Production: A Comparison between Iran and Other Upper Middle-Income Countries." *Health Policy and Technology* 9 (3): 335–47.

Mohamadi, Efat, Amirhossein Takian, Alireza Olyaeemanesh, Arash Rashidian, Ali Hassanzadeh, Moaven Razavi, and Sadegh Ghazanfari. 2020. "Health Insurance Benefit

Package in Iran: A Qualitative Policy Process Analysis." *BMC Health Services Research* 20 (1): 722.

Mohammadi, Effat, Ahmad Reza Raissi, Mohsen Barooni, Massoud Ferdoosi, and Mojtaba Nuhi. 2014. "Survey of Social Health Insurance Structure in Selected Countries; Providing Framework for Basic Health Insurance in Iran." *Journal of Education and Health Promotion* 29 (3): 116.

MoHME (Islamic Republic of Iran, Ministry of Health and Medical Education). 2020. "Implementation Process for Reviewing and Determining the Level and Coverage of the Basic Health Insurance Package in the Country." Secretariat of the Supreme Council of Health Insurance.

Mohtasham, Farideh, Reza Majdzadeh, and Ensiyeh Jamshidi. 2017. "Hospital-Based Health Technology Assessment in Iran." *International Journal of Technology Assessment in Health Care* 33 (4): 529–33.

Mohtasham, Farideh, Bahareh Yazdizadeh, Zahra Zali, Reza Majdzadeh, and Sima Nedjat. 2016. "Health Technology Assessment in Iran: Barriers and Solutions." *Medical Journal of the Islamic Republic of Iran* 30: 321.

Moradi, Najmeh, Arash Rashidian, Shirin Nosratnejad, Alireza Olyaeemanesh, Marzieh Zanganeh, and Leila Zarei. 2019. "Willingness to Pay for One Quality-Adjusted Life Year in Iran." *Cost Effectiveness and Resource Allocation* 17 (1): 1–10.

Mounesan, Leila, Saharnaz Nedjat, Reza Majdzadeh, Arash Rashidian, and Jaleh Gholami. 2013. "Only One-Third of Tehran's Physicians Are Familiar with 'Evidence-Based Clinical Guidelines.'" *International Journal of Preventive Medicine* 4 (3): 349–57.

NIHR (Iran's National Institute of Health Research). 2023. "A Snapshot on the Health of the Islamic Republic of Iran." https://nihr.tums.ac.ir/ZbAso.

Nosratnejad, Shirin, Arash Rashidian, Mohsen Mehrara, Ali Akbari Sari, Ghadir Mahdavi, and Maryam Moeini. 2014. "Willingness to Pay for Social Health Insurance in Iran." *Global Journal of Health Science* 6 (5): 154.

Nouhi, Mojtaba, Rob Baltussen, Seyed Sajad Razavi, Leon Bijlmakers, Mohammad Ali Sahraian, Zahra Goudarzi, Parisa Farokhian, et al. 2022. "The Use of Evidence-Informed Deliberative Processes for Health Insurance Benefit Package Revision in Iran." *International Journal of Health Policy and Management* 11 (11): 2719–26.

Pileroudi, Sirous, Kamel Shadpour, and Hassan Vakil. 1981. *Overview of Health and Medical Education.* Tehran: Training Campus of Ministry of Health.

Rahbari Bonab, Maryam, Reza Majdzadeh, and Fatemeh Rajabi 2023. "A Cross-Country Study of Institutionalizing Social Participation in Health Policymaking: A Realist Analysis." *Health & Social Care in Community*, April 20, 2023. https://doi.org/10.1155/2023/1927547.

Sajadi, Haniye Sadat, Elham Ehsani-Chimeh, and Reza Majdzadeh. 2019. "Universal Health Coverage in Iran: Where We Stand and How We Can Move Forward." *Medical Journal of the Islamic Republic of Iran* 33: 9.

Sajadi, Haniye Sadat, Fateme Gholamreza Kashi, and Reza Majdzadeh. 2020. "Identifying National Health Priorities: Content Analysis of the Islamic Republic of Iran's General Health Policies (GHPs)." *World Medical & Health Policy* 12 (2): 123–36.

Sajadi, Haniye Sadat, Hamidreza Safikhani, Alireza Olyaeemanesh, and Reza Majdzadeh. 2024. "Challenges in Institutionalizing Evidence-Informed Priority Setting for Health Service Packages: A Qualitative Document and Interview Analysis from Iran." *Health Research Policy and Systems* 22 (110): 1–13.

Sajadi, Haniye Sadat, Stephen Gloyd, and Reza Majdzadeh. 2021. "Health Must Be a Top Priority in the Iran Nuclear Deal." *The Lancet* 397 (10289): 2047–48.

Sajadi, Haniye Sadat, Zahra Goodarzi, Amirhossein Takian, Efat Mohamadi, Alireza Olyaeemanesh, Farhad Hosseinzadeh Lotfi, Hamid Sharafi, et al. 2020. "Assessing the Efficiency of Iran Health System in Making Progress towards Universal Health Coverage: A Comparative Panel Data Analysis." *Cost Effectiveness and Resource Allocation* 18 (1): 1–11.

Sajadi, Haniye Sadat, Mohamed Jama, and Reza Majdzadeh. 2023. "Institutionalisation Is a Vital Element for Fairness of Priority Setting in the Package Design if the Target Is Universal Health Coverage; Comment on 'Evidence-Informed Deliberative Processes for Health Benefits Package Design–Part II: A Practical Guide.'" *International Journal of Health Policy and Management* 12 (Continuous): 1–4.

Sajadi, Haniye Sadat, and Reza Majdzadeh. 2019. "From Primary Health Care to Universal Health Coverage in the Islamic Republic of Iran: A Journey of Four Decades." *Archives of Iranian Medicine* 22 (5).

Sajadi, Haniye Sadat, Farkhondeh Alsadat Sajadi, Maryam Yaghoubi, and Reza Majdzadeh. 2022. "Informal Payments for Outpatient Health Care: Country-Wide Evidence from Iran." *Medical Journal of the Islamic Republic of Iran* 36 (1): 409–15.

Soucat, Agnes, Ajay Tandon, and Eduardo Gonzales Pier. 2023. "From Universal Health Coverage Services Packages to Budget Appropriation: The Long Journey to Implementation." *BMJ Global Health* 8 (Suppl 1): e010755.

Takian, Amirhossein, Azam Raoofi, and Sara Kazempour-Ardebili. 2020. "COVID-19 Battle during the Toughest Sanctions against Iran." *The Lancet* 395 (10229): 1035.

WHO (World Health Organization). 2020a. "PHC Country Profile: Islamic Republic of Iran." Fact sheet, WHO, Regional Office for the Eastern Mediterranean. http://www.emro.who.int/images/stories/phc/iran_phccp.pdf?ua=1.

WHO (World Health Organization). 2020b. *Principles of Health Benefits Packages.* Geneva: WHO.

World Bank. 2022. "Islamic Republic of Iran." Country Overview. https://www.worldbank.org/en/country/iran/overview, accessed December 17, 2023.

World Bank. 2023. *Open and Inclusive: Fair Processes for Financing Universal Health Coverage.* Washington, DC: World Bank.

Yazdani, Shahram, and Mohammad-Pooyan Jadidfard. 2017. "Developing a Decision Support System to Link Health Technology Assessment (HTA) Reports to the Health System Policies in Iran." *Health Policy and Planning* 32 (4): 504–15.

Yazdizadeh, Bahareh, Safoura Shahmoradi, Reza Majdzadeh, Shila Doaee, Mohammad Bazyar, Aghdas Souresrafil, and Alireza Olyaeemanesh. 2016. "Stakeholder Involvement in Health Technology Assessment at National Level: A Study from Iran." *International Journal of Technology Assessment in Health Care* 32 (3): 181–89.

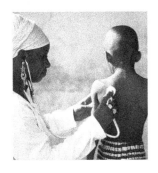

9

Priorities and Health Packages in Reforming the Nigerian Health System: Experience from the Lancet Nigeria Commission

Ibrahim Abubakar, Blake Angell, Tim Colbourn, Obinna Onwujekwe, and Seye Abimbola

ABSTRACT

Nigeria is projected to become the third most populous nation globally by 2100, which will place increasing pressure on the nation's health systems and necessitate widespread reform to ensure Nigerians have widespread access to affordable, quality health care. The Lancet Nigeria Commission built a case for targeted and high-value investment to support that goal and achieve substantial health gains through several highly cost-effective priority areas for health investment based on analyses of the local burden of disease, prevailing measures of cost-effectiveness, and a prioritization process involving key health system stakeholders. Specifically, the Commission undertook an analysis of existing literature, policies, programs, and governance frameworks, and used the OneHealth Tool[1] and the Lives Saved Tool[2] to project health and cost effects. It identified high–net gain areas including maternal and child health. The Commission's recommendations on health reform have had significant influence on national legislation to mandate health insurance and to create a Vulnerable Group Fund. Building on those early achievements will require health care system reform that leverages the strengths of the system and works within the realities of the complex, federalized system but still meaningfully and sustainably overcomes the limitations previously restricting population health outcomes and access to care. Significant scope remains for further development through carefully directed investment, particularly in primary care, health promotion, and interventions to improve the social determinants of health.

INTRODUCTION

The United Nations projects that Nigeria, with Africa's largest economy and population, will become the third most populous nation in the world by 2100 (UN DESA 2019). Although a nation of great promise, Nigeria must urgently address a series of challenges to reach its true potential. Nigeria experiences the worst outcomes in the world across several health and social outcomes such as malaria (WHO 2018), under-five mortality,[3] and the number of children out of school (World Bank 2022). Health expenditure remains low by global standards, and the health system is beset by a myriad of challenges. Recent analysis comparing Nigeria to other West African countries with similar or lower gross domestic product per capita and investment in health suggests that the country has room to increase both the efficiency of current levels of health spending and the overall envelope of investments (Angell et al. 2022). An increase in domestic funding is also essential to allow a gradual weaning from donor support.

The Lancet Nigeria Commission (LNC) drew together a multidisciplinary group of leading experts to develop evidence-based recommendations to strengthen Nigeria's health system and achieve universal health coverage (UHC) in the country (Abubakar et al. 2022). The LNC calls for "a new social contract centred on health to address Nigeria's need to define the relationship between the citizen and the state" (Abubakar et al. 2022, 1156). For Nigeria to achieve that goal, the LNC recommends a prevention agenda at the heart of health policy using a whole-of-government approach and community engagement. The large inequality between urban and rural areas, and between different regions of the country, requires equitable delivery of health, social welfare, education, and employment. The COVID-19 pandemic also exposed vulnerabilities in health security, which will require a whole system assessment of the investment needs, including for manufacturing capacity of essential health products, medicines, and vaccines.

This chapter draws on the expertise and expands the analysis of the LNC to build the case for targeted and high-value investment to achieve substantial gains in population health and health care for Nigerians. It focuses on the policy implications of the LNC's work, highlighting the links between the findings of the analyses, existing policy initiatives in Nigeria, and the reforms the LNC argues are necessary to propel Nigeria to UHC. There is a scarcity of robust local data to inform policy and investment decision-making in Nigeria (Abubakar et al. 2022). The LNC report and this chapter seek to begin filling that gap, presenting the case and priorities for targeted investment to progress the country toward reaching its potential. The chapter outlines the process through which priorities were set, the sources of data and tools used, and examples of care packages that will support UHC. Properly implementing those packages will require widespread health system and financing reform, and the chapter presents several recommendations to sustainably achieve that reform.

Overview of the Nigerian Health System

The inherently complex Nigerian health system involves three different levels of government, each responsible for the provision of different levels of care. Public funding is split between the federal government (53 percent), state governments (27 percent), and local governments (20 percent); as stated earlier, however, the overall level of funding devoted to health remains low by global standards. Wide inequities exist across the nation along with an imbalance between revenue-raising potential (dominated by the federal government) and the responsibilities of service provision for the other levels of government. On top of public funding, a substantial private sector also provides care to Nigerians, characterized by high out-of-pocket costs.

Recent reforms, notably the passing of the National Health Insurance Authority (NHIA) Act 2022, build on reforms from recent decades that have aimed at improving health care coverage and population health across Nigeria. Those earlier reforms include the establishment and implementation of the National Health Insurance Scheme (NHIS) in the late 1990s and early 2000s; the National Strategic Health Development Plan (NSHDP I), introduced in 2010 and prioritizing eight key areas for further health system reforms (later adopted in NSHDP II); the National Health Act of 2014, which introduced the Basic Health Care Provision Fund (BHCPF), a mechanism for the national government to finance health care provision at the state level; and, more recently, the introduction of the Essential Health Care Package designed to outline key services the population should be able to access. Despite gains through those programs, UHC remains elusive. Several shortcomings have hindered the impact of the reforms; the chapter outlines those shortcomings and develops recommendations to feasibly move the country toward UHC.

PRIORITY-SETTING PROCESS

The priority-setting recommendations emerged from an evidence-based, multistage process led by the LNC. The Commissioners had expertise and experience in the diverse disciplines required to shape national health policy, including public health and epidemiology, political science, history, health economics, health policy and systems research, public policy, sociology, demography, law, anthropology, and health systems.

Ownership and Governance

The LNC ensured representation with respect to gender and local origin, included a range of political and health policy views among experts based within and outside Nigeria, and consulted with a diverse group of policy stakeholders to provide insight into the challenges of delivering health and health care in Nigeria. It set a 10-year time frame for all analyses, looking beyond the life span of the current Nigerian government, to ensure relevance to current and future administrations in Nigeria.

Although some Commissioners had roles within government and public agencies, the process took place outside government, and the LNC does not hold formal power to implement the recommendations. Nevertheless, the government has already adopted some of the LNC's recommendations.

Scope and Content

The LNC sought to generate and synthesize evidence to inform policy and program implementation and with a view to building a strengthened health system that meets the needs of all Nigerians. The process occurred over the following four stages used to generate final recommendations:

1. The LNC reviewed Nigerian history with a focus on the health system to understand current structures and systems by rooting them in precolonial, colonial, and modern-day trends and events.
2. It conducted a comprehensive analysis of the country's disease burden to identify the major causes of morbidity and mortality using the best available data.
3. It analyzed policy documents (health-specific and broader intersectoral policies that influence health beyond health care) and health system factors to identify key challenges and suggest systems-level leverage points for potential intervention.
4. It combined health and economic analyses to generate evidence on the most cost-effective combination of interventions to achieve health goals given Nigeria's disease burden and summarized approaches to improve health financing.

Criteria Used

The LNC's work was underpinned by the core values of fairness, equity, pragmatism, and evidence-driven approaches. Given the youth of the Nigerian population, the LNC's stated priorities include prevention and keeping young Nigerians healthy. The LNC conducted extensive analyses of Nigeria's disease burden and compared population health outcomes to those in neighboring nations to determine areas where the Nigerian system was underperforming and to identify cost-effective, sustainable reform options. An e-Delphi process was conducted in late 2020 with 23 Commissioners and Nigerian health policy makers to identify the key conditions and risk factors most important to address to improve population health in Nigeria (described in detail in the supplementary appendix in Abubakar et al. 2022). That group prioritized key conditions and risk factors using four criteria:

1. The *magnitude of need*, to assess how important an issue the condition or risk factor was to the Nigerian population and health system
2. *Available knowledge*, to assess the importance of further knowledge of the burden of the condition for the Nigerian population and health system
3. *Leverage*, to assess the potential for the LNC's work in this area to contribute to strengthening Nigeria's health system
4. *Equity*, to assess whether work to address the specific condition or risk factor would likely also act to reduce disparities across the population.

The group then presented respondents with a prioritized list of all conditions and risk factors, and asked them to either agree with the ranking or alter it to match their own priorities. The process resulted in the prioritization of 11 conditions and five risk factors considered particularly important to the Nigerian health system (table 9.1).

Table 9.1 Final List of Prioritized Conditions and Risk Factors, Nigeria

Condition group	Rank from prioritization process	DALY-based ranking
Maternal and neonatal conditions	1	1
Cardiovascular diseases	2	6
Diabetes and chronic kidney diseases	3	14
Neglected tropical diseases and malaria	4	4
Respiratory infections and tuberculosis	5	3
Neoplasms	6	11
Mental disorders	7	10
Enteric infections	8	2
Transportation injuries	9	16
Nutritional deficiencies	10	12
HIV/AIDS and sexually transmitted infections	11	5
Risk factors		
Child and maternal malnutrition	1	1
Unsafe water, sanitation, and handwashing	2	2
High systolic blood pressure	3	4
Air pollution	4	3
High fasting plasma glucose	5	6

Sources: Prioritization rankings come from Abubakar et al. 2022; DALY-based rankings use data from Institute for Health Metrics and Evaluation, Global Burden of Disease Study 2019, https://ghdx .healthdata.org/gbd-2019.
Note: DALY = disability-adjusted life year.

Accountability and Transparency Measures

Given that the LNC's work lay outside government and that the LNC had no authority over the implementation of recommendations, its work did not incorporate specific accountability mechanisms. Nevertheless, the LNC's review of current Nigerian policy settings identified several existing measures:

- *Federal and state budgets.* The development of annual health budgets by the Federal Ministry of Health (FMoH) and some state ministries of health was preceded by the development of Medium Term Sector Strategies, which attracted broad-based participation, including by civil society organizations (CSOs), in order to help ensure that annual budgets are used to buy essentials covered by the basic Health Benefits Package (HBP) Nigerians should receive (refer to the third bullet item in this list). Unfortunately, the Medium Term Sector Strategy process is not very active or well established. Nevertheless, the published annual budgets give CSOs and other stakeholders the framework to monitor the contents of the budget and the implementation, and Nigeria's Open Treasury portal (https://opentreasury.gov.ng) enables them to monitor the HBP within FMoH's annual budget.

- *Social health insurance and other risk protection mechanisms.* The recent passage of the NHIA Act in 2022, based on the recommendation of the LNC (Adebowale-Tambe 2022), provides a further potential source of funds through the establishment of a Vulnerable Group Fund and mandatory health insurance for formally employed persons. A broad-based participatory mechanism will likely be used to develop a cost-effective HBP that assures value for money when deployed by the schemes. The existence of the law provides a governance framework, but ensuring transparent, efficient, and equitable use of the extra funds to cover the target population groups will require development of accountability mechanisms.

- *HBP under the BHCPF.* A broad-based technical working group—composed of government, CSOs, and development partners—led the development of the benefit package. The main implementing agencies at the federal level (the National Primary Healthcare Development Agency [NPHCDA], NHIS, and FMoH) are striving to create awareness about the HBP gateways among health care providers and consumers. The NHIA, through the NHIS gateway of the BHCPF and implemented by subnational (state) social health insurance schemes, purchases services from primary health care centers, a practice based on the agreed HBP of the BHCPF. The HBP was circulated for review, debated, and approved by the National Council on Health, which draws participation from all health sector leaders in Nigeria. It has an accountability framework, which involves both the public and private sectors in ensuring that the purchase of HBP follows the stipulated guidelines. The accountability framework is currently undergoing revision to address some practical issues with implementation of the BHCPF. It is also envisaged that the accountability framework will encompass the monitoring of health workers' presence and productivity, because absenteeism of frontline health workers can undermine the use of the fund. The FMoH has developed a capacity-building and awareness program on the BHCPF to further inform implementers, other decision-makers, and CSOs about the BHCPF's salient features, including the HBP. The current implementation of the BHCPF as a vertical program, however, does not align with the law that established it. That law envisioned integration of the BHCPF into the normal activities of the NHIS, NPHCDA, and their equivalents in states and local governments. Verticalization of the BHCPF has negative implications for efficiency and the amount of benefits the fund can buy.

- *NHIS Formal Sector Social Insurance Programme (FSSHIP).* Development of the initial HBP of the FSSHIP of the NHIS (now the NHIA) used a broad participatory method, involving academics, health insurance companies, NHIS staff, physician groups, and others. Although subsequent revisions of the HBP of the FSSHIP have not followed such a broad-based approach, the NHIA regularly informs citizens and their accredited providers about the summary contents of the HBP, delineating the benefits to be provided or purchased at primary, secondary, and tertiary levels of care. With the passage of the NHIA Act 2022, that mechanism will need to be updated.

- *State Social Health Insurance Schemes.* The State Social Health Insurance Schemes, found at subnational levels, try to follow the steps taken by the NHIA in developing its HBP and creating accountability mechanisms for monitoring the provision and consumption of the HBP.
- *Other special financial risk protection interventions.* Examples include the Free Maternal and Child Health programs, especially the defunct National Health Insurance Scheme–Millennium Development Goals/Maternal and Child Health and Subsidy Reinvestment and Empowerment Programme/Maternal and Child Health Project programs that had HBPs developed using broad-based participatory co-creation methods involving both the public and private sectors. In some states and local councils, implementation of HBPs also involves community entities such as Ward Development Committees and Village Development Committees. Some also have adjunct accountability frameworks on paper.
- *NSHDP I and NSHDP II, State Strategic Health Development Plans I and II, and Federal Strategic Health Development Plans I and II.* The decision of which interventions/activities to include in NSHDP I, and especially in NSHDP II, followed a prioritization mechanism that ensured that the 10 Nigerian health system building blocks focused on key interventions to protect population health. In addition to priority-setting and consensus meetings with key stakeholders in the health sector to arrive at many priority interventions and activities, the process also used the OneHealth Tool to cost the interventions and activities, and model their potential benefits, to arrive at the final lists of benefits included in the plans. NSHDP II (2018–22) will soon undergo evaluation in preparation for the development of NSHDP III.
- *Non-Communicable Diseases and Injuries (NCDI) Poverty Commission priority setting.* In 2022, the NCDI Poverty Commission embarked on a detailed priority-setting process to arrive at an HBP on NCDI for the country. The HBP prioritization proceeded through ordered steps—following the NCDI poverty analytical framework that focuses on equity, cost-effectiveness, and value for money—to arrive at a draft HBP for NCDI.

ANALYSES AND TOOLS

A variety of analyses, undertaken using the best data available, informed the work of the LNC.

Data Sources

The LNC relied heavily on the Global Burden of Diseases, Injuries and Risk Factors Study 2019,[4] which provides ongoing estimates of the mortality and morbidity burden attributable to a wide array of conditions and exposure to risk factors in all countries (Murray et al. 2020; Vos et al. 2020). In addition to using those estimates, the LNC undertook bespoke data collection and assessed the quality of existing data to inform future disease burden estimates. It used population-level data (demographic surveillance sites and census information), national facility–based databases (DHIS2), surveys and surveillance databases (such as Surveillance Outbreak Response Management and Analysis System [SORMAS], the Nigeria HIV/AIDS Indicator and Impact Survey, and NPHCDA immunization coverage data), and morbidity and mortality records requested from hospitals across the country.[5]

The process of collating the data had its challenges, beginning with identifying where the data were situated and requesting permission to access the data, because of limited institutional memory and frequent leadership changes. Although some organizations were confused as to the rightful guardian of the data, others had several custodians with numerous channels to permission, each of whom had to consent to the release of data. Approval processes were therefore complex and slow. Even when data existed, as in many health facilities, the data were not captured using electronic medical record systems, leading to data that were often incomplete and marred with inaccuracies. Furthermore, despite having approval from the National Health Research Ethics Committee, the LNC had to follow different guidelines for different organizations before receiving data. Reluctance on the part of some institutions to share data arose because of concerns about opportunities to publish their own data, costs of extracting data, and apprehensions about privacy and data misuse.

Tools and Methods

The LNC undertook several reviews of the literature to summarize the best evidence available on Nigeria-relevant disease burden and priorities and health system reform to inform subsequent data analysis and modeling. It used the OneHealth Tool to project health system costs under different scenarios as specified under NSHDP II.

Because the e-Delphi process and the analysis of Nigerian health policy and burden of disease highlighted maternal and child health as a key priority, the LNC conducted specific analysis to assess the potential effect of investment targeting a package of cost-effective interventions to address that priority. The LNC used the Lives Saved Tool (LiST) to dynamically project the health and cost effects between 2021 and 2030 of three scenarios of policy intervention: (1) baseline (no improvements in intervention coverage), (2) moderate increased investment (defined as linear progress to 20 percent increased coverage of interventions relative to baseline), and (3) universal coverage (defined as linear progress to 90 percent coverage of interventions). The supplementary appendix to Abubakar et al. (2022) provides further details of the interventions included, LiST, and the projection methods.

SUMMARY OF ANALYSIS FINDINGS

The Basic Minimum Package of Health Services (BMPHS) aims to achieve fully functional primary health care facilities in Nigeria—with at least one in each political ward (with average population of about 23,000 per ward) by 2026, seven years after its launch via the Basic Health Care Provision Fund distributed by the federal government.[6] The package also aims for at least three fully equipped secondary facilities and a national ambulance service in each of Nigeria's 37 states by 2024. It includes a set of preventive, protective, promotive, curative, and rehabilitative services including basic emergency obstetric and newborn care. As of October 2021, 6,287 primary health care facilities, representing 68 percent of political wards, had been authorized to receive funds.[7] Box 9.1 outlines ongoing work on health benefits package design for primary health care in Nigeria.

Box 9.1

Health Benefits Package Design for Primary Health Care in Nigeria

Ongoing work by the National Primary Health Care Development Agency seeks to design a feasible benefits package for Nigeria's Ward Health Service (Oritseweyimi et al. 2023). The agency is using a framework for health benefits package design that considers the incremental cost-effectiveness ratio of the services currently provided by the Ward Health Service and the services that could be provided, and how those ratios relate to a cost-effectiveness threshold for current health spending in Nigeria of US$214 per disability-adjusted life year averted. The incremental cost-effectiveness ratios of interventions and services were obtained from the Tufts database;[a] when such data for interventions in Nigeria were not available, the analysis used data from countries deemed similar to Nigeria.

The emerging findings of this work indicate that overcoming supply and demand constraints to increase coverage of Ward Health Service interventions in primary health care in Nigeria have large net health and monetary benefits, on the order of approximately US$1 billion per 10 percent increase in primary health care use and up to about US$15 billion at 100 percent use—US$9 billion more than at the current 44 percent use (Oritseweyimi et al. 2023).

Further work is required to investigate the equity implications of increasing coverage, particularly with regard to scaling up interventions close to the cost-effective threshold, given that interventions included in health benefits coverage should be available for all those expected to use services (up to 100 percent coverage). Such work needs to consider the costs and benefits of broader health system strengthening efforts including recruiting, training, paying, and retaining health workers, and building and maintaining new health facilities. Overall, the work should guide investment decisions as health budgets increase to meet the large unaddressed primary health care needs of Nigeria's population.

a. Tufts Medical Center, Center for the Evaluation of Value and Risk in Health, "GH CEA Registry," https://cevr.tuftsmedicalcenter.org/databases /gh-cea-registry.

The comprehensive burden of disease analysis highlighted several key priorities for the Nigerian system (Angell et al. 2022). Outcomes for children under 5 years and maternal mortality remain poor in Nigeria, with children under 5 years bearing most of the nation's mortality burden. In contrast, outcomes for adults over 50 years, particularly men over 50 years, are among the best in West Africa. Those relatively good outcomes, however, are threatened by a growing burden of noncommunicable diseases that account for an increasing proportion of the total disease burden for older population groups (figure 9.1). Preventing such diseases early will be essential to ensure that scarce health care resources are not unduly diverted away from overcoming the burden of maternal and child mortality and that the already stretched health care system can meet the needs of the population.

Figure 9.1 Proportion of DALYs Attributable to Diseases, by Age Group, Nigeria, 2019

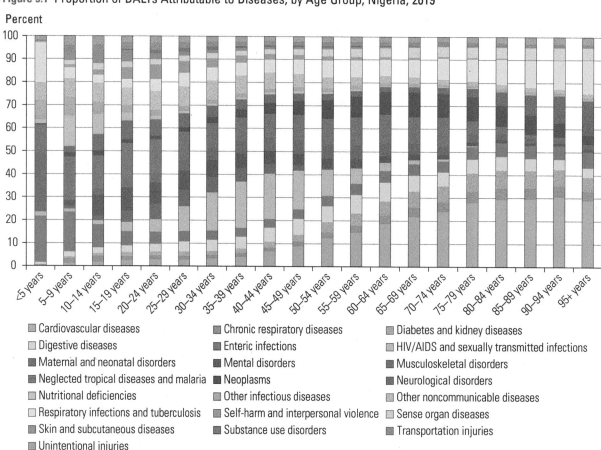

Source: Institute for Health Metrics and Evaluation, Global Burden of Disease Study 2019, https://ghdx.healthdata.org/gbd-2019.

Note: DALYs = disability-adjusted life years.

Following the NSHDP II (FMoH 2018b), the LNC costed provision of all health program areas[8] at US$2–US$3 and all health system strengthening[9] at US$17–US$27 per capita per year during 2021–30 for a moderate scale-up scenario of coverage increase of 17.5 percent during 2018–22 extrapolated to 2030. An aggressive scale-up scenario extrapolation of a 30 percent increase during 2018–22 to 2030 would cost US$19–US$29 per capita per year for all program areas and US$19–US$30 for health system strengthening. Achieving those scenarios would entail massive increases in health expenditure, especially government health expenditure (only US$11.85 per capita in 2019), given that three-quarters of health spending in Nigeria is out of pocket (Abubakar et al. 2022).

The LNC's analysis of scaling up maternal, newborn, and child health services found that an additional US$64 per capita for the period 2021–30, or US$10.5 per capita in 2030 at 90 percent coverage of services, could avert a total of 309,000 maternal deaths, 967,000 newborn deaths, and 2.61 million child deaths (Abubakar et al. 2022). Those numbers represent highly cost-effective spending: given a total population ranging from 206 million in 2021 to 263 million in 2030, the approximately 4 million lives saved over the decade are saved at a cost of about US$600 each. Because most lives saved are newborn babies or children with their whole lives ahead of them, that cost translates to less than US$15 per disability-adjusted life year averted. Such increased health spending—despite requiring an almost doubling of current government health expenditure just for maternal and newborn health—should be affordable because it represents only about 0.5 percent of Nigeria's gross domestic product per capita of US$2,097 in 2020.

Linking to Service Delivery Reforms

A Healthcare Reform Committee (HRC), chaired by the Vice President, has been inaugurated with a remit to lead the development of a people-centric health care system—fundamental for Nigeria's socioeconomic development. The HRC had a six-month timeline to deliver its outputs but faced delays due to political and other considerations. At the time of writing, the HRC secretariat had completed consultation with stakeholders and worked closely with state governments and the Federal Capital Territory to outline actions needed at all levels of government and in communities to improve health. The LNC report provides data and information to inform the HRC's recommendations. Even with the ongoing nature of the system reforms process in the country, and the LNC's lack of power over implementation, the country has already adopted several LNC recommendations; for example, the NHIA Act 2022 includes requirements to mandate basic health insurance, to pool risks, and to create a vulnerable group fund to be financed partly by BHCPF. Further, initiatives have been incorporated by the ongoing work of Commissioners with several HRC subcommittees, and the LNC continues to engage with the new government to pursue further implementation.

To strengthen domains for action and policy in Nigeria's health system, the LNC proposes a reformed setup of centrally determined (albeit with active involvement of a broad range of health system stakeholders) but locally delivered systems. The reform will require that Nigeria digitize its health system; thoughtfully centralize standards; pool and streamline resources; improve supply chains, local manufacturing, and data management while localizing production of basic products and allocation decisions; define basic health services packages to align with local risk factors; and implement modes of community service delivery sensitive to socio-cultural norms.

Centralization and Localization

In a large, diverse, and federally governed country like Nigeria, careful calibration of a centrally determined cost-effective HBP with flexibility in its local implementation is essential. For example, although a federal entity, NPHCDA, is designing the HBP for Nigeria's Ward Health Service, the state governments (through state primary health care boards/agencies) will implement the HBP in each state. The BHCPF itself is centrally legislated (by the federal parliament) and coordinated (by federal entities NHIA and NPHCDA), but is implemented by state governments (again, through their state primary health care boards/agencies). More broadly, certain health system functions must not only be centrally determined but also be centrally financed—especially those functions that benefit from national uniformity or economies of scale. For example, implementing a national initiative such as the BHCPF requires having nationally uniform information systems to inform its design and monitor its ongoing implementation. As such, the federal government must bear the costs of developing and providing central guidelines and forms (paper-based and electronic) with resources for adaptations to suit different subnational levels and local contexts; the costs of training and mentoring; and the costs of personnel to ensure data collection and quality assurance. Similarly, developing and providing national quality of care guidelines, improving the health commodities supply chain system, and strengthening logistics and quality assurance of border transactions on importation will require central efforts. These examples of functions that require centralization mean the federal government must take on costs and responsibilities.

Nevertheless, the central government can only do so much, especially given its distance from local needs and preferences in as large and diverse a country as Nigeria. Subnational governments must play a major role in the adaptation and implementation of national benefits packages, systems, guidelines, and standards. Although the federal government may provide support at early stages of implementation (because doing so is efficient and sets a good example), it may phase out and means-test such support over time, based on the level of available financial and technical resources in each state.

Linking to Financing Mechanisms

For Nigeria's health system to deliver UHC will require health financing reform. The recent passage of the NHIA Act 2022 presents an ambitious framework that if implemented will allow a substantial rise in the funds available to the Nigerian health sector. Specific elements of the act include mandatory health insurance for all residents of Nigeria irrespective of employment status, additional powers for NHIA to regulate and integrate schemes, a specific mandate to promote UHC, expanded options for organizations to act as third-party administrators but with limited fund management function, and the establishment of a Vulnerable Group Fund. The act mentions numerous sources of potential funding for the Vulnerable Group Fund, including levies and new taxes. The recent amendment of the Finance Act to allow taxation of sugar-sweetened beverages should provide further revenue.

Implementation of the act should prioritize increasing government funding for health, improving resource management through strategic purchasing, and creating a more robust benefit package. The new legislation provides the statutory basis to establish strong systems for oversight and regulation of providers such as health maintenance organizations. Ultimately, improving financial risk protection and the effectiveness of health financing mechanisms, such as social health insurance, in Nigeria will require addressing implementation bottlenecks in the three health financing functions: revenue mobilization, pooling, and purchasing. An evidence-based and systematic process should guide the development of government annual health budgets to ensure collective use of funds to achieve set goals and targets—for example, achieving some of the health-related targets of the Sustainable Development Goals.

Options for Revenue Mobilization

Fiscal space for increased domestic funding of health services requires increases in overall government revenue and increasing the share of government resources devoted to the health sector. Nigeria's current overreliance on oil revenue for foreign exchange exposes the country to continuous financial shocks. Health system actors will have to negotiate for increased allocation to the health sector, even when the overall government revenue increases, because the Ministry of Finance may decide to allocate the increased resources to other sectors of the economy.

The country could improve health spending by instituting a dedicated predetermined budget at the federal and state levels, outside of the electoral cycle, and with mechanisms to ensure it is spent efficiently and equitably. Ensuring equity in the distribution of resources and setting of health priorities will require making the budget public and subject to independent auditors. Increasing states' internally generated revenue would also lower their dependence on federal funding and could refocus priorities on internal needs in determining health spending if states allocate a good proportion of the increased resources to the health sector. A transparent, public process for assigning and using grants from international donor partners, subject to independent regular audits, is also needed. Nigeria established the BHCPF in 2014 to address some of those issues, financing it through an annual federal government grant of not less than 1 percent of the Consolidated Revenue Fund, grants from external donors, and other sources. The NHIA will administer 50 percent of the funds to provide basic health services to citizens and for subsidy payments to state insurance agencies to provide health care to people who cannot afford premium payments. The NHIA Act 2022 complements and potentially increases the revenue available and should provide the basis for far-reaching reform to reach Nigeria's goal of UHC.

Reducing the burden and financial risk of health care spending by individuals, families, and communities will therefore require dramatic provision of and access to pooled funding (insurance) or prepaid government provision of health care. Pooling is the health financing function whereby collected health revenues are transferred to purchasing organizations, which manage revenues and distribute risks. Nigeria should strive to develop large pools because having small, scattered, and uncoordinated pools will not lead to efficient and equitable financial risk protection. However, in the case of multiple pools—such as the various State Social Health Insurance Schemes, the FSSHIP, free programs funded by the budget, community-based health insurance schemes, and private health insurance—the country can achieve risk equalization via mechanisms such as a dedicated fund and health reinsurance, under the leadership of the FMoH, the National Council of Health, and the Nigeria Governors Forum.

Alternatively, mandatory social insurance for health could be levied, though it too would need to be done equitably to guard against increasing inequality and resulting health, social, and economic harms. Additionally, the country will need to find solutions for barriers to coverage of those working in the informal sector and the unemployed (Onwujekwe et al. 2019). Levying taxes and social insurance is also difficult because most work in Nigeria takes place in the informal sector. However, as in other countries like Ethiopia and India, should UHC become an election issue both nationally and at the state level, concerted advocacy and community engagement efforts from committed institutions and CSOs could provide creative approaches to facilitate UHC.

To further improve pooling and management of revenue, the federal, state, and local governments should ensure the development and institutionalization of efficient, equitable, and transparent fund management systems. Development partners should move from their current opaque systems to ensure the pooling of donor funds that will be transparently managed. The government, through the health and finance ministries, should ensure harmonization and alignment of donor funding to health with national policies, strategies, and priorities. Third-party funds pooling agents can be public, quasi-public, or private entities depending on the context and preferences of the different levels of government.

Furthermore, the federal government needs to revise the benefit package so that every citizen has social health insurance coverage, implemented with strict oversight and regulation of health maintenance organizations. It should also increase the awareness and benefits of social health insurance. At regular intervals, NHIA's implementation strategy should undergo review to fast-track and improve the level of coverage among informal and formal sector workers, with government covering the poorest Nigerians, in order to provide universal financial risk protection and reduce both out-of-pocket spending and the proportion of expenditure it covers. Federal and state-specific strategies should address context-related challenges of individual states (such as the inability to reallocate funds into FSSHIP).

In keeping with the recommendation to localize certain aspects of health services provision, it is important to allocate more funds at the state and local government levels for purchasing health services, with evidence-based, strategic, and appropriately tracked spending to ensure efficient use of resources and the removal of financial barriers to access by reducing out-of-pocket expenditure in both absolute and relative terms (Hirose et al. 2018). Innovative strategies are also needed to enable potential beneficiaries, especially in the informal sector, to better comprehend and accept the concept of prepayment methods for financing health care. Such strategies can also ensure that all formal sector employees have adequate information about the FSSHIP. State and local governments can establish a tax-based health-financing mechanism targeted at vulnerable groups, the poorest, and those working in the informal sector of the economy to accelerate progress toward UHC. Health insurance schemes in Ghana and in Anambra State offer lessons about potential strategies to expand health insurance coverage among informal sector workers (Abubakar et al. 2022).

Monitoring and Evaluation

NSHDP II was accompanied by a comprehensive monitoring and evaluation plan agreed by all stakeholders involved in developing NSHDP II (FMoH 2018a). The monitoring and evaluation plan set indicators and targets covering all the main areas of health and programming addressed in NSHPD II. The data collected on those indicators, and analysis assessing the progress of NSHDP II, including a long-awaited Joint Annual Review midterm review, have not yet been published. Embedding the use of monitoring and evaluation of the plan in the health policy system requires further attention.

LIMITATIONS AND FUTURE DIRECTIONS

Despite clear priorities for the health system, and the financing opportunities provided in the NHIA Act 2022, the Finance Act needs to be modified to generate some of the revenue to support the Vulnerable Group Fund. The NHIA Act, a federal law, should be domesticated in all states for national implementation. Otherwise, the whole burden of implementing the law, including providing health insurance for 83 million people, will fall entirely on the federal government.

New financing approaches must be undertaken with simultaneous reform of governance and increased probity in the use of revenue. Health is not immune to the widespread corruption that affects other sectors in Nigeria. Nigeria needs holistic and participatory accountability systems that track not only supplies and financial management systems but also the human resources for health required to ensure efficient use of available funds, and that citizens receive the services they need when they need them.

A critical test of the reforms currently in their embryonic stage is whether the government newly elected in 2023 adopts and implements positive changes. Nigeria's last change of leadership allowed the partial implementation of the Health Act 2014 by the previous government. It is possible that future political cycles and the next government will continue to implement those reforms. Beyond specific health system changes, major population health can be achieved only with concrete and substantial action outside the health sector, which requires an all-of-government approach.

LESSONS LEARNED

The future of health in Nigeria will be determined by the ability of political leaders to learn from past failures and successes to identify and implement locally appropriate priorities to address the many health challenges facing the population. The priority setting for health in Nigeria makes clear the overly donor-dependent nature of the process for formulating national development plans such as NSHDP II. Without donor funding and coordination of the process, such plans may not happen—as suggested by lack of a published midterm review of NSHDP II or any movement on a new plan. Political leaders in Nigeria urgently need to chart a course for locally led and driven policy formulation and implementation, with donors playing a supportive role.

The LNC's experience shows the importance of involving the main actors in the health policy space in Nigeria so that their ownership of the work takes it forward. At the same time, ensuring that priority setting sufficiently covers everyone's health needs requires truly engaging the public through a bottom-up consultation process. Local and national ownership of the policy agenda, engagement with policy makers in formulating recommendations, and public engagement are essential to guarantee the success of health prioritization and the ultimate impact on population health.

NOTES

1. Avenir Health, "OneHealth Tool," https://www.avenirhealth.org/software-onehealth.
2. For more on the Lives Saved Tool, refer to its website https://www.livessavedtool.org.
3. World Health Organization, "Child Mortality (Under 5 Years)," https://www.who.int/news-room/fact-sheets/detail/levels-and-trends-in-child-under-5-mortality-in-2020 (accessed August 1, 2022).
4. Institute for Health Metrics and Evaluation, Global Burden of Disease Study 2019, https://ghdx.healthdata.org/gbd-2019.
5. For more information about DHIS2, refer to the University of Oslo's DHIS2 web page, https://dhis2.org; for more information about the Nigeria HIV/AIDS Indicator and Impact

Survey, refer to its website, https://naiis.ng; for more information about SORMAS, refer to the SORMAS Foundation website, https://sormas.org.

6. NPHCDA, "Basic Health Care Provision Fund (BHCPF)," https://nphcda.gov.ng/bhcpf/ (accessed January 13, 2023).

7. NPHCDA, "Basic Health Care Provision Fund (BHCPF)."

8. Maternal and reproductive health, child health, immunization, adolescent health, malaria, tuberculosis, HIV/AIDS, nutrition, water, sanitation and hygiene, noncommunicable diseases, mental health, neglected tropical diseases, health promotion and social determinants of health, emergency hospital services, public health emergencies, and preparedness and response.

9. Program activity costs, human resources, infrastructure, logistics, medicines, commodities and supplies, health financing, health information systems, and governance.

REFERENCES

Abubakar, I., S. L. Dalglish, B. Angell, O. Sanuade, S. Abimbola, A. L. Adamu, I. M. O. Adetifa, et al. 2022. "The *Lancet* Nigeria Commission: Investing in Health and the Future of the Nation." *The Lancet* 399 (10330): 1155–200. https://doi.org/10.1016/S0140-6736(21)02488-0.

Adebowale-Tambe, N. 2022. "UPDATED: Buhari Signs Health Insurance Bill into Law." *Premium Times*, May 19, 2022. https://www.premiumtimesng.com/news /headlines/531087-updated-buhari-signs-health-insurance-bill-into-law.html.

Angell, B., O. Sanuade, I. M. Adetifa, I. N. Okeke, A. L. Adamu, M. H. Aliyu, E. A. Ameh, et al. 2022. "Population Health Outcomes in Nigeria Compared with Other West African Countries, 1998–2019: A Systematic Analysis for the Global Burden of Disease Study." *The Lancet* 399 (10330): 1117–1129. https://doi.org/10.1016/S0140-6736(21)02722-7/.

FMoH (Nigeria, Federal Ministry of Health). 2018a. *Monitoring and Evaluation Plan for the Second National Strategic Health Development Plan 2018–2022*. Abuja: Federal Government of Nigeria. https://ngfrepository.org.ng:8443/handle/123456789/4209.

FMoH (Nigeria, Federal Ministry of Health). 2018b. *Second National Strategic Health Development Plan 2018–2022*. Abuja: Federal Government of Nigeria. https://www .premiumtimesng.com/news/headlines/531087-updated-buhari-signs-health-insurance -bill-into-law.html?tztc=1.

Hirose, A., I. O. Yisa, A. Aminu, N. Afolabi, M. Olasunmbo, G. Oluka, K. Muhammad, and J. Hussein. 2018. "Technical Quality of Delivery Care in Private- and Public-Sector Health Facilities in Enugu and Lagos States, Nigeria." *Health Policy and Planning* 33 (5): 666–74. https://doi.org/10.1093/heapol/czy032.

Murray, C. J., A. Y. Aravkin, P. Zheng, C. Abbafati, K. M. Abbas, M. Abbasi-Kangevari, F. Abd-Allah, et al. 2020. "Global Burden of 87 Risk Factors in 204 Countries and Territories, 1990–2019: A Systematic Analysis for the Global Burden of Disease Study 2019." *The Lancet* 396: 1223–49. https://doi.org/10.1016/S0140-6736(20)30752-2.

Onwujekwe, O., N. Ezumah, C. Mbachu, F. Obi, H. Ichoku, B. Uzochukwu, and H. Wang. 2019. "Exploring Effectiveness of Different Health Financing Mechanisms in Nigeria; What Needs to Change and How Can It Happen?" *BMC Health Services Research* 19: 1–13.

Oritseweyimi, O., S. Martina, O. Otokpenb, M. A. Adbullahic, and H. G. Pama. 2023. "Optimizing Health Investments through Health Benefit Package Modelling: A Case Study of the Nigerian Ward Health System." National Primary Care Development Agency. Unpublished.

UN DESA (United Nations, Department of Economic and Social Affairs, Population Division). 2019. *World Population Prospects 2019—Volume 1: Comprehensive Tables*. New York: United Nations. https://www.un.org/development/desa/pd/sites/www.un.org .development.desa.pd/files/files/documents/2020/Jan/un_2019_wpp_vol1_comprehensive -tables.pdf.

Vos, T., S. S. Lim, C. Abbafati, K. M. Abbas, M. Abbasi, M. Abbasifard, M. Abbasi-Kangevari, et al. 2020. "Global Burden of 369 Diseases and Injuries in 204 Countries and Territories, 1990–2019: A Systematic Analysis for the Global Burden of Disease Study 2019." *The Lancet* 396: 1204–22. https://doi.org/10.1016/S0140-6736(20)30925-9.

WHO (World Health Organization). 2018. "High Burden to High Impact: A Targeted Malaria Response." WHO, Geneva. https://www.who.int/publications/i/item/WHO-CDS-GMP-2018.25.

World Bank. 2022. "Nigeria Development Update June 2022: The Continuing Urgency of Business Unusual." World Bank, Washington, DC. https://documents1.worldbank.org/curated/en/099740006132214750/pdf/P17782005822360a00a0850f63928a34418.pdf.

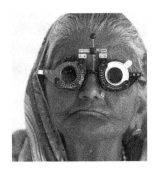

10

India's Transformational Ayushman Bharat Health System Reforms

Ajay Tandon, Sheena Chhabra, Guru Rajesh Jammy, Basant Garg, Sudha Chandrashekar, and Shankar Prinja

ABSTRACT

The world's most populous country as of 2023, India is expected to be the world's third-largest economy by 2030. India has made much progress on improving key population health outcomes, but several challenges remain, such as relatively high levels of out-of-pocket spending and inequalities in effective coverage; emerging new challenges include a rapidly growing burden from noncommunicable diseases and increasing risk factors related to climate change. To further improve outcomes, India is implementing several potentially transformational reforms including Ayushman Bharat Health and Wellness Centers to bolster provision of comprehensive primary health care at frontline public facilities and the Ayushman Bharat Pradhan Mantri Jan Arogya Yojana, a tax-financed noncontributory health insurance scheme that provides inpatient care at public and empaneled private hospitals to more than 500 million poor and near-poor individuals. In addition to detailing those two reforms, this chapter summarizes the process the country used to identify and adopt benefit packages under the reforms.

INTRODUCTION

With a population of 1.4 billion in 2023, India is the world's most populous country and by 2030 is expected to be its third-largest economy. With an estimated national income of US$2,380 in 2022, India is classified by the World Bank as a lower-middle-income country. In recent decades, the country has made notable progress on sustaining rapid economic growth as well as on reducing poverty. At two children per woman, the total fertility rate is now below replacement level

(IIPS and ICF 2021). Significant improvements in key health outputs such as routine immunization, antenatal care, skilled birth attendance, and institutional deliveries have occurred.[1] Despite its significant improvements in outputs, the country has had relatively mixed progress on population health outcomes. At 26 infant deaths per 1,000 live births, infant mortality rates are worse than in neighboring countries such as Bangladesh, Bhutan, and Nepal.[2] India's maternal mortality ratio of 103 deaths per 100,000 live births is still higher than the 2030 Sustainable Development Goal target of 70. Almost one-fifth of all households in the country reported using more than 10 percent of their budget on out-of-pocket (OOP) spending for health; consequently, an estimated 65 million individuals are pushed into poverty annually (WHO and World Bank 2021). Enormous inequalities underlie the average or poor performance on health outcomes: the poor and Scheduled Caste/Scheduled Tribe populations—that is, those people belonging to officially designated disadvantaged socioeconomic groups—have significantly worse access to health services and outcomes. Additional risk factors due to climate change are rapidly emerging.

India is currently in the midst of implementing several transformational reforms, realizing the vision laid out in its 2017 National Health Policy (NHP), which recognized four major trends affecting the country's health system: (1) improvements in maternal and child health alongside a growing burden from noncommunicable diseases (NCDs) and an unfinished agenda related to infectious diseases; (2) emergence of a robust health industry; (3) high rates of new and deeper impoverishment due to dependence on OOP financing for health; and (4) availability of enhanced "fiscal space" due to sustained economic growth (MoHFW 2017). Most notably, the 2017 NHP called for a paradigm shift in primary health care—from limited and selective care to provision of comprehensive services at frontline public facilities along with appropriate forward and backward referral links. For secondary and tertiary care, NHP emphasized the need for a move from input-based financing to output-based strategic purchasing from both public and private providers.

NHP 2017's vision was realized in 2018 with initiation of the first stage of Ayushman Bharat reforms comprising two distinct subcomponents, Ayushman Bharat Health and Wellness Centers[3] (AB-HWCs) and the Pradhan Mantri Jan Arogya Yojana (PM-JAY). The AB-HWC reforms include upgrading of existing frontline public primary health care infrastructure into HWCs and creating a new layer of HWCs catering to the urban poor. That new layer of HWCs provides diagnostic tests, free essential medicines, and other comprehensive primary health care services including those to address NCDs. PM-JAY provides tax-financed noncontributory health insurance coverage for a package of inpatient secondary and tertiary hospital care to more than 500 million poor and near-poor individuals up to a maximum annual limit of 500,000 rupees, or Re, (about US$6,000) per eligible family at government and empaneled private hospitals.

The remainder of the chapter discusses in further detail the process and nature of amendment to services and benefits that are being implemented under AB-HWC and

PM-JAY reforms, including whether and how explicitly cost-effectiveness criteria were used to inform the design and implementation of these reforms. The next section provides an overview of India's health system. The following sections detail reforms related to AB-HWC and PM-JAY. The final section concludes with a summary.

HEALTH FINANCING, SERVICE DELIVERY, AND GOVERNANCE OF INDIA'S HEALTH SYSTEM

India has a three-tiered federal governance system, with a center, 28 states, and 8 centrally administered union territories. Below the states are local government bodies (both urban and rural). India's central government levies corporate, income (excluding agricultural income), wealth, and customs taxes; union excise duties (including on petrol, diesel, crude oil, tobacco, and sugar); and the goods and services tax. It shares 41 percent of central tax receipts—that is, all taxes collected excluding proceeds from surcharges and cesses, net of collection costs—with states based on an allocation formula. The center also receives nontax revenues from dividends and profits from public enterprises, interest receipts, regulatory charges, user charges, and license fees, among others.

In addition to receiving transfers from the center, states also generate own-source tax revenues from the goods and services tax, vehicle taxes, stamps and registrations, property taxes, taxes on agricultural income, and state excise duties (including on alcohol and petroleum products). Sources of state-level nontax revenues are similar to those at the center; some states that are rich in natural resources also raise nontax revenues from sources such as petroleum and mining. Local government bodies—in addition to receiving transfers from the center and the state—can also levy property taxes, profession taxes, and entertainment taxes, among others, but have relatively low own-source tax collection.

Health is a "state subject" in India, implying that states have the primary responsibility for implementing health programs; two-thirds of all public expenditure for health occurs at the state level. The central government plays a stewardship role and influences the direction of reforms by providing vision, guidelines, and cofinancing via several centrally sponsored schemes, which are special purpose cofinancing arrangements to implement programs to attain national goals including for health. Public sector health care delivery channels use a three-tier model of primary, secondary, and tertiary care facilities with the referral hierarchy in the same order. Primary health care facilities in rural areas include subhealth centers, primary health care centers, and community health centers; in urban areas these centers are designated as urban primary health care centers and urban community health centers. Secondary health care delivery facilities include subdistrict hospitals and district hospitals. Tertiary care delivery facilities are either medical college hospitals or other super-specialty hospitals. In addition to the public sector, India has many private facilities; in many states, the utilization of health care services is higher in the private than in the public sector.

Financing of AB-HWC occurs through the existing architecture of the National Health Mission of the Ministry of Health and Family Welfare (MoHFW), a centrally sponsored scheme whereby the central and state governments cofinance implementation using a 60:40 ratio (that is, 60 percent from the center and 40 percent from the state); smaller and hilly states enjoy a cofinancing ratio of 90:10, and union territories a ratio of 100:0. PM-JAY is implemented with the same cofinancing arrangements but operates as a separate centrally sponsored scheme with overall coordination and implementation oversight by the National Health Authority (NHA), an attached office of MoHFW, at the central level and by state health agencies at the state level. Whereas the National Health Mission makes outpatient primary and some elements of secondary care available universally at public health care facilities, PM-JAY focuses on provision of certain day-care treatments and inpatient secondary and tertiary care at public and empaneled private hospitals for India's poor and near-poor population (figure 10.1). Three states/union territories (Delhi, Odisha, and West Bengal) have opted not to implement PM-JAY; instead, they implement their own-financed versions of the health insurance scheme. Other states like Andhra Pradesh, Assam, Chhattisgarh, Karnataka, Kerala, Maharashtra, Meghalaya, Nagaland, Rajasthan, Tamil Nadu, and Uttarakhand have expanded population and benefits coverage beyond the minimum required under PM-JAY.

Figure 10.1 Summary of India's Ayushman Bharat Reforms

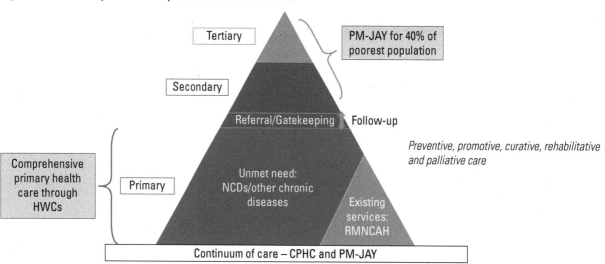

Source: Lahariya 2020.

Note: CPHC = comprehensive primary health care; HWCs = health and wellness centers; NCDs = noncommunicable diseases; PM-JAY = Pradhan Mantri Jan Arogya Yojana; RMNCAH = reproductive, maternal, newborn, child, and adolescent health.

AB-HWC and PM-JAY reforms build upon previous iterations of policy shifts implemented beginning in 2005 with the introduction of the National Rural Health Mission to improve reproductive, maternal, newborn, child, and adolescent health outcomes and to bridge rural-urban inequalities. In 2013, the National Rural Health Mission and its urban sub-mission counterpart were combined and renamed the National Health Mission. PM-JAY builds upon and expands the Rashtriya

Swasthya Bima Yojana scheme launched by the Ministry of Labor in 2008 to provide 36 million families below the poverty line with tax-financed noncontributory inpatient care up to an annual coverage of Re 30,000 (about US$400) per family at public and empaneled private facilities for mostly secondary care.

In 2021, Ayushman Bharat reforms expanded further under the Pradhan Mantri Ayushman Bharat Health Infrastructure Mission, which includes financing for additional investments for improving pandemic preparedness in light of COVID-19 as well as establishment of a new layer of frontline urban health and wellness centers in urban slum areas catering to catchment populations of 15,000–20,000. The Fifteenth Finance Commission—complementing the Pradhan Mantri Ayushman Bharat Health Infrastructure Mission—provides financing to local government bodies for bolstering provision of comprehensive primary health care in rural and urban areas along with strengthening Block Public Health Units (MoHFW 2021). In addition, the Ayushman Bharat Digital Mission is developing the necessary digital ecosystem for linking providers and patients digitally and introducing electronic health records.

At 1.35 percent of gross domestic product in 2019/20, public spending on health in India remains relatively low, a result of the low priority given to health in central and state budgets (NHSRC 2023). Despite remaining low as a share of gross domestic product, levels of public financing for health have increased over the last several years to more than Re 2,000 in 2019/20, primarily because of robust economic growth. Nevertheless, India remains one of the most privatized health systems in the world in terms of both health financing and service delivery. Almost 73 percent of outpatient use and 58 percent of all inpatient use occur at private facilities (MoSPI 2020). Regulation of the private sector remains weak in terms of quality and prices charged for services. Private OOP spending—at just over half of all health spending—represents the largest source of financing for health. The high levels of OOP spending reflect the widespread use of private sector services, such as for outpatient-level medicines and diagnostics, as well as constraints related to supply-side readiness and responsiveness at government facilities.

COMPREHENSIVE PRIMARY HEALTH CARE VIA HEALTH AND WELLNESS CENTERS

AB-HWC reforms are expanding the package of primary care services to include, among others, NCD management at frontline public facilities across India. One foundational element of these reforms is the new role of HWCs in providing comprehensive primary health care that aims to reduce "time to care" to less than 30 minutes and to decrease preventable morbidity and mortality. HWCs provide an expanded package of 12 services, up from an existing package of 6 services (table 10.1). Most progress to date involves expanding one additional package—screening and management of NCDs—at HWCs and three additional packages on health education—eating right, staying fit, and doing yoga.

The upgraded frontline HWCs—subhealth centers and primary health care centers that have been upgraded to HWCs in rural areas, upgraded urban primary health care centers, and the new layer of urban HWCs catering to a smaller catchment population—are staffed by a primary health care team headed by a community health officer and supported by a team of two multipurpose health workers (at least one of whom is female) as well as three to five Accredited Social Health Activists (ASHAs). They provide preventive, promotive, curative, and rehabilitative care through outreach visits to communities and households, at the HWCs themselves, and through upward referrals to community health centers and urban community health centers as well as district and other hospitals.

The first converted HWC was launched in Jangla village in Bijapur district in the state of Chhattisgarh in April 2018; as of December 1, 2022, the country had more than 150,000 HWCs in operation. One of the primary objectives of each HWC is to create population-based household lists and undertake registration of all individuals and families residing within its catchment area. ASHAs conduct home visits to ensure screening and encourage risk factor modification, counseling, and adherence to treatment. Although termed honorary volunteers, ASHAs receive activity-based compensation and incentives. From the perspective of surveillance for infectious diseases, ASHAs and other frontline workers also fill out Form S, the reporting form for syndromic surveillance under India's Integrated Disease Surveillance Program.

Table 10.1 Service Provision through India's HWCs

Services through SHCs and PHCs	Services added as part of HWCs
General outpatient care for acute simple illnesses and minor ailments	Screening and management of NCDs
Family planning and other reproductive health services	Screening and basic management of mental health ailments
Neonatal and infant health care services	Care for common ophthalmic and ear, nose, and throat problems
Care in pregnancy and childbirth	Basic dental health care
Childhood and adolescent health care services	Geriatric and palliative health care services
Services for communicable diseases under national health programs	Basic trauma and emergency medical services

Source: Lahariya 2020.

Note: HWCs = health and wellness centers; NCDs = noncommunicable diseases; PHCs = primary health care centers; SHCs = subhealth centers.

One primary motivation behind India's HWC reforms was the recognition that NCDs represent the largest source of morbidity and mortality in the country and that addressing NCDs at frontline primary health care facilities is both necessary and cost-effective. In 2019, NCDs accounted for 58 percent of the overall burden of disease, whereas in 1990 they accounted for only 29 percent (figure 10.2). Neonatal disorders were responsible for the largest share of the overall disease burden, causing 9 percent of all disability-adjusted life years lost because of morbidity and premature mortality in 2019—although that share represents a decline from 14 percent in 1990 (table 10.2). Ischemic heart disease has rapidly increased to the second-highest position, followed by chronic obstructive pulmonary disease. The share of diabetes in the overall burden of disease has also risen since 1990. Although its share has slowly declined, tuberculosis remains among the top 10 contributors to the burden of disease.

In terms of risk factors, particulate matter pollution now poses the largest risk for health (table 10.3). Additional risk factors related to urbanization and lifestyle changes—high systolic blood pressure, high fasting plasma glucose, high body mass index, and high LDL cholesterol—also feature prominently among the top 10 risk factors contributing to the country's overall disease burden. Within India, the states of Chhattisgarh, Uttar Pradesh, Assam, Madhya Pradesh, and Odisha have the highest per capita burden of disease (and the highest shares due to reproductive, maternal, newborn, child, and adolescent health and to communicable conditions). Goa, Kerala, and Tamil Nadu, have the highest burden from NCDs, which account for more than two-thirds of the overall disease burden in those states.

Figure 10.2 Overall Burden of Disease, by Health Area, India, 1990–2019, percent

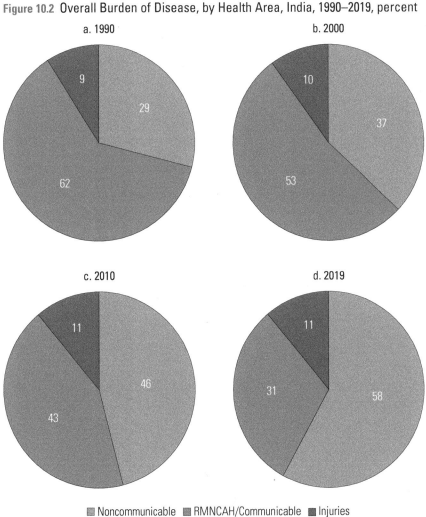

a. 1990

b. 2000

c. 2010

d. 2019

■ Noncommunicable ■ RMNCAH/Communicable ■ Injuries

Source: Indian Council of Medical Research, Public Health Foundation of India, and Institute of Health Metrics and Evaluation, "Disease Burden Initiative in India," https://www.healthdata.org/research -analysis/health-by-location/disease-burden-initiative-india.

Note: RMNCAH = reproductive, maternal, newborn, child, and adolescent health.

Table 10.2 Top 10 Diseases/Conditions, India, 1990–2019

Rank in 2019	Diseases/conditions	DALYs share (%)			
		1990	2000	2010	2019
1	Neonatal disorders	14	14	12	9
2	Ischemic heart disease	3	4	6	8
3	Chronic obstructive pulmonary disease	2	3	3	5
4	Diarrheal diseases	10	9	6	4
5	Lower respiratory infections	10	8	6	4
6	Stroke	2	2	3	4
7	Tuberculosis	5	5	4	3
8	Road injuries	2	3	3	3
9	Diabetes mellitus	1	1	2	3
10	Dietary iron deficiency	2	2	2	2

Source: Indian Council of Medical Research, Public Health Foundation of India, and Institute of Health Metrics and Evaluation, "Disease Burden Initiative in India," https://www.healthdata.org/research-analysis/health-by-location/disease-burden-initiative-india.

Note: DALYs = disability-adjusted life years.

Table 10.3 Top 10 Risk Factors, India, 1990–2019

Rank in 2019	Risk factors	DALYs share (%)			
		1990	2000	2010	2019
1	Particulate matter pollution	13	12	12	11
2	Low birth weight, short gestation	17	15	13	9
3	High systolic blood pressure	3	5	6	8
4	High fasting plasma glucose	2	3	4	7
5	Smoking	4	4	5	6
6	High body mass index	1	1	3	4
7	High LDL cholesterol	2	2	3	4
8	Unsafe water source	9	7	5	3
9	Alcohol use	2	2	3	3
10	Kidney dysfunction	1	2	2	3

Source: Indian Council of Medical Research, Public Health Foundation of India, and Institute of Health Metrics and Evaluation, "Disease Burden Initiative in India," https://www.healthdata.org/research-analysis/health-by-location/disease-burden-initiative-india.

Note: DALYs = disability-adjusted life years.

Other factors motivating HWC reforms included reducing the need for secondary and tertiary care by providing screening, early detection, and treatment of common NCDs like hypertension and diabetes as close to communities as possible. Government guidelines for population-level screening of those common NCDs estimate that over half of all conditions can be managed at the primary care level (NHSRC 2018). Before the HWC reforms, NCD clinics conducted opportunistic screening for common NCDs at the district and community health center levels. In addition, glucose monitoring was supposed to have been implemented at primary health care centers and subhealth centers in 2012 for all those above 30 years of age and all pregnant women. Despite those programs, screening rates for NCDs remain extremely low in the country, and most people with hypertension and diabetes do not know or do not receive treatment. For instance, only 1.9 percent of women ages 30–49 had ever been screened for cervical cancer and only 0.9 percent had been screened for breast cancer or oral cancer (IIPS and ICF 2021). Only 1.2 percent of men in the same age group reported ever being screened for oral cancer. Over 80 percent of the population that is hypertensive is not aware or not on treatment; and over 90 percent of those with impaired blood glucose were in a similar predicament—either unaware or not on treatment (IIPS and ICF 2021).

Supply-side readiness problems at both private and public primary health facilities compound the issue: studies have identified gaps in terms of availability of essential medicines, technologies, and training of human resources for NCDs (Krishnan et al. 2021). Under the latest set of reforms, population-based screening has replaced opportunistic screening, with all men and women above the age of 30 screened annually for hypertension and diabetes and every five years for three cancers (oral, breast, and cervical). MoHFW guidelines mention that screening for women over 40 has a better "yield" for breast cancer but that screening of those over 30 was implemented for ease of operational management; however, the guidelines make no specific references to studies with supporting evidence (NHSRC 2018).

In terms of the priority-setting process under AB-HWC, an MoHFW task force that studied the 2014 rollout of comprehensive primary health care submitted its findings in 2015 (MoHFW 2015). That task force included representatives from MoHFW, state governments, academia, think tanks, and nongovernmental organizations. It also included representatives from the World Bank and the World Health Organization. The 2017 NHP subsequently adopted the task force's 2015 findings, and the rollout of HWCs began in 2018.

In making recommendations for expanding the benefit packages to include frontline screening for NCDs, the task force referred to studies that demonstrated the burden and cost benefits in the Indian context. For instance, MoHFW's cancer screening guidelines report that breast, cervical, and oral cancers account for almost one-third of all cancers in India, making them a public health priority. Regarding screening and early detection of cancers, MoHFW guidelines reference a World Bank working paper (Mahal, Karan, and Engelgau 2010) estimating the likelihood of incurring catastrophic hospitalization expenditure—that is, OOP spending that represents a relatively large share of the household budget—at 160 percent higher for cancer than for communicable diseases. The same study found the incidence of catastrophic expenditures for cancers to be nearly double when compared to expenditures for accidents and cardiovascular diseases. MoHFW did not conduct a full assessment of costs and benefits or report them in its guidelines, but the decision to roll out frontline NCD reforms implies the expectation of improvements in financial risk protection. Although they do not provide or reference specific numbers, the guidelines also note that all three cancers have good survival rates if detected early, implying cost-effectiveness. For oral cancer screenings, the guidelines reference a cluster-randomized trial to prioritize screenings among tobacco users (Sankaranarayan et al. 2005).

As part of the national rollout, MoHFW's Department of Health Research commissioned a study to look at health technology assessment of three different strategies for cervical cancer screening: (1) visual inspection with acetic acid (VIA); (2) Papanicolaou test (PAP smear); and (3) human papillomavirus DNA test every 3, 5, or 10 years among women ages 30–65 in India (Chauhan et al. 2020). The study recommended a strategy of VIA screening every 5 years, estimating that the cost-effectiveness of VIA screening would require a minimum 30 percent of screened positive patients and a lifetime risk of at least 0.7. In terms of equity, the study estimated much higher reductions in cervical cancer cases and subsequent mortality gains among the poorest one-third of the population. It also estimated better financial risk protection for the poor in terms of estimated reductions in OOP treatment costs. Overall cost-effectiveness analysis took a societal perspective including costs of implementing the intervention and costs averted among households due to early detection.

MoHFW also commissioned a health technology assessment to examine the economic case for implementing population-based screening programs for diabetes and hypertension as envisioned under AB-HWC, including for assessing which age groups to target and determining cost-effectiveness at different screening frequencies (Kaur et al. 2021). The study used incremental costs per quality-adjusted life year resulting from various implementation scenarios. It derived costing information from the government's National Health System Cost Database and the Costing of Health Services in India (CHSI) study.[4] The study found that, by itself, population-level screening for diabetes and hypertension was not a cost-effective strategy for India. However, when combined with provision of treatment of the conditions as envisioned under AB-HWC, screening programs were cost-effective. Providing treatment at HWCs to even 20 percent of newly diagnosed patients for uncomplicated diabetes or hypertension would make screening interventions cost-effective for people ages 30–65 at either a three-year or five-year frequency. Providing treatment to 70 percent of newly diagnosed patients—up from the 4 percent that currently receive treatment—would make annual population screening cost saving, according to the study (Kaur et al. 2021).

Several government guidelines and training materials note equity considerations, especially the positive impact of the availability of comprehensive primary health care at frontline facilities in terms of helping improve access for screening, especially for women and the poor. Without that access, many people would have to forgo at least a day's wages to access preventive and promotive care for several conditions included in the comprehensive primary health care package of services. The government's training module for medical officers mentions that "primary and secondary prevention of chronic diseases and their common risk factors provide the most sustainable and cost-effective approach to chronic disease prevention and control" but does not provide any explicit references (NCDC 2017, 1).

TAX-FINANCED HOSPITALIZATION INSURANCE FOR THE POOR AND NEAR-POOR UNDER PM-JAY

In complementing AB-HWC reforms, PM-JAY focuses on expanding access to inpatient secondary and tertiary care for India's poor and near-poor population. Unlike AB-HWC reforms, designed to cover everyone, PM-JAY targets the bottom 40 percent of India's population (more than 500 million individuals) as identified by the 2011 Socio-Economic Caste Census and based on deprivation criteria in rural areas and occupational categories in urban areas (table 10.4). Those families that were eligible for Rashtriya Swasthya Bima Yojana, the precursor to PM-JAY, were automatically eligible for PM-JAY. In addition, people in rural areas living in households with no adult members ages 16–59, living in female-headed households with no adult male members ages 16–59, and meeting other such criteria were deemed eligible. In urban areas, deprivation criteria were based on employment: domestic workers, drivers, conductors, and other such categories of workers were eligible. Some households—for example, those paying income taxes, those with refrigerators, those with at least one member employed by the government, and so on—were automatically ineligible for the scheme.[5]

Table 10.4 Deprivation Criteria for PM-JAY Eligibility, India

Rural	Urban	Ineligible
Only one room with kucha walls and kucha roof	Rag picker	Households having motorized 2-, 3-, or 4-wheeler/fishing boat
No adult members ages 16–59	Beggar	Households having mechanized 3- or 4-wheeled agricultural equipment
Female-headed households with no adult male members ages 16–59	Domestic worker	Households having Kisan Credit Card with credit limit above Re 50,000
Disabled member and no able-bodied adult member	Street vendor, cobbler, hawker, other service provider working on streets	Household member is a government employee
Scheduled Caste/Scheduled Tribe households	Construction worker, plumber, mason, labor, painter, welder, security guard	Households with nonagricultural enterprises registered with government
Landless households deriving income from manual casual labor	Coolie or other head-load worker	Any member of household earning more than Re 10,000 per month
Households without shelter	Sweeper, sanitation worker, mali	Households paying income tax
Destitute/living on alms	Home-based worker, artisan, handicrafts worker, tailor	Households paying professional tax
Manual scavenger families	Transportation worker, driver, conductor, helper to drivers and conductors, cart puller, rickshaw puller	House with three or more rooms with pucca walls and roof
		Owning at least 7.5 acres of land with at least one piece of irrigation equipment
Primitive tribal groups	Shop worker, assistant, peon in small establishment, helper, delivery assistant, attendant, waiter	Owning a refrigerator; owning 5 acres or more of irrigated land for two or more crop seasons
Legally released bonded labor	Electrician, mechanic, assembler, repair worker, washerman, chowkidar	Owning a landline phone; owning more than 2.5 acres of irrigated land with one piece of irrigation equipment

Source: NHA 2021a.

Note: PM-JAY = Pradhan Mantri Jan Arogya Yojana.

NHA, as the apex body for implementing PM-JAY, has the responsibility for providing policy and strategic direction to PM-JAY and for providing guidelines to states on all aspects including beneficiary authentication, health benefit packages, standard treatment guidelines, hospital empanelment, claim adjudication, and grievance management. NHA is also responsible for providing a strong information technology backbone to ensure that all processes—from beneficiary identification to claim settlement—are paperless and can be conducted online using the PM-JAY IT platform. NHA, as an attached office of MoHFW, has full functional autonomy with a governing board chaired by the Union Minister for Health and Family Welfare and whose member secretary is the NHA's chief executive officer. State health agencies implement PM-JAY at the state level and have the flexibility to do so under either an "assurance/trust" mode (that is, the agency purchases health services directly from providers) or an "insurance" mode (the agency contracts an insurance company to purchase health services from providers on its behalf) or using a combination of the two modes (for example, using insurance mode up to a certain threshold and trust/ assurance mode above that). NHA provides guidelines on various processes of the scheme with flexibility for state-level implementation.

The program's initial health benefit packages (HBP 1.0) provided coverage for a total of 1,393 secondary and tertiary care procedures, included 1 surgical procedure classified as "unspecified," and covered 8 medical specialties and 16 surgical specialties.[6] In order to define HBP 1.0, a Technical Committee established in 2016 by MoHFW's Directorate General of Health Services initiated the process by collecting and analyzing data on prevalent packages throughout the country (refer to figure 10.3 for a summary of the entire process). The Technical Committee included representatives from state governments, central government hospitals, state government–funded health insurance schemes, clinical and health financing experts, industry representatives, quality control bodies, the Central Drugs Standard Control Organization, the National Institution for Transforming India (NITI Aayog, the main think tank for the government of India), the World Bank, and the World Health Organization. The Technical Committee's terms of reference included development of a comprehensive list of hospitalization packages, identification of packages at potential risk of misuse and identification of strategies to minimize misuse, development of criteria for empanelment of providers, establishment of preauthorization modalities, and delineation of strategies for ensuring quality of care.

Thirteen subgroups—composed of clinical specialists, insurance experts, and other relevant stakeholders identified by the Technical Committee—developed a preliminary HBP list. The subgroups also reviewed existing evidence on prices from state and central government insurance programs and from available costing studies before finalizing recommendations. In 2018, following the announcement of the launch of PM-JAY, MoHFW reconvened the Technical Committee to review the recommendations of the subgroups. After that review, NITI Aayog reviewed the contents of HBP 1.0 in consultation with MoHFW's Department of Health Research using a four-pronged strategy for finalization of reimbursement rates: (1) a rapid survey of public and private hospitals across different cities, (2) a comparison of insurance data with reimbursement rates from central and state government health insurance schemes, (3) expert consultations convened by NITI Aayog and the Department of Health Research to seek recommendations on inclusion or exclusion of packages and appropriateness of reimbursement rates, and (4) private sector stakeholder consultations to seek feedback on the benefit packages list as well as rates.

The national committee under the chairpersonship of NITI Aayog and MoHFW reviewed the recommendations of experts and other stakeholders, and finalized the list of 1,393 packages and reimbursement rates. The committee based its prioritization primarily on existing use patterns, clinical effectiveness of interventions, and burden of disease. Primary criteria appear to have been to define and finance packages that cover diseases with high incidence and prevalence as well as those that contribute to high OOP expenditure (NHA 2020).

Figure 10.3 PM-JAY Benefit Packages Design Process, India

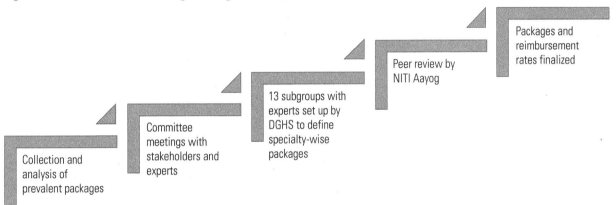

Source: Adapted from NHA 2020.

Note: DGHS = Directorate General of Health Services; NITI Aayog = National Institution for Transforming India; PM-JAY = Pradhan Mantri Jan Arogya Yojana.

In November 2019, PM-JAY's HBP was refined and expanded (and renamed HBP 2.0): the number of procedures increased to 1,573, reimbursement rates rose for 270 packages and fell for 57 packages, 237 new packages were added, 554 packages were discontinued, and 43 stratified packages were adopted (NHA 2022).[7] Several factors prompted the update of HBP 1.0. Prominent among those factors was feedback from private providers that reimbursements did not cover costs for several packages, thereby resulting in lower-than-expected empanelment of private hospitals as well as low participation in provision of the packages among private hospitals that did empanel. Whereas public hospitals are cofinanced with government budgetary allocations, private hospitals were not. In addition, different packages offered within HBP 1.0 as well as some already covered under separate national health programs had some overlaps and inconsistencies.[8] HBP 2.0 included additional diseases and conditions not covered earlier, such as heart catheterization, chronic hepatitis, diabetic foot, triple valve procedure, and gastrectomy. HBP 2.0 also helped identify specific procedures to be reserved for certain types of hospitals (for example, public or tertiary hospitals) to reduce fraud and help ensure provision of services at the appropriate level.

NHA led the rationalization process by constituting eight specialty committees that reviewed the packages, using CHSI data and holding consultations with top public hospital experts regarding specialties for which CHSI data were not available (Prinja et al. 2021). In addition, the review of oncology packages for four subspecialties (surgical, medical, radiation, and pediatric) was conducted by Tata Memorial Hospital, an autonomous grant-in-aid institution under the overall administrative control of the Department of Atomic Energy and that provides comprehensive cancer care. The governing body approved the NHA review committee recommendations for updating to HBP 2.0 based on the inputs from specialty committees, state consultations, and Tata Memorial Hospital (for oncology packages), and the suggestions of the 24 specialist committees (constituted under HBP 1.0). HBP 2.0 also marked the introduction of various new concepts including cross-specialty packages, stratified packages, add-on packages, packages with multiple procedures, and dynamic-priced packages (refer to annex 10A for additional details).

In 2021, HBP 2.0 underwent two additional revisions, HBP 2.1 and HBP 2.2. The overall package now comprises 1,670 procedures. NHA made the update with support from state health agencies, the All India Institute of Medical Sciences, Christian Medical College, the Department of Health Research, PGIMER Chandigarh, and the World Bank. It also consulted with the Association of Healthcare Providers India, Confederation of Indian Industry, and Federation of Indian Chambers of Commerce and Industry, among others. The interim review introduced a new specialty of organ and tissue transplants, which consisted of renal and corneal transplant procedures (NHA 2021b).

SUMMARY AND CONCLUSIONS

This chapter has summarized some of the potentially transformational Ayushman Bharat reforms currently being implemented across India. Their implementation mechanisms represent one of the unique aspects of those reforms. One set of reforms aims to bolster frontline provision of comprehensive primary health care by public sector facilities under the AB-HWC program, including and especially for addressing the rising NCD burden. A second complementary program provides tax-financed noncontributory health insurance coverage for inpatient care at public and empaneled private hospitals targeting more than 500 million poor and near-poor individuals. Although it is too soon to assess the impact of the programs, their underlying intent is to emphasize prevention, promotion, and early detection as well as to improve financial risk protection from high OOP spending, especially for the poor and vulnerable. It remains to be seen whether the country will take steps toward greater integration of both programs—formally or otherwise—to ensure provision of health services across the entire care continuum.

India's use of health technology assessment is still at a nascent stage. Nevertheless, at least for the case of the AB-HWC program, cost-effectiveness criteria combined with information on the changing burden of disease appear to have helped inform the design of comprehensive primary health care services. The government commissioned several studies to assess the localized cost-effectiveness of proposed interventions and referenced global evidence in determining the choice of additional services to be included.

PM-JAY has also expanded coverage to include a comprehensive and wide-ranging inpatient benefit packages; however, the formal use of health technology assessment appears to have been limited to date. A Health Financing and Technology Assessment unit, currently under establishment at NHA, should help ensure future formalization of the health technology assessment process. The unit evaluates existing and newer interventions to refine the health benefit packages and undertake other strategic purchasing decisions. Greater use of value-based pricing methods is also expected to inform the inclusion of new packages and pricing decisions.

ANNEX 10A. NEW CONCEPTS INTRODUCED IN HBP 2.0

The following explanations are adapted from NHA (2022).

Cross-specialty packages. These packages fell under the purview of more than one specialty in HBP 1.0 wherein the practice was to write the package under every concerned specialty, resulting in unnecessary repetition/duplication. In HBP 2.0, such packages are defined under one specialty and marked as cross-specialty packages, and the names of other relevant specialties are mentioned against such procedures so that those specialties can also use the procedures.

Stratified packages. Some packages may involve different treatment modalities for the same or similar procedures (for example, type of anesthesia, surgical approach, unilateral/bilateral application, and etiology). The rates of these stratified packages may or may not be the same, or one of the packages will have an additional treatment modality used along with the basic procedure. These kinds of packages are labeled as stratified procedures, and the stratification criteria are defined in detail along with the financial implications, if any.

Add-on packages. Certain packages can be booked with a primary package at 100 percent reimbursement, contrary to the principle of 100 percent reimbursement of the primary package and 50 percent reimbursement of the secondary package under HBP 1.0. These packages are defined as add-on packages.

Stand-alone packages. Packages identified as stand-alone packages cannot be booked with any other package.

Packages with multiple procedures. Some of the packages consist of a group of procedures. In view of the need to capture separately the different procedures covered under a single package, the packages were further divided into respective procedures as required.

Follow-up packages. Some procedures require prolonged or multiple follow-up care beyond the limit of 15 days included in a package. For such procedures, the specialist committees included some follow-up packages that can be booked only if there is documented history of treatment covered under the primary package. The follow-up packages are aligned with their specific primary packages.

Static-priced packages. Procedures for which there is either no usage of implants/high-end consumables or usage of a definitive number and type of implants are defined as static-priced procedures. (Note: In HBP 2.0, the implant rates were separately configured.)

Dynamic-priced packages. Procedures for which variable numbers and types of implants/high-end consumables are used are defined as dynamic-priced procedures. The cost of implant(s) will be added to this price. (Note: In HBP 2.0, the implant rates were separately configured.)

ACKNOWLEDGMENTS

The authors are grateful to Dinesh Nair, Trina Haque, and peer reviewers Agnes Couffinhal and Somil Nagpal for helpful inputs.

NOTES

1. According to 2019–21 National Family Health Survey-5 data, 76 percent of children ages 12–23 months were fully vaccinated, 58 percent of pregnant women had at least four antenatal care visits, skilled birth attendance was 89 percent, and the institutional delivery rate was 89 percent (IIPS and ICF 2021).
2. Based on 2023 data from the World Bank DataBank, World Development Indicators, https://databank.worldbank.org/source/world-development-indicators.
3. Health and Wellness Centers have recently been branded as Ayushman Arogya Mandirs.
4. The CHSI study was the first nationally representative costing survey in India. Its costing methodology followed standard principles using an economic perspective so that it could identify, measure, and account for all resources used for delivering a service—regardless of who pays. CHSI data came from both public and private hospitals—a total of 52 public health facilities including 13 public tertiary care hospitals and 39 district hospitals providing secondary care—across 13 states. The study used a top-down approach to calculate unit costs because of the unavailability of data on the use of input resources required for providing services based on the morbidity profile of patients. To calculate the unit cost of various surgical interventions in operation theatres, however, the study used a bottom-up approach.
5. Some states such as Chhattisgarh, Karnataka, and Maharashtra use ration cards for targeting.
6. States have the option to expand coverage beyond that specified by the central government using own-source revenues. For example, the state of Tamil Nadu provides additional coverage for outpatient diagnostics and additional inpatient high-end packages not covered by PM-JAY. Some states such as Himachal Pradesh have also expanded population coverage beyond the target population specified by the central government using own-source revenues.

7. Sixty-one percent of package prices increased whereas 18 percent saw a decline. Nearly 42 percent of HBP 1.0 packages were estimated to be priced at less than half of the true cost of provision; that proportion is estimated to have declined to 20 percent with HBP 2.0.
8. For example, tubectomy and vasectomy packages were discontinued under PM-JAY because the National Family Welfare Program already provides these services.

REFERENCES

Chauhan, Akashdeep Singh, Shankar Prinja, Radhika Srinivasan, Bavana Rai, J. S. Malliga, Gaurav Jyani, Nidhi Gupta, and Sushmita Ghoshal. 2020. "Cost Effectiveness of Strategies for Cervical Cancer Prevention in India." *PLoS One* 15 (9): e0238291. https://doi.org/10.1371/journal.pone.0238291.

IIPS (International Institute for Population Sciences) and ICF. 2021. *National Family Health Survey (NFHS-5), 2019–21: India*. Mumbai: IIPS.

Kaur, Gunjeet, Akashdeep Singh Chauhan, Shankar Prinja, Yot Teerawattananon, Malaisamy Muniyandi, Ashu Rastogi, Gaurav Jyani, et al. 2021. "Cost-Effectiveness of Population-Based Screening for Diabetes and Hypertension in India: An Economic Modelling Study." *The Lancet Public Health* 7 (1): e65-e73. https://doi.org/10.1016/S2468-2667(21)00199-7.

Krishnan, Anand, Prashant Mathur, Vaitheeswaran Kulothungan, Harshal Ramesh Salve, Sravya Leburu, Ritvik Amarshand, Baridalyne Nogkynrih, et al. 2021. "Preparedness of Primary and Secondary Health Facilities in India to Address Major Noncommunicable Diseases: Results of a National Noncommunicable Disease Monitoring Survey (NNMS)." *BMC Health Service Research* 21 (1): 757. https://doi.org/10.1186/s12913-021-06530-0.

Lahariya, Chandrakant. 2020. "Health & Wellness Centers to Strengthen Primary Health Care in India: Concept, Progress and Ways Forward." *Indian Journal of Pediatrics* 87 (11): 916–29. https://link.springer.com/article/10.1007/s12098-020-03359-z.

Mahal, A., A. Karan, and M. Engelgau. 2010. "The Economic Implications of Non-Communicable Disease for India." World Bank/HNP Discussion Paper, World Bank, Washington, DC.

MoHFW (India, Ministry of Health and Family Welfare). 2015. "Report of the Task Force on Comprehensive Primary Health Care Rollout." Government of India, New Delhi. https://nhsrcindia.org/sites/default/files/2021-03/Report%20of%20Task%20Force%20on%20Comprehensive%20PHC%20Rollout.pdf.

MoHFW (India, Ministry of Health and Family Welfare). 2017. *National Health Policy*. New Delhi: Government of India. http://cdsco.nic.in/writereaddata/National-Health-Policy.pdf.

MoHFW (India, Ministry of Health and Family Welfare). 2021. "Operational Guidelines for Pradhan Mantri Health Infrastructure Mission." Government of India, New Delhi. https://nhsrcindia.org/sites/default/files/FINAL%20PM-ABHIM__15-12-21.pdf.

MoSPI (India, Ministry of Statistics and Program Implementation). 2020. "Health in India." Government of India. https://mospi.gov.in/sites/default/files/publication_reports/NSS%20Report%20no.%20586%20Health%20in%20India.pdf.

NCDC (National Centre for Disease Control). 2017. "Training Module for Medical Officers for Prevention, Control and Population Level Screening of Hypertension, Diabetes and Common Cancer (Oral, Breast & Cervical)." Government of India, New Delhi. https://nhsrcindia.org/sites/default/files/2021-06/Module%20for%20MOs%20for%20Prevention%2CControl%20%26%20PBS%20of%20Hypertension%2CDiabetes%20%26%20Common%20Cancer.pdf.

NHA (India, National Health Authority). 2020. "Journey from HBP 1.0 to HBP 2.0." Government of India, New Delhi. https://pmjay.gov.in/sites/default/files/2020-01/Journey-from-HBP-1.0-to-HBP-2.0.pdf.

NHA (India, National Health Authority). 2021a. "Ayushman Bharat PM-JAY IEC Guidelines 2021-22, Version 2.0." Government of India, New Delhi. https://nha.gov.in/img/resources/1623-NHA-IEC-Guidelines-3-01-21.pdf.

NHA (India, National Health Authority). 2021b. *National Health Benefit Package 2.2: User Guidelines*. New Delhi: Government of India. https://nha.gov.in/img/resources/HBP -2.2-manual.pdf.

NHA (India, National Health Authority). 2022. *Ayushman Bharat Pradhan Mantri Jan Arogya Yojana, Health Benefit Package Manual Part 1*. New Delhi: Government of India.

NHSRC (India, National Health Systems Resource Centre). 2018. "Ayushman Bharat Comprehensive Primary Health Care through Health and Wellness Centers: Operational Guidelines." Government of India, New Delhi. https://www.nhm.gov.in /New_Updates_2018/NHM_Components/Health_System_Stregthening/Comprehensive _primary_health_care/letter/Operational_Guidelines_For_CPHC.pdf.

NHSRC (National Health Systems Resource Centre). 2023. "National Health Accounts: Estimates for India 2019-20." Government of India, New Delhi. https://nhsrcindia.org /sites/default/files/2023-04/National%20Health%20Accounts-2019-20.pdf.

Prinja, Shankar, Maninder Pal Singh, Kavitha Rajsekar, Oshima Sachin, Praveen Gedam, Anu Nagar, Balram Bhargava, and CHSI Study Group. 2021. "Translating Research to Policy: Setting Provider Payment Rates for Strategic Purchasing under India's National Publicly Financed Health Insurance Scheme." *Applied Health Economics and Health Policy* 19 (3): 353–70. https://pubmed.ncbi.nlm.nih.gov/33462775/.

Sankaranarayan, Rengaswamy, Kunnambath Ramadas, Gigi Thomas, Richard Muwonge, Somanathan Thara, Babu Mathew, Balakrishnan Rajan, and Trivandrum Oral Cancer Screening Study Group. 2005. "Effect of Screening on Oral Cancer Mortality in Kerala, India: A Cluster-Randomized Trial." *The Lancet* 365 (9475): 1927–33. https://pubmed.ncbi .nlm.nih.gov/15936419/.

WHO (World Health Organization) and World Bank. 2021. *Global Monitoring Report on Financial Protection in Health 2021*. Washington, DC: World Bank. https://openknowledge .worldbank.org/handle/10986/36723.

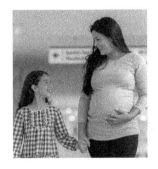

11

Evolution of Health Benefits Packages in Colombia: Thirty Years of Successes and Failures

Marcela Brun Vergara and Javier Guzman

ABSTRACT

Since the 1990s, health benefits packages in Colombia have undergone significant transformations. This chapter outlines the progression of priority setting in Colombia, categorized into three distinct periods marked by substantial reforms, commencing with a major overhaul of the health care sector in 1993. Each of those periods presented both advantages and disadvantages, stemming from varying institutional arrangements, processes, and methodologies. The most notable shift occurred when Colombia transitioned from a positive list of specific services to an approach that covers all services and technologies, except those explicitly set out in a restricted negative list. The evolution of Colombia's health care system offers valuable insights for low- and middle-income countries seeking to establish evidence-based priority-setting mechanisms.

INTRODUCTION

Colombia is an upper-middle-income country with an estimated population of 51.6 million as of 2021 (DANE 2020).[1] Since the 1990s, the country has made substantial progress on social and economic indicators. Gross domestic product per capita reached US$6,418.1 in 2021,[2] life expectancy increased from 69 years in 1989 to 77 years in 2019 (DANE 2021), multidimensional poverty decreased from 29.7 percent in 2010 to 16 percent in 2021 (DANE 2022a), and the country's Human Development Index score improved from 0.610 in 1990 to 0.752 in 2021.[3]

Nevertheless, inequality remains high. The Gini coefficient for Colombia barely changed between 2009 and 2021 (54.3 and 52.3, respectively), and yawning gaps between urban and rural areas persist. In 2021, departments such as Chocó and La Guajira had poverty rates above 60 percent, whereas Cundinamarca and Caldas had rates of 22.8 percent and 28.4 percent, respectively (DANE 2022b). Current estimates also suggest that about 60 percent of the workforce is employed in the informal economy (DANE 2022c).

In 1993, Colombia embarked on a major health sector reform.[4] The country introduced mandatory universal social health insurance financed through a combination of payroll contributions and general taxation. The reform introduced competition into both insurance and the provision of care through a managed care model, and it created a contributory regime (CR) for those able to pay as well as a fully subsidized regime (SR) for the poor. Central to the health sector reform and the priority-setting process was the introduction of a health benefits package (HBP) that included promotive, preventive, curative, rehabilitative, and palliate health services.

This chapter describes and reviews the evolution of HBPs in Colombia since the major health sector reform in 1993. The chapter first describes the main achievements and challenges associated with the reform after nearly 30 years of implementation. It then describes the institutional and governance arrangements, processes, methodologies, and implementation pathways Colombia has used to design and update HBPs, as well as successes, failures, advantages, and disadvantages associated with different approaches used over time. Finally, it reflects on lessons learned, main challenges, and future perspectives.

THIRTY YEARS OF REFORM

Since 1993, Colombia has made remarkable progress toward universal health coverage, financial risk protection, and equitable access, regardless of people's ability to pay. Coverage increased from 29 percent of the population in 1995 to 99 percent in 2021 (figure 11.1), out-of-pocket expenditure fell from 52 percent in 1993 to about 15 percent in 2019, and all citizens within the system are entitled to an equal basket of services. Data from 2019 show that Colombia's out-of-pocket expenditure (14.86 percent) is low relative to the average for Latin America and the Caribbean (28.35) and similar to the average for Organisation for Economic Co-operation and Development countries (13.86 percent).[5]

Figure 11.1 Health Coverage of Colombia's Population, by Type of Coverage, 1995–2021

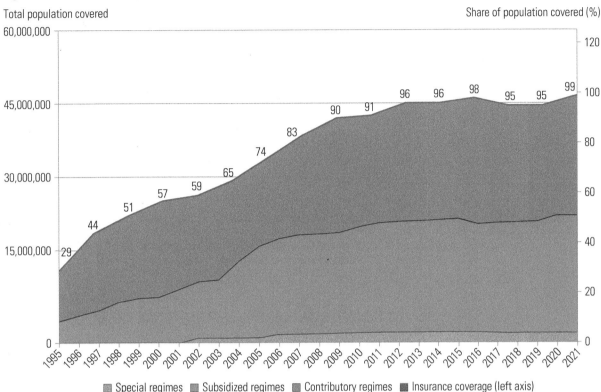

Source: Adapted from MoHSP 2023.

Despite those impressive achievements, the Colombian health system faces significant challenges including financial sustainability, regional and urban-rural inequities, and an imbalance between primary and specialized care. Insurers, mostly private but heavily regulated, often do not manage clinical and financial risk appropriately; and poor employment contracts, inefficient payments systems, and lack of infrastructure in some areas hamper quality of care, especially at the primary health care level. Colombia spent about US$16.6 billion[6] (or 8 percent of gross domestic product) on health in 2021, much more than it spent before the reform in 1993 or even a decade earlier (figure 11.2), but not enough to meet current demands. The country has an estimated current annual budgetary deficit of US$1.1 billion, mainly associated with a very generous interpretation of the right to health enshrined in statutory laws since 2015. According to Colombian law, every health technology and health service must be covered by the system, except in very specific circumstances (refer to discussion in the subsection on Period 3).

Figure 11.2 Health Expenditure as Share of GDP, Colombia, 2000–21

Health expenditure (% of GDP)

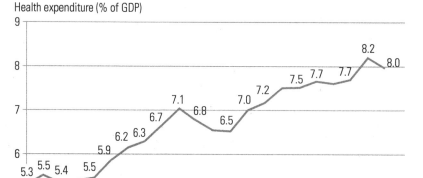

Source: World Bank DataBank, "Colombia," https://data.worldbank.org/country/colombia?name _desc=false. GDP expressed in constant 2015 US dollars.

HEALTH BENEFITS PACKAGE EVOLUTION SINCE THE REFORM OF 1993

The way the Colombian health care system makes decisions on coverage—what to cover, and at what cost—has evolved over the past 30 years. The changes result from key decisions made by the three branches of the Colombian government: the Congress, the Executive branch, and the Constitutional Court (refer to figure 11.3). Interestingly, and contrary to the experience of other middle-income countries, the Constitutional Court has played a major role in determining the content and the processes by which the Executive branch decides on HBPs. For example, in 2008, the Court ruled that the Executive branch had to unify the HBPs in the CR and SR as stated in the health sector reform law, and it established a deadline of a year for the Executive branch to do so.[7] The Court also mandated the Executive branch to regularly update the HBPs in a participatory, transparent, and evidence-based manner.

The history of HBPs in Colombia in the past 30 years can be divided into three main periods, based on the shape of the HBP, governance arrangements (that is, who made what decisions), processes followed (that is, criteria used for inclusion or exclusion, stakeholder participation, transparency, and so on), and methodologies considered to inform coverage decisions and implementing mechanisms. The first period began in 1993, when Colombia passed the major health sector reform, and continued to 2007, when the country established the Health Regulation Commission (Comisión de Regulación en Salud, or CRES) and the Constitutional Court issued its major ruling on the right to health. The second period went from 2007 to 2011, when the Ministry of Health and Social Protection (MoHSP) took several responsibilities from CRES and established a new Advisory Commission. The final period, from 2011 onward, includes a key milestone—the passage by Congress of a Statutory Law establishing the right to health as a fundamental human right.[8] This chapter describes the key features of the three periods, their major outcomes, and the pros and cons of each institutional arrangement.

Figure 11.3 Colombia's HBP Regulatory Milestones for Health, 1993–2021

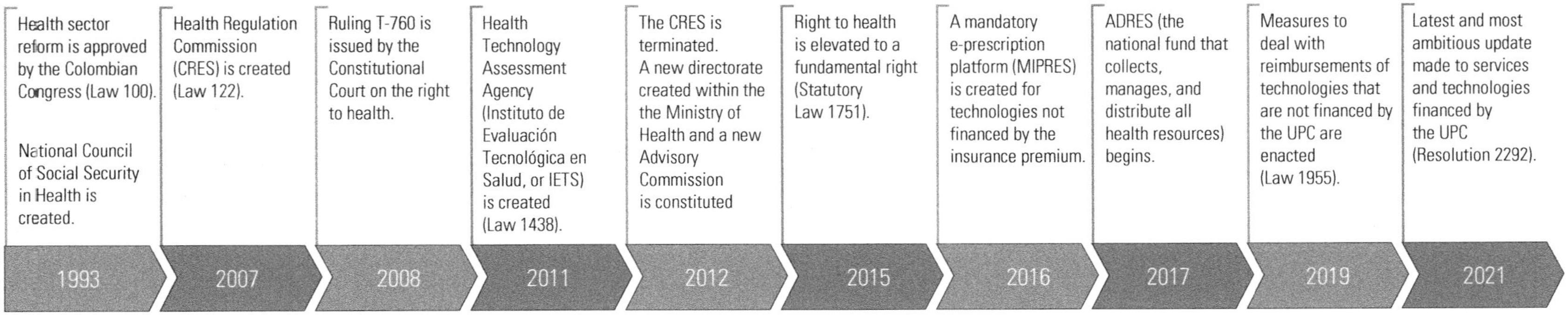

1993	2007	2008	2011	2012	2015	2016	2017	2019	2021
Health sector reform is approved by the Colombian Congress (Law 100). National Council of Social Security in Health is created.	Health Regulation Commission (CRES) is created (Law 122).	Ruling T-760 is issued by the Constitutional Court on the right to health.	Health Technology Assessment Agency (Instituto de Evaluación Tecnológica en Salud, or IETS) is created (Law 1438).	The CRES is terminated. A new directorate created within the the Ministry of Health and a new Advisory Commission is constituted	Right to health is elevated to a fundamental right (Statutory Law 1751).	A mandatory e-prescription platform (MIPRES) is created for technologies not financed by the insurance premium.	ADRES (the national fund that collects, manages, and distribute all health resources) begins.	Measures to deal with reimbursements of technologies that are not financed by the UPC are enacted (Law 1955).	Latest and most ambitious update made to services and technologies financed by the UPC (Resolution 2292).

Source: Original figure created for this publication.

Note: UPC = Unidad de Pago por Capitación (premium).

Colombia's HBP evolution provides several lessons for low- and middle-income countries interested in institutionalizing evidence-based priority-setting processes and pursuing universal health coverage. In 30 years, the country went from having two explicit HBPs, with benefits linked to the ability to contribute, to covering in theory everything for everyone, excluding just a narrow negative list of services and health technologies.

Period 1: Two Explicit HBPs and a Multistakeholder Decision-Making Body (1993–2007)

This first period began in 1993 when the Colombian Congress approved the health sector reform and implementation started. A cornerstone of the reform involved guaranteeing a package of health services for both the CR and the SR.

Governance and institutional arrangements. A collegiate body, the National Social Security Council in Health (CNSSS), had responsibility to boost the system in administrative and financial matters. The CNSSS was very inclusive, consisting of representatives from all interest groups (table 11.1).

Table 11.1 CNSSS Members According to Colombia's Law 100 of 1993

Permanent members (voice and vote)	Advisers (no vote)
• Chair: Minister of Health	• One representative from the National Academy of Medicine
• Minister of Labor and Social Security, or Vice Minister	• One representative from the Colombian Medical Federation
• Minister of Finance and Public Credit, or Technical Vice Minister	• One representative from the Colombian Association of Medical Schools
• Two representatives from state and municipal governments	• One representative from the Colombian Hospital Association
• Two representatives from employers, one of whom will represent small and medium companies	• One representative from the Faculties of Public Health
• Two representatives from workers, one of whom will represent pensioners	
• One representative from insurers	
• One representative from providers	
• One representative from health professionals	
• One representative from associations of health services users in the rural sector	

Source: Congress of the Republic of Colombia, Law 100 of 1993, https://www.funcionpublica.gov.co/eva/gestornormativo/norma.php?i=5248.
Note: CNSSS = National Social Security Council in Health.

CNSSS made decisions on the content of the HBPs, as well as on several other matters ranging from criteria for identifying beneficiaries to the value and destination of contributions to the system. A few years after the creation of CNSSS, it established an ad hoc technical secretariat, the Technical Committee on Medicines, which later became the Medicines and Technology Evaluation Committee. Both committees were coordinated by the Ministry of Health, consisted of ad honorem members, and had the mandate to evaluate any health technology considered for inclusion. Because the committees did not have proper funding or all the expertise needed, their efforts were unsuccessful.

Processes followed. The design of the initial HBPs did not follow a systematic, transparent, or participatory process. The HBP for the contributing members of the system was based on the tariff manual used by the Social Security Institute, an insurer covering private workers before the reform. CNSSS made the decision after rejecting a proposal developed by a team of world-class experts and based on cost-effectiveness criteria, doing so because the proposal contained fewer benefits than previously provided by the Social Security Institute and because of doubts about the robustness of the data used.

During the period 1993–2007, CNSSS updated the HBPs marginally, by including new health technologies, 12 times. Moreover, CNSSS established a taxonomy for medical procedures, the Single Classification of Health Procedures, which helped the council consider or include certain health technologies into the HBPs It made decisions by single majority voting, with the Minister of Health casting a tie-breaking vote when necessary.

Shape of the HBP. CNSSS established two separate explicit lists of inclusions or HBPs: a larger package known as the Mandatory Health Plan (Plan Obligatorio de Salud, or POS) for contributing members of the system, and a smaller publicly subsidized HBP, known as POS-S (Plan Obligatorio de Salud–Subsidiado), which covered about 50 percent of the interventions included in the POS for the lower-income population. When establishing the two regimes and HBPs, CNSSS intended to progressively expand the breadth of POS-S, such that by 2000 it would be equal to the POS. Regrettably, it did not meet that lofty goal because of reduced growth in contributing members and initial projections of public revenue. Beneficiaries also used legal claims that forced their insurers to pay for health services not included in the POS or POS-S packages.

HBP implementation. Since passage of the health sector reform, HBPs have been translated into actual health care delivery through the premium or UPC (Unidad de Pago por Capitación). The UPC is paid every year to insurers to provide the services included in HBPs. At first, CNSSS calculated the UPC for both regimes on the basis of available funds, guided by annual increments in minimum wages. It initially calculated the UPC for the SR as a fixed percentage (50 percent) of the UPC for the CR, mainly because it lacked reliable information to calculate a separate premium. Since 2004, it has calculated the UPC for the CR actuarially, considering the frequency of use and the costs reported by insurers. CNSSS introduced UPC adjustments by level of care, age, sex, and geography (box 11.1). It also determined the level of copayments for both regimes.

In the period 1993–2007, Colombia made notable improvements in expanding coverage, particularly among the poorest segments of the population. Nevertheless, during those first two decades of implementation, increasing investment in new and expensive interventions threatened both the sustainability and the equitable distribution of health services. Less than 1 percent of payments for new drugs covered people in the poorest quintile of society, whereas 70 percent of those payments covered drugs for the two richest quintiles (Gaviria 2014).

Major pros and cons. In theory, CNSSS provided an inclusive platform for discussion and a participatory decision-making process. All relevant stakeholders had a seat at the table and were invited to air their concerns and suggestions. In practice, however, effective participation was not easy for certain groups: workers and users, especially, were underrepresented because the government and employers had the most seats and votes (Martínez 2015). Moreover, CNSSS had too many functions, tensions existed between CNSSS and the Ministry of Health over responsibilities, and limits and regulations were not appropriately developed and enforced, in part because regulated parties also acted as regulators.

Additionally, the processes followed by the CNSSS had serious shortcomings in relation to using evidence, ensuring transparency, and following standardized methods with clear criteria for decision-making. Despite the creation of technical committees starting in 1997, the committees were not set up for success and failed to provide the rigor needed.

Period 2: Unified HBP, Gradual Dilution of HBPs and Creation of a Decision-Making Body Attached to the Ministry of Social Protection (2007–11)

CNSSS was eliminated as a decision-making body in 2007 and its functions transferred to CRES. CRES was created as part of Law 1122 of 2007,[9] the first health reform passed by Congress to modify the system since 1993. The new law aimed to improve the system's finances, improve the flow of resources, and clarify roles and responsibilities of the Ministry of Social Protection,[10] especially in relation to regulation and enforcement, among other key objectives.

Governance and institutional arrangements. CRES, created as a technical institution with regulatory functions and attached to the Ministry of Social Protection, had responsibility for defining the HBP, establishing the value of the UPC for each regime, and determining copayments. It consisted of five full-time experts (the Commissioners) and two Ministers, the Minister of Finance and Public Credit and the Minister of Social Protection. Under Law 1122 of 2007, CRES had its own budget and its own staff who supported the Commissioners.

Processes followed. As CRES was being established and before it was fully functional, the Constitutional Court issued a seminal ruling that clarified the right to health and provided instructions to the Executive branch. The Court mandated that CRES unify the HBPs (POS and POS-S), initially for children and later for adults, and develop a participatory, transparent, and evidence-based process to comprehensively update the HBP immediately and then annually. That action by the Court arose in response to a wave of litigation to enforce the right to health, with citizens filing tens of thousands of tutelas[11] or writs before judges to protect their fundamental constitutional rights. Those writs became a systemic problem associated with the lack of clarity, regulation, and transparency in the Colombian health system at the time. Citizens filed writs to get insurers to pay for health technologies not included in the HBPs, which was particularly out of date for the SR. Writs reached record numbers in 2008—more than 35 writs for every 10,000 people (Restrepo-Zea, Casas-Bustamante, and Espinal-Piedrahita 2018) (figure 11.4).

In response to the ruling, CRES conducted a comprehensive update of the HBPs in 2009. As part of that update, it designed new mechanisms for stakeholder participation and commissioned health technology assessments. Stakeholders including insurers, providers, and users no longer took part in the decision-making process, as they had with CNSSS, but were consulted on key stages of the process. CRES also improved transparency, especially regarding the benefits covered by the system, and launched an app, POS Pópuli, that allowed anyone to search for and identify what health services were covered. The app won many awards, including a prize for best web- and mobile-based government application.

Figure 11.4 Health Writs Filed in Colombia, 1999–2019

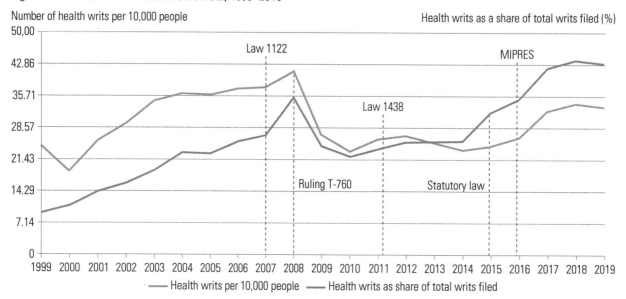

Number of health writs per 10,000 people

Health writs as a share of total writs filed (%)

Source: Adapted from Restrepo-Zea, Casas-Bustamante, and Espinal-Piedrahita 2018 and unpublished information from Jairo Humberto Restrepo Zea.
Note: Law 1122 of 2007 was the first reform of Law 100 of 1993, and Law 1438 of 2011 was the second; both attempted to improve the health system by introducing new rules and concepts such as primary care. The T-760 ruling was the most important ruling at its time, with an enormous impact on what until then citizens knew as PBS (positive list), introducing the need to change the understanding of the right to health and the ambition of a negative list instead. The statutory law elevated health as a fundamental right and, among other things, established the HBP as a negative list. HBP = health benefits package; MIPRES = Mi Prescripción, an obligatory system to prescribe nonincluded benefits to patients.

Shape of the HBP. CRES began the unification of HBPs in response to the ruling. Initially, it unified the packages for children younger than 12 years but then progressively unified the packages for all ages. Also, CRES clarified the content of the HBPs and determined the general rules for the system to deal with technologies not included in the HBPs. It determined that those technologies could be reimbursed ex post by a separate fund if approved by the technical-scientific committees within insurers.

HBP implementation. Unifying both HBPs led to important adjustments to the SR UPC. Although the UPC calculation method did not change, UPC values were significantly adjusted to consider the additional services included in the HBPs. Ex post adjustments were also designed to balance asymmetries associated with the number of patients insured with some high-cost conditions such as renal failure.

Major pros and cons. The creation of CRES, as an autonomous institution with technical capacity and mechanisms for more expeditious decision-making, brought important advances to the system. CRES incorporated evidence from health technology assessments into the decision-making process and provided new vehicles for stakeholder participation.

Compared to CNSSS, CRES had more autonomy and a degree of separation from regulated parties that allowed it to be a better regulator. However, the relationship with the Ministries of Social Protection and Finance made CRES to some extent subject to their power and influence. Some authors associate that influence with the low profile of Commissioners and the fact that CRES decisions were tied to the financial balance of the system, which in turn made it subject to the decisions of the Ministry of Finance (Martinez 2015).

Period 3: Elimination of Explicit HBPs and a New Institutional Framework Based on the Right to Health (2011–23)

In 2011, Law 1438 created a new Health Technology Assessment (HTA) Agency, the Instituto de Evaluación Tecnológica en Salud (IETS), as part of the second reform to the system since 1993.[12] Its creation came as a response to the wave of litigation to enforce the right to health, the institutional and technical limitations of CRES, and the international move to establish HTA agencies. IETS was established as a nonprofit organization, governed by a board of public and private entities including the Ministry of Health; the Administrative Department of Science, Technology and Innovation; the National Institute of Health; the National Institute of Drug and Food Surveillance; and the Colombian Association of Medical Schools. It was created to generate evidence to support decision-making within the health system, especially in relation to the HBP and Standard Treatment Guidelines.

In addition to the creation of the HTA Agency, Decree 2562 of 2012 eliminated CRES and established a new directorate (Dirección de Regulación de Beneficios, Costos y Tarifas del Aseguramiento en Salud, or DRBCTAS) within the MoHSP. Decision-making was also transferred to the MoHSP, and created an Advisory Commission to the Ministry on issues related to benefits, costs, and tariffs.[13]

In 2015, Congress passed the third reform to the health system since 1993 when it established the right to health as an autonomous fundamental human right. The law, known as Statutory Health Law 1751, linked that right to public health interventions and health services, and established that financial or fiscal sustainability could not become a barrier to fully exercising the right to health.[14] It mandated the Executive to move from marginally expanding the HBP with inclusions to assuming that the HBP covered all health services and interventions except in specific circumstances.

Governance and institutional arrangements. Since 2012, the Minister of Health and Social Protection, following the advice of an Advisory Commission (Comisión Asesora de Beneficios, Costos y Tarifas, or CABCT), makes decisions related to the HBP. CABCT consists of the Minister of Health and Social Protection, the Minister of Finance and Public Credit, the Director of the National Planning Department, a delegate from the Presidency, and the Director General of IETS.[15] It makes decisions through consensus; to date, the Minister has always followed the Commission's advice.

The new directorate created in 2012 within the MoHSP (DRBCTAS) functions as the technical and administrative secretariat of CABCT. MoHSP/DRBCTAS works in coordination with IETS to build the evidence necessary for the Advisory Commission to make decisions. Representatives from the other members also provide technical contributions before formal submission and decision-making take place. CABCT may invite other stakeholders to its sessions to participate without voting rights.

Processes followed. After the elimination of CRES in 2012 and until full implementation of the Statutory Health Law in 2017, the process to update the HBP aimed at including new health technologies in the package and occurred at least every two years as mandated by law. Stakeholders including clinicians, users, and the pharmaceutical industry nominated health technologies not included in the HBP and therefore not included in the UPC calculation. MoHSP/DRBCTAS then implemented a topic selection process to determine the technologies that would be assessed; IETS conducted the HTAs, focusing on comparative effectiveness and budget impact; and CABCT appraised the evidence and issued a recommendation to the Minister on the basis of the appraisal (figure 11.5). The topic selection process and appraisal used explicit criteria including weights, built after a long participatory process. The HTA followed methodological guidelines developed by IETS, with stakeholder participation primarily conducted during the technical assessment and before the MoHSP/DRBCTAS submitted the evidence to the Commission.

Upon implementation of the Statutory Health Law in 2017, however, the process changed completely to focus on exclusions rather than inclusions. Decision-making on how the system would finance health technologies not explicitly included in the HBP and financed through the UPC continued to use an abridged form of the old process. Nevertheless, a negative list following an exclusion process was the goal.

Figure 11.5 Health Technology Assessment Process and Key Actors before Colombia's 2015 Statutory Health Law

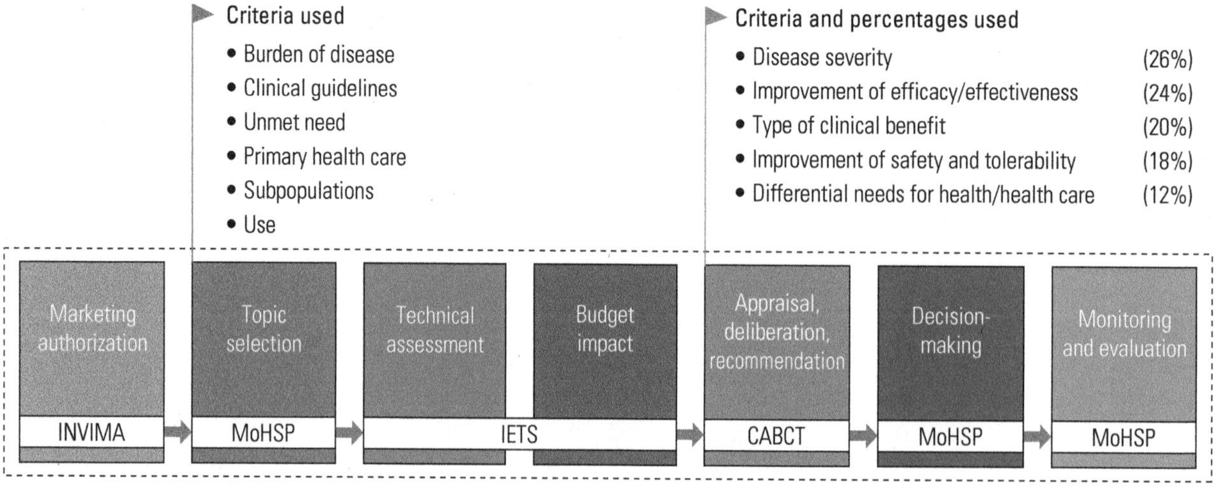

▶ Criteria used
- Burden of disease
- Clinical guidelines
- Unmet need
- Primary health care
- Subpopulations
- Use

▶ Criteria and percentages used
- Disease severity (26%)
- Improvement of efficacy/effectiveness (24%)
- Type of clinical benefit (20%)
- Improvement of safety and tolerability (18%)
- Differential needs for health/health care (12%)

| Marketing authorization | Topic selection | Technical assessment | Budget impact | Appraisal, deliberation, recommendation | Decision-making | Monitoring and evaluation |
| INVIMA | MoHSP | IETS | | CABCT | MoHSP | MoHSP |

Source: Gutiérrez et al. 2015.

Note: CABCT = Comisión Asesora de Beneficios, Costos y Tarifas; IETS = Instituto de Evaluación Tecnológica en Salud; INVIMA = Instituto Nacional de Vigilancia de Medicamentos y Alimentos; MoHSP = Ministry of Health and Social Protection.

MoHSP/DRBCTAS established the exclusion process following the clear mandate included in the Statutory Health Law, which required a scientific and technical process that would also be participatory, public, and transparent. Potentially affected groups would also have to be consulted before decisions on exclusions were made. Following on these requirements, MoHSP/DRBCTAS established a four-step process of nomination, evaluation, consultation, and adoption and publication (box 11.2). The evaluation now focuses on establishing the rationale for exclusion, using six potential reasons included in the Statutory Health Law, summarized as follows: the health technology (1) is indicated for cosmetic purposes, (2) does not have scientific evidence on safety and efficacy, (3) does not have scientific evidence on clinical effectiveness, (4) has not been authorized by the regulatory agency, (5) is still under clinical development, or (6) is not available in the country.

Box 11.2

Exclusion Process Phases for Colombia's Health Benefits Packages

1. **Nomination and prioritization.** Stakeholders including the Ministry of Health and Social Protection and medical associations nominate technologies for exclusion. The Ministry's directorate (Dirección de Regulación de Beneficios, Costos y Tarifas del Aseguramiento en Salud, or DRBCTAS) prioritizes nominations using criteria such as public health interest, population affected, and budgetary impact.
2. **Analysis.** The Health Technology Asessment Agency (Instituto de Evaluación Tecnológica en Salud, or IETS) with participation of independent experts from health care associations, the National Academy of Medicine, and associations of schools with different health care programs, among others, assesses and appraises the information collected and makes recommendations on whether to exclude the health technology. Decisions are made by consensus.
3. **Consultation.** Potentially affected patients and the public are consulted through virtual surveys, events, and the Mi Vox-Pópuli app.
4. **Adoption and publication.** The Ministry of Health and Social Protection adopts, publishes, and implements the recommendation made during the analysis and verified during the consultation.

Source: Colombia, Ministry of Health and Social Protection, Resolution 330 of 2017, https://www.minsalud.gov.co/Normatividad_Nuevo/Resolución%200330%20de%202017.pdf.

Shape of the HBP. The HBP evolved from a positive list with inclusions, as established by Resolution 5261 of 1994, to a package that, in theory, covers everything for everyone, excluding a negative list of 18 procedures and 55 medicines, according to Resolution 2273 of 2021.[16] Since the time of CRES to 2020, technologies included in the HBP were financed ex ante through the UPC, whereas excluded technologies were reimbursed ex post by a separate fund if certain approvals were met. However, since March of 2020, with the implementation of Law 1955 of 2019, any technology not explicitly included in the UPC calculation is also covered ex ante by a prospective budget cap mechanism.[17] Insurers calculate budgets caps on the basis of the historical spending on, and the number of patients receiving, the health technology. The number of technologies included in the UPC has increased steadily; in 2022, 97 percent of procedures and almost 94 percent of medicines approved and available in Colombia were financed through the UPC (MoHSP 2022a) (table 11.2).

Table 11.2 Included/Excluded Medicines and Procedures, by Financing Mechanism, Colombian Health Benefits Package

Financing mechanism	Number of procedures covered	Share of procedures (%)	Number of medicines covered	Share of medicines (%)
UPC	9,197	96.87	61,056	93.64
Budget caps	275	2.90	4,079	6.26
Exclusions	18	0.19	55	0.10
Other	4	0.04	10	0
Total	9,494	100	65,200	100

Sources: MoHSP 2022a; Colombia, Ministry of Health and Social Protection, Resolution 2273 of 2021, https://www.minsalud.gov.co/sites/rid/Lists/BibliotecaDigital/RIDE/VP/RBC/informe-actualizacion-ts-upc.zip; Colombia, Ministry of Health and Social Protection, Resolution 2292 of 2021, https://www.minsalud.gov.co/Normatividad_Nuevo/Resolución%20No.%202292%20de%202021.pdf.

Note: UPC = Unidad de Pago por Capitación.

HBP implementation. The UPC continues to be calculated actuarially, considering the frequency and severity of the health services covered in the HBP historically, adjusted by level of care, age, sex, and geographical area. The UPC calculation uses the loss ratio method, which seeks to find the necessary increase on current premiums to ensure balance of the fundamental insurance equation, in addition to incurred but not reported and incurred but not enough reserve adjustments. MoHSP/DRBCTAS conducts those analyses using information reported by insurers. Over time, this directorate within the MoHSP has become incredibly good at collecting relevant data and calculating and adjusting the insurance premium.

As expected, and in alignment with the gradual expansion of health services included in HBPs, the UPC has grown substantially in the past 30 years. In 2022, UPC averaged Col$1,109,221.20 (US$246.00) for the CR and Col$964,807.20 (US$214.00) for the SR.[18] By comparison, in 1995 and 1996 when the two regimes were first established,[19] UPCs averaged Col$141,600.00 (US$31.46) for the CR and Col$108,464.00 (US$24.10) for the SR.

Age and sex adjusters are now defined in 14 groups as opposed to 7 in the past. Geographic adjusters are defined in four categories, based on access to health care services and supply conditions. Insurers for Indigenous people get an extra 4.81 percent, which covers traditional medicines and procedures. The high-cost disease ex post adjusters have evolved, now making adjustments for chronic kidney disease, HIV, hemophilia, and 11 types of cancers, based on prevalence and health outcomes (MoHSP 2022b).

Major pros and cons. Colombia established a more stable, coherent, and mature priority-setting system, especially in the first part of the period. Positive developments included the creation of IETS, the HTA Agency; MoHSP/DRBCTAS, the directorate within the MoHSP responsible for carrying out clear, specific stages of the process; and CABCT, the commission responsible for making the final recommendations to the Minister of Health. Over time, these institutions have also become stronger. For example, IETS has conducted about 200 budgetary impact analyses and 50 economic evaluations in the 10 years since its creation (IETS 2022).

Separation of key roles and responsibilities between those conducting the evaluation, those appraising the evidence, and those making the decisions was fully established. Methods to evaluate potential inclusions became more robust by the end of the first part of the period. Finally, transparency and stakeholder participation continued to improve to some degree in some stages, but the Executive branch had sole decision-making authority.

Despite that progress, the system did not fully incorporate the concept of opportunity cost, and economic evaluations including cost-effectiveness analysis were rarely conducted or used to make coverage decisions, inform price negotiations, or incentivize quality improvements. IETS also could not receive funds directly from the national budget, depending instead on funds linked to projects financed by MoHSP and the Ministry of Finance. The absence of direct funding from the national budget undermined the institution and had adverse repercussions on its interactions with other stakeholders in the priority-setting process, including MoHSP. This situation also impeded the growth of organizational capabilities and the retention of skilled staff.

In the second part of the period, the implementation of the Statutory Law substantially changed the concept and goal of the priority-setting system. On the positive side, it provided clarity to all stakeholders on the mandate to protect and deliver on the right to health (users now knew insurers could not deny health services not listed in the HBP); protected medical autonomy (health care professionals could prescribe the best care for their patients without additional bureaucratic and administrative barriers); reduced transaction costs (patients did not need to go to court or through lengthy approvals to access care); and empowered insurers to better manage clinical and financial risk (insurers got all the funding ex ante and no longer had to rely on ex post reimbursement).

Nevertheless, questions on financial feasibility remain because neither health care expenditure nor the premium paid to insurers increased to cover a scenario whereby, in theory, all services covered would translate into services that patients actually receive. Furthermore, because the criteria mandated by law limit the process for exclusions, making it typically slower and more cumbersome than the process for introducing new technologies, insurers are now more exposed to increased, early demand for high-cost technologies and interventions. That challenge persists even though the Colombian regulatory agency, INVIMA, experiences delays in reviewing and granting marketing authorization for new technologies. In response to that new reality, some insurers might have imposed access barriers or resorted to implicit rationing or low quality of care. Implicit rationing coupled with lack of essential services in some regions and the risk of favoring new, high-cost technologies in urban areas might lead to increased inequity. Finally, overall value for money might have decreased, with funds spent on services that do not provide the biggest benefit for society (that is, there is no signaling on essential, cost-effective interventions and cost-effectiveness can't be used as a criterion for the negative list).

LESSONS LEARNED, MAIN CHALLENGES, AND FUTURE PERSPECTIVES

Since 1993, the Colombian health system has used explicit priority setting via an HBP as a key policy instrument for improving coverage and working toward universal health coverage. The Colombian government successfully used HBPs to determine what services it would make available to whom, calculate the premium paid to insurers, and signal priority services to clinicians and patients. Over time, institutional arrangements became clearer and more stable, and processes and methodologies more robust. Because insurers could not always adequately deliver the services included in the HBPs, the system could not ensure timely delivery of an equal basket of services regardless of type of affiliation. In addition, as Colombians grew richer and embraced the right to health, knowledge of and exposure to new health technologies increased, and a very strong human rights framework was established in the country, explicit priority setting in the form of an HBP no longer represented a viable option. The Constitutional Court and the Congress mandated that the Executive branch move away from explicit priority setting and HBPs to delivering on the idea that the system will cover every health technology and health service, except in very limited circumstances.

That move has made explicit a clear tension between two views. The first embraces health as a fundamental human right and, when taken to the extreme, argues that health care must be guaranteed regardless of funds available and financial considerations. The second view argues that the funding available must determine what services the system covers and that allocative efficiency or value for money should be maximized for any given budget envelope. Colombia has already leaned toward the former, and key challenges such as financial sustainability, weak primary health care, and access to quality care in remote, poorer regions remain. The country will need alternative policy options to maximize health benefits, improve health outcomes within current health expenditure, and guarantee that the system delivers on the promise of universal health care and health as a fundamental human right within existing financial means.

The alternative policy options are imperfect, and no country can possibly offer access to all available health technologies and services. Agreeing on the need to have limits and the process to decide on coverage—what's covered, by whom, and at what cost—is essential for Colombian society. Unfortunately, those decisions mean explicit priority setting at the central level, which Colombia opted to leave behind a few years ago. Amid that backdrop, potential policy options for Colombia include the following:

- *Strengthening priority setting at lower levels within the system.* In the absence of a centralized priority-setting process including HTAs, insurers and health care providers could conduct their own evaluations and make their own decisions regarding what products and services to procure, prescribe, and pay for, and at what price. Although suboptimal and less efficient, that move could increase health care quality and make these stakeholders better stewards of public funds. Insurance, hospital, and medical associations and networks could play a vital role in running these processes on behalf of or with their members, which would reduce duplication and increase reach and impact (Giedion et al. 2018).
- *Implementing alternative processes to deal with high-cost but low-value health technologies.* Although MoHSP cannot conduct or use economic evaluation to exclude products on cost-effectiveness grounds, it should apply such methodologies for other purposes, including price regulations and negotiations, and developing standard treatment guidelines and protocols. MoHSP would benefit from deploying horizon scanning and early negotiation techniques, such as managed entry agreements, to avoid high-cost products from entering the Colombian market without adequate stewardship. It could also apply co-payments to services and technologies with low health value to signal the market and dissuade demand.
- *Deploying alternative options for funding insurers.* Colombia should put in place adequate incentives to encourage insurers to manage clinical and financial risk better and deliver high-value quality care. Incentives could include incorporating outcome-based indicators and conditions to change the way the UPC is calculated. In addition, better ex post adjustments could reduce risk asymmetries and address risk concentration in the populations covered by certain insurers.
- *Increasing efficiency in the system.* The country should tackle productive inefficiencies or inefficiencies in the form of excess costs in producing a given output. Demand aggregation and centralized procurement of expensive technologies; increased use of generic and biosimilar medicines; tackling waste, corruption, and fraud; and so on would help the system achieve more health services and better outcomes for the money.
- *Improving monitoring and evaluation.* Systematically and routinely measuring the services provided, and the quality of such services, would help MoHSP measure

effective coverage, identify and address implicit rationing, or signal inadequate or inefficient consumption patterns. MoHSP already collects information on services provided (to calculate the UPC) but needs to capture additional attributes and improve data quality and timeliness.

- *Strengthening stakeholder participation.* Along with improvements in engaging stakeholders in certain processes such as determining exclusions, it is vital to increase their effective engagement in fundamental discussions such as the financial sustainability of the system, the importance of maximizing health benefit, and the need to incorporate new technologies at adequate prices.

In early 2023, the Colombian government introduced a significant health care reform bill to the Colombian Congress, with primary objectives centered on expanding health care access in rural areas, prioritizing preventive and primary care, and enhancing fund management. Despite widespread agreement on those objectives, considerable controversy surrounds the proposed strategies for their achievement. The reform suggests significant alterations to various aspects of the Colombian health care system, including the transition to a National Health System with a single public insurer, increased support for public health care provision through funding for public hospitals, and the establishment of more primary health care clinics throughout the country. In terms of priority setting, the reform proposes to revive the CNSSS, a participatory body established after the 1993 reform, as described at the outset of this chapter, and integrate IETS into the government. The reform does not propose other changes concerning the processes and methodologies for defining health care benefits. It does, however, embrace the perspective that views health as a fundamental human right despite budgetary constraints.

Because the government does not possess the majority vote, the fate of the health reform's approval by Congress remains uncertain. Consequently, the draft reform will probably need to undergo amendments to secure successful approval.

CONCLUSION

Over the past three decades, priority setting in Colombia has undergone a significant evolution. The country has established more transparent and stable governance arrangements while refining and strengthening its institutions and processes. During that transformative period, Colombia shifted its approach from explicit priority setting, featuring a positive list of health services, to an inclusive approach covering all services and technologies except those explicitly set out in a restrictive negative list. The transition brought about certain advantages but also significant drawbacks, particularly concerning financial sustainability and value for money.

Colombia's progression offers valuable lessons for low- and middle-income countries aiming to establish evidence-based priority-setting mechanisms. The successes and failures in Colombia's journey can serve as instructive insights for ongoing and future discussions on achieving universal health coverage.

NOTES

1. United Nations Development Programme, Human Development Reports—Colombia, https://hdr.undp.org/data-center/specific-country-data#/countries/COL (accessed February 12, 2023).
2. World Bank DataBank, "Colombia," https://data.worldbank.org/country/colombia?name_desc=false. Gross domestic product expressed in constant 2015 US dollars.
3. United Nations Development Programme, Human Development Reports—Colombia.
4. Congress of the Republic of Colombia, Law 100 of 1993, https://www.funcionpublica.gov.co/eva/gestornormativo/norma.php?i=5248.
5. World Bank DataBank, "Colombia."
6. Government of Colombia, ADRES, Managed Resources Unit (URA), "Quotes," https://www.adres.gov.co/nuestra-entidad/informacion-financiera/unidad-de-recursos-administrados-ura/presupuesto.
7. Constitutional Court of Colombia, Decision T-760-08. Fundamental right to health, https://www.corteconstitucional.gov.co/english/Decision.php?IdPublicacion=9345.
8. Congress of the Republic of Colombia, Statutory Law 1751, https://www.minsalud.gov.co/Normatividad_Nuevo/Ley%201751%20de%202015.pdf.
9. Congress of the Republic of Colombia, Law 1122 of 2007, https://www.minsalud.gov.co/sites/rid/Lists/BibliotecaDigital/RIDE/DE/DIJ/ley-1122-de-2007.pdf.
10. The Ministry of Social Protection resulted from a merger of the Ministry of Health and the Ministry of Labor between 2002 and 2011.
11. The 1991 Constitution created a Constitutional Court, together with mechanisms such as the *tutela* (protection writ) to protect individual rights, and greatly enhanced the public's access to the courts through unfettered standing and lack of procedural requirements (Yamin and Parra-Vera 2009).
12. Congress of the Republic of Colombia, Law 1438 of 2011, https://www.minsalud.gov.co/Normatividad_Nuevo/LEY%201438%20DE%202011.pdf.
13. Colombia, Ministry of Health and Social Protection (MoHSP), Decree 2562 of 2012, https://www.minsalud.gov.co/sites/rid/Lists/BibliotecaDigital/RIDE/DE/DIJ/Decreto-2562-de-2012.pdf.
14. Congress of the Republic of Colombia, Statutory Law 1751.
15. Colombia, MoHSP, Decree 2562 of 2012.
16. Colombia, Ministry of Health and Social Protection, Resolution 5261 of 1994, https://www.minsalud.gov.co/Normatividad_Nuevo/RESOLUciÓN%205261%20DE%201994.pdf; Colombia, MoHSP, Resolution 2273 of 2021, https://www.minsalud.gov.co/Normatividad_Nuevo/Resolución%20No.%202273%20de%202021.pdf.
17. Congress of the Republic of Colombia, Law 1955 of 2019 (article 240), https://www.funcionpublica.gov.co/eva/gestornormativo/norma.php?i=93970.
18. This gap is explained by different administrative efforts as the insurers in the CR manage sick leave compensations.
19. Although approved in December 1993, the SR did not begin until 1996.

REFERENCES

DANE (Colombia, Departamento Administrativo Nacional de Estadística, National Department of Statistics). 2020. Serie nacional de población por área, para el periodo 2018–2070. Government of Colombia, Bogotá. https://www.dane.gov.co/index.php/estadisticas-por-tema/demografia-y-poblacion/proyecciones-de-poblacion.

DANE (Colombia, Departamento Administrativo Nacional de Estadística, National Department of Statistics). 2021. Proyecciones y retroproyecciones de población con base CNPV 2018. Government of Colombia, Bogotá. https://www.dane.gov.co/index.php/estadisticas-por-tema/demografia-y-poblacion/proyecciones-de-poblacion.

DANE (Colombia, Departamento Administrativo Nacional de Estadística, National Department of Statistics). 2022a. "Multidimensional Poverty 2021." Government of Colombia, Bogotá. https://www.dane.gov.co/index.php/estadisticas-por-tema/pobreza-y -condiciones-de-vida/pobreza-multidimensional.

DANE (Colombia, Departamento Administrativo Nacional de Estadística, National Department of Statistics). 2022b. "En 2021, en el total nacional la pobreza monetaria fue 39,3% y la pobreza monetaria extrema fue 12,2%." Press release, April 26, 2022. https://www.dane.gov.co/files/investigaciones/condiciones_vida/pobreza/2021 /Comunicado-pobreza-monetaria_2021.pdf.

DANE (Colombia, Departamento Administrativo Nacional de Estadística, National Department of Statistics). 2022c. "En diciembre de 2021, la tasa de desempleo en el total nacional fue 11,0% y en el total 13 ciudades y áreas metropolitanas fue 11,6%." Press release, January 31, 2022. https://www.dane.gov.co/files/investigaciones/boletines/ech/ech /CP_empleo_dic_21.pdf.

Gaviria, A. 2014. "Prices of New Medicines Threaten Colombia's Health Reform." *Finance & Development* 51 (4).

Giedion, U., M. Distrutti, A. L. Muñoz, D. M. Pinto, and A. M. Díaz. 2018. "La priorización en salud paso a paso: cómo articulan sus procesos México, Brasil y Colombia." Monografía del BID 596, Inter-American Development Bank. https://publications.iadb.org/en /la-priorizacion-en-salud-paso-paso-como-articulan-sus-procesos-mexico-brasil-y -colombia.

Gutiérrez, C., Ú. Giedion, A. L. Muñoz, and A. Ávila. 2015. Serie de notas técnicas sobre procesos de priorización en salud: nota 2: un enfoque sistemático. Nota técnica del BID 838. https://publications.iadb.org/en/publication/15424/serie-de-notas-tecnicas-sobre -procesos-de-priorizacion-en-salud-nota-2-un-enfoque.

IETS (Instituto de Evaluación Tecnológica en Salud). 2022. Hitos en 10 años. Unpublished manuscript.

Martínez, Alberto. 2015. "La Comisión de Regulación en Salud: crónica de un final anunciado." *Revista de Salud Pública* 17 (4): 626–35.

MoHSP (Ministry of Health and Social Protection). 2022a. Informe de la actualización de los servicios y tecnologías de salud financiados con recursos de la UPC año 2022. https://www.minsalud.gov.co/sites/rid/Lists/BibliotecaDigital/RIDE/VP/RBC/informe -actualizacion-ts-upc.zip.

MoHSP (Ministry of Health and Social Protection). 2022b. Estudio de suficiencia y de los mecanismos de ajuste del riesgo para el cálculo de la Unidad de Pago por Capitación para el año 2022: recursos para garantizar la financiación de tecnologías y servicios de salud en los regímenes Contributivo y Subsidiado." https://www.minsalud.gov.co/sites/rid/Lists /BibliotecaDigital/RIDE/VP/DOA/estudio-suficiencia-upc-2022.pdf.

MoHSP (Ministry of Health and Social Protection). 2024. "Insurance Behavior." https://www .minsalud.gov.co/proteccionsocial/Regimensubsidiado/Paginas/coberturas-del-regimen -subsidiado.aspx.

Restrepo-Zea, J. H., L. P. Casas-Bustamante, and J. J. Espinal-Piedrahita. 2018. "Universal Coverage and Effective Access to Health Care: What Has Happened in Colombia Ten Years after Sentence T-760?" *Revista de Salud Pública* 20 (6): 670–76.

Yamin, A. E., and O. Parra-Vera. 2009. "How Do Courts Set Health Policy? The Case of the Colombian Constitutional Court." *PLoS Medicine* 6 (2): e1000032.

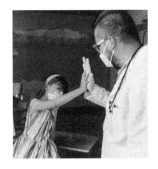

12

The Rise and Fall of Priority Setting in Mexico: Lessons from a Health Systems Perspective

Eduardo González-Pier, Mariana Barraza-Lloréns, and Jaime Sepúlveda

ABSTRACT

Mexico's Seguro Popular, launched in 2004, provided expanded health access and financial protection to uninsured Mexicans (41 percent of the population) through two health benefits packages, comprising 294 essential and 66 high-cost interventions. The Seguro Popular, however, was repealed in 2020. This chapter focuses on the importance of priority setting in health and the benefits of increasing access through health benefits packages while acknowledging the relevance of sustainability, providing valuable lessons for other countries. By paving an ordered way to make and legitimize coverage decisions, priority setting strengthens health systems, enhances its performance, and informs pathways to universal health coverage, with investment in human capital and institutional development yielding significant gains that should not be underestimated.

INTRODUCTION

With a population of 127 million and per capita income of US$10,046, Mexico stands as a large upper-middle-income country and the second-largest economy in Latin America and the Caribbean. It also ranks favorably on the Human Development Index (0.758). Life expectancy at birth increased substantially after 1970; although progress slowed from the early 2000s, life expectancy reached close to 75 years before the pandemic hit in 2020.[1] Health challenges have rapidly transitioned from infectious to noncommunicable diseases and injuries;

for example, Mexico now has the largest share of overweight or obese population among Organisation for Economic Co-operation and Development countries. Access to quality care, measured by population coverage through an explicit health benefits package (HBP), has improved substantially since 2003 because of the Seguro Popular (SP, or Popular Health Insurance) reforms. Nevertheless, the health system has remained chronically underfunded with health spending averaging 5.4 percent of gross domestic product over the past two decades, roughly half of which is paid out of pocket (box 12.1). Consequently, Mexico has 2.4 doctors, 2.9 nurses, and 1.0 bed per 1,000 population, less than one-third the comparable numbers in Organisation for Economic Co-operation and Development countries. The most pressing challenge looking forward is to provide sustainable access to quality care to a rapidly ageing population without exposing them to excessive catastrophic spending (OECD 2021).

Box 12.1

Key Features of Mexico's Health System

Mexico's health system dates from 1943, and its main feature has been institutional fragmentation resulting in coexisting publicly funded health care subsystems. Whereas salaried employees have access to social security institutions, the remaining 50 percent of the population is served by other public institutions, including 32 decentralized services run by state governments alongside federally run general hospitals and high-specialty centers.

Only 30 years ago, a double burden of disease characterized the country's health needs landscape. Noncommunicable diseases were just emerging, and communicable diseases and maternal, neonatal, and nutrition-related conditions were the leading causes of morbidity and mortality, especially in poor populations. Mexicans now live 75 years on average, and an increasing burden of noncommunicable diseases—mainly cardiovascular conditions and diabetes—drives population health needs. Many of those diseases are linked to a high prevalence of overweight and obesity. Slightly less than 75 percent of adults (ages 20 and older) are overweight or obese, and 20 percent of children are obese.

Total health spending as a share of gross domestic product has increased from 4.2 percent in 2000 to 6.1 percent in 2020. Despite its increase, that share still falls behind the average of Organisation for Economic Co-operation and Development countries (9.7 percent in 2020). In addition, public budgets fund only half of total health spending. The rest comes mainly from out-of-pocket spending and, to a minimal extent, from private health insurance.

Sources: Organisation for Economic Co-operation and Development, OECD Data Explorer, Health Expenditure and Financing, https://data-explorer.oecd.org/?fs[0]=Topic%2C1%7CHealth%23HEA%23%7CHealth%20expenditure%20and%20financing%23HEA_EXP%23&pg=0&fc=Topic&bp=true&snb=4; Shamah-Levy et al. 2021.

Mexico has a long tradition of using explicit priority setting to inform health coverage expansion, starting with international efforts to develop disease priorities in the 1990s and culminating in the 2003 creation of the SP. Soon after the launch of the landmark *World Development Report 1993: Investing in Health* (World Bank 1993), which promoted the use of burden of disease and cost-effectiveness to define a set of essential health care interventions, the Mexican Health Foundation (Funsalud), a health policy think tank, proposed a series of reforms. Those reforms included an essential HBP of cost-effective interventions to tackle the double burden of infectious diseases and emerging noncommunicable diseases (Frenk 1994). That approach meant a break from previous policy trends—which focused largely on ad hoc supply-side strategies to extend access to health care—to a more equitable and rational resource allocation process to steer supply-related efforts to increase coverage in deprived areas (González-Pier et al. 2006).

The Funsalud proposal found fertile ground in 2000, when the political commitment of a newly elected presidential administration allowed Mexico to shift its health policy aims to reach universal health coverage (UHC), driven by the excessive burden placed on families to access essential health care through out-of-pocket expenditures.[2] The 2000 World Health Report flagged the high level of catastrophic spending among Mexican families, ranking the country 144th for fairness in financial contributions (53rd World Health Assembly 2000). Evidence supporting advocacy efforts included an analysis of catastrophic and impoverishing spending across health conditions and associated interventions needed to deliver targeted financial protection to vulnerable population groups. Access to timely and quality cancer care for children—including medicines—emerged as a flagship set of interventions to be included in the purposely designed Catastrophic Spending Protection Fund (Fondo de Protección para Gastos Catastróficos, FPGC). The Ministry of Health (MoH) secured Ministry of Finance (MoF) funding, and Congress amended the General Health Law to launch the SP in 2004.

For 16 years—overlapping four presidential administrations—the SP provided expanded health access and financial health protection to previously uninsured Mexicans. The reform involved a new financial architecture including federal and state government contributions to fund the delivery of two HBPs: one package of 91 essential interventions, covering about 90 percent of the leading causes of demand in primary care and general hospitalization, and a package of 6 high-cost/high-specialty interventions clusters (González-Pier et al. 2006). Population coverage, and thus incremental funding, was phased in over a seven-year period. The arrival of a new presidential administration in late 2018 withdrew political support, and the SP was repealed on January 1, 2020. By then, the SP provided coverage to 52 million Mexicans (41 percent of the total population), the number of essential interventions had increased to 294, and the number of high-cost interventions had grown to 66 in nine broad disease clusters (CNPSS 2019).

This chapter aims to illustrate the life cycle of explicit priority setting in health in the context of the Mexican experience. It encompasses more than 30 years of policy progression starting in the early 1990s when MoH introduced the explicit definition of a set of cost-effective interventions to support the national vaccination campaigns and tackle maternal, newborn, and child mortality under a context of highly limited resources. It continues to 2020 with the dismantling of the SP alongside the two explicitly defined HBPs. For nearly 30 years, HBPs guided health coverage expansion paths. The story of the rise and fall of HBPs in Mexico provides valuable lessons to other countries at different stages of maturity of HBP design and implementation. Understanding accomplishments and shortfalls of explicit priority setting and the elements of sustainability can help guide efforts for UHC reforms. The benefits of targeted policy to increase access to health services through HBPs, particularly through the SP, are plenty and have been documented elsewhere (Frenk et al. 2006; Knaul et al. 2012; Knaul et al. 2023). This chapter is intended to provide a critical but constructive reflection of the key role of explicit priority setting and HBPs, from a health system and long-term perspective.

PRIORITY-SETTING PROCESS

Health inequalities—resulting from disparities in socioeconomic determinants, health financing, and access to quality care in a fragmented health care system—have long been a concern in Mexico. Those inequalities have led to significant disparities in health outcomes, with a nine-year difference in life expectancy at birth between the poorest municipality in the southern state of Guerrero and the affluent suburbs of the northern city of Monterrey (CONAPO 2019).

In 2000, health financing disparities translated into an average level of public per capita spending 2.1 times higher for the insured through social security than for the uninsured. Furthermore, federal expenditure per capita across the 32 states was 6.1 times higher in the state with the highest expenditure than in the one with the lowest. Differences in state per capita contributions to health care in the same year were even more dramatic, more than 100 times higher in the state with the highest expenditure than in that with the lowest (Knaul et al. 2012). It is in this context that continuing efforts to increase health care access and reduce health financing gaps across regions and populations have taken place over the last 30 years.

First encounters with explicit priority setting started in the early 1990s, when MoH led continuing efforts to improve children's health by building upon previously successful universal vaccination campaigns and the use of interventions—notably oral rehydration salts. Those efforts resulted in a package of highly cost-effective interventions embedded into National Health Weeks taking place twice per year and dedicated to children's health. From that experience emerged the notion that vertical programs could offer a first step to coverage expansion through a "diagonal approach" (box 12.2).

Box 12.2

The Diagonal Approach to Health Care

The medical literature has long debated which approach to delivering health interventions—a vertical program or a horizontal program—is more effective. Vertical programs refer to focused, proactive, disease-specific interventions on a massive scale, whereas horizontal programs refer to more integrated, demand-driven, resource-sharing health services. The debate represents a false dilemma because both interventions need to coexist in what could be called a diagonal approach, that is, the proactive, supply-driven provision of a set of highly cost-effective interventions that bridge health clinics and homes.

Mexico has a long tradition of prioritizing interventions with great impact on population health. Several cost-effective public health interventions implemented since 1985 explain the rapid declines in child mortality, particularly from diarrheal diseases in infants. Public health intervention packages included a series of cost-effective interventions of expanded immunization vaccine schemes, oral rehydration salts, micronutrients such as vitamin A and zinc, deworming with albendazole, and so on. Those interventions started as vertical programs and were later scaled up through National Health Weeks and finally mainstreamed into health benefits packages aiming toward universal health coverage, a strategy exemplifying the diagonal approach. Such incremental implementation of multiple public health interventions could be thought of as the equivalent of a public health "polypill."

Source: Sepúlveda et al. 2006.

Later, in 1996, MoH revisited the notion of an explicit intervention package as part of the Program for Extension of Coverage (Programa de Ampliación de Cobertura, PAC). At the time, MoH had resumed the devolution of health care provision to the states that had started in 1987 but lost momentum soon after as states pushed back because of budget uncertainty and political considerations. The new conditional transfers to deliver a package of basic services proposed under PAC provided policy incentives to strengthen stewardship in the devolved states. Covering 34 health care interventions in 13 different categories of community-based and preventive personal care, PAC was then adopted as the health component of the internationally recognized poverty alleviation conditional cash transfer program PROGRESA. PAC matured as a centrally managed program, but by 2001 it was evident that 34 covered interventions could not sufficiently support the chronically underserved, rural, and poor target populations (González-Pier et al. 2006) (box 12.3).

Box 12.3

Essential Interventions Covered by Mexico's Program for Extension of Coverage

The Program for Extension of Coverage (Programa de Ampliación de Cobertura) deemed essential those interventions that were high impact, low cost, technically feasible, and aligned to a restricted budget envelope. Within its scope, the package allowed the addition of other services according to regional priorities (for example, malaria, onchocerciasis, and dengue). The core of the essential package consisted of community-based and preventive interventions, community participation for self-care, and actions of collective benefit, in addition to health promotion and education and health care interventions. The package grouped interventions in the following 13 categories:

1. *Basic sanitation at the family level.* Control of harmful fauna, home water disinfection, sanitary disposal of garbage and excreta, and health education

2. *Family planning.* Orientation and distribution of contraceptive methods, identification of the population at risk, referral for IUD application, tubal ligation or vasectomy, cervical-vaginal cytology and infertility management, and education and health promotion

3. *Prenatal, delivery, postpartum, and newborn care.* Identification of pregnant women, prenatal consultations, application of tetanus toxoid, iron and folic acid supply, promotion of breastfeeding, identification and referral of women with high-risk pregnancy, family planning counseling, eutocic delivery care, immediate newborn care, screening and referral of newborns with problems, application of the Sabin and BCG vaccines to newborns, postpartum care, and health education

4. *Surveillance of child nutrition and growth.* Identification of children under five years of age, diagnosis, follow-up of the child without malnutrition, follow-up of the child with malnutrition, nutritional diagnosis, nutritional guidance, referral and counterreferral, training for mothers, micronutrient delivery, and health education

5. *Immunizations.* Vaccine administration and health promotion and education

6. *Case management of diarrhea at home.* Education and training for mothers, treatment of cases, distribution and use of rehydration serum sachets, referral of complicated cases, and health education

7. *Antiparasitic treatment for families.* Periodic administration of antiparasitics to the family and health education

8. *Management of acute respiratory infections.* Training for mothers, specific treatment, referral for treatment, and health education

9. *Prevention and control of pulmonary tuberculosis.* Identification of coughers, primary treatment, study of contacts and protection measures, reinforced treatment, and health education

10. *Prevention and control of arterial hypertension and diabetes mellitus.* Detection, diagnosis, treatment, and control of arterial hypertension; screening, diagnosis, treatment, and control of diabetes mellitus; and health education in arterial hypertension and diabetes mellitus

11. *Accident prevention and initial injury management.* First aid in case of wounds, burns, dislocations, unexposed fractures, open fractures, and poisonings; case referral; and health education and promotion

box continues next page

The introduction of the SP in 2003 built on Funsalud's 1994 reform proposals and World Health Organization evidence of Mexico's poor performance in financial protection. Funsalud's costed package of essential interventions extended previous ones and aligned cost-effective interventions with the leading causes of demand for health care services, mainly in primary care and general hospitalization settings.

Presidential political commitment was crucial in proposing a reform of the General Health Law to Congress in 2003. In 2000, for the first time in 70 years, a democratically elected president from an opposition party took office, allowing for the opportunity to translate the democratic principles of inclusiveness, equity, and citizenship-based rights into health reform. Along this line, the SP aimed to level the financial contributions and access to health care interventions across population groups, ensuring that access to health care depends on citizenship and not on employment status.

The introduction of HBPs under the SP involved building on previous HBP experience and a series of additional preparatory analyses undertaken by MoH. They included an in-depth analysis of supply-driven delivery of health interventions supported by line-item budget allocations at both federal and state levels, and the learnings of a pilot program in five states. The pilot helped refine the essential interventions package and secure buy-in from other states, informing discussions with MoF and members of Congress. During the negotiation of the reform in Congress and with state governors, political commitment was obtained by linking additional funding to the responsibility for enrolling the target population and delivering interventions covered in both packages.

The SP aimed at covering the uninsured 50 percent of the Mexican population (who had no access to social security). During a seven-year rollout period, population coverage was to be increased gradually alongside additional financial resources. Enrollment went up from 5.3 million in 2004 to 51.8 million in 2011, or 45 percent of the total population at the time. Over the following years, annual enrollment remained above 50 million, reaching a maximum of 57.3 million in 2014 (CNPSS 2019).

The SP had a financial tripartite scheme set into law, which included contributions from the federal and state governments and, to a lesser extent, from beneficiaries. All budgetary allocations to states were based on enrolled families according to prenegotiated rollout targets. To improve financial equity, the federal government would support the scheme with the same per-family contribution it had allocated to the population covered under the Mexican Institute of Social Security (Instituto Mexicano del Seguro Social). Using local revenues, states were required to contribute with a smaller per capita allocation in exchange for matching funds from the federal MoH. Those matching funds were adjusted using a formula that considered health needs, among other criteria. In theory, families would be charged a small means-tested co-insurance premium. Families from the poorest three income deciles were exempt; in practice, most SP beneficiaries did not pay into the system. Although allocations were initially set according to enrolled families, the rules changed in 2010 partly because of strategic gaming from some states that had room to modify the way they accounted for families.[3] In 2010, funding rules were redefined on a per-person basis to increase transparency and accountability (Knaul et al. 2012).

SP beneficiaries automatically had access to the coverage of two supplementary HBPs: the Universal Catalogue of Essential Interventions (Catálogo Universal de Intervenciones Esenciales en Salud, CAUSES) and the interventions covered through FPGC. Funding for CAUSES came from combined federal and state per capita allocations, except for an 8 percent share kept at the central level to fund FPGC. Financial rules and content revision of both packages occurred through separate processes. Those responsibilities fell under the SP National Commission (Comisión Nacional de Protección Social en Salud) run by the federal MoH that oversaw the SP in coordination with the 32 states.

Both CAUSES and FPGC packages covered personal health care interventions but followed different criteria for priority setting and processes for inclusion and revision mechanisms. CAUSES's guiding principles to include interventions followed mostly health-maximizing criteria informed by burden of disease and cost-effectiveness considerations with a resulting focus on primary care and general hospitalization. By contrast, FPGC focused on high-cost or high-specialty interventions that exposed families to financial hardship, but it followed less technically strict considerations. FPGC was also prone to pressures from a mix of political actors, social organizations, health professionals, and industry associations but was kept in check by hard financial feasibility constraints informed by actuarial studies. Both processes were supported by technical work, including costing, budget impact, or full health technology assessments developed by internal teams comprising budget officials and health system experts or external technical advisers. Collegiate bodies within MoH made and sanctioned decisions. Notably, although both HBPs largely guided service delivery of state health care networks and federal hospitals, a considerable yet unquantified volume of care fell outside the scope of the explicitly defined benefits packages, thus reflecting the fact that service providers need to respond to pressures not accounted for in HBPs, such as the need to continue providing care available before packages were in place, services provided to promote medical training, or those justified under a research protocol.

The pilot program costed and implemented a basic package of 78 interventions that aligned essential interventions covered earlier through PAC and PROGRESA and integrated other federally run vertical programs. That initial pilot package provided the basis for the definition and costing of CAUSES.[4] Eventually, CAUSES included 294 interventions (figure 12.1), covering most causes of demand in primary care and nearly 95 percent of all causes of admissions in general hospitals (González-Pier et al. 2006; Knaul et al. 2012).[5] State health services had responsibility for the direct delivery of CAUSES to the population enrolled in the SP. CAUSES included relatively low-cost and high-volume interventions, and the financial risk associated with budget holding could be diversified at the state level. In contrast, because of FPGC's focus on providing financial protection by covering high-cost/high-specialty interventions—including for some health conditions of low incidence but high financial risk—FPGC resources were retained and managed at the federal level to reimburse providers on a per case basis. The underlying rationale was to diversify the financial risk at the national level.

Figure 12.1 Evolution of Mexico's HBPs in the Context of the Seguro Popular, by Number of Interventions, 2004–20

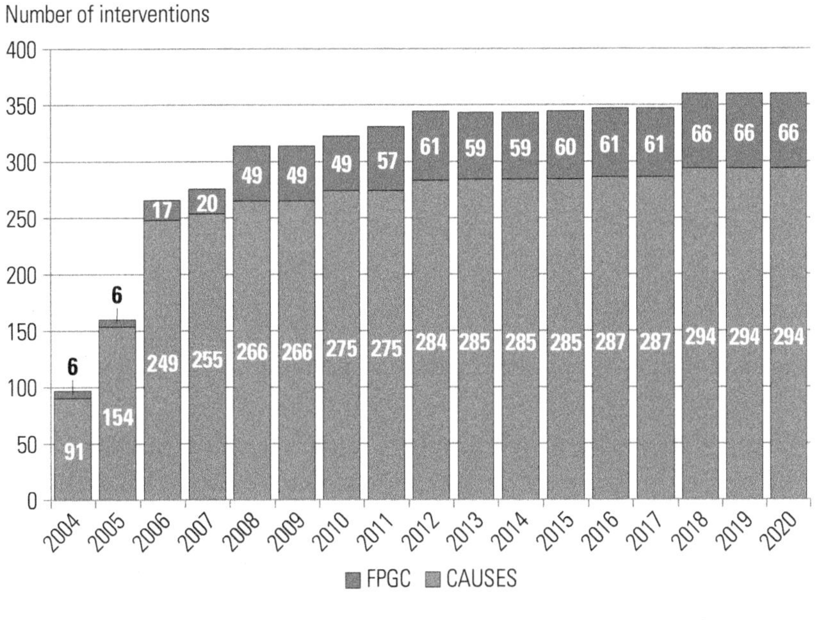

Number of interventions

FPGC ■ CAUSES

Source: Adaptation based on Knaul et al. 2012 and annual reports from the SP National Commission (Comisión Nacional de Protección Social en Salud).

Note: CAUSES = Catálogo Universal de Intervenciones Esenciales en Salud (Universal Catalogue of Essential Interventions); FPGC = Fondo de Protección para Gastos Catastróficos (Catastrophic Spending Protection Fund); HBPs = health benefits packages.

FPGC exemplifies the budget and delivery challenges countries face when expanding interventions beyond essential services. After the launch of FPGC in 2004 with six conditions and treatments (cervical/uterine cancer, acute lymphoblastic leukemia, prematurity, neonatal sepsis, respiratory distress syndrome, and ambulatory antiretroviral therapy), political pressure led to the inclusion of 66 conditions by 2019. In practice, having accumulated significant reserves over the initial implementation phase, FPGC became the main mechanism through which demands for coverage were channeled. That dynamic generated explicit choices and budget impact analysis in a more orderly fashion, yet concerns remain about how effectively the inclusion process balanced political and technical arguments. Political pressure—in some cases by organized patient groups and on inclusiveness grounds—led to the addition of some interventions; addition of others relied more on the technical arguments, including financial protection for both individuals and public institutions (CNPSS 2019; Lozano and Garrido 2015).

In some cases, covered interventions have legitimately and successfully increased financial protection, such as with various oncology treatments, including for children's cancers. In other cases, the need to balance inclusion demands with financial resources has resulted in age limits that contain the financial risk for public institutions but are hard to explain to society, especially procedures such as kidney transplants for illnesses that affect individuals throughout their lives. For years, pressure to include hemodialysis and end-stage renal disease coverage for the uninsured kept mounting without resulting in a clear decision. At 16.8 percent of adults, Mexico's prevalence of diabetes is one of the largest in the world (Basto-Abreu et al. 2021). Given the poor rates of controlled diabetic patients, chronic renal disease is one of the leading causes of mortality among Mexicans. However, coverage of replacement therapy for end-stage renal disease without limits would have resulted in significant crowding out effects for other interventions because no additional funding was anticipated for the SP. Thus, discussions mostly centered on the age threshold and criteria to cover renal transplants. In 2011, the intervention was finally included but only for individuals under 18 years old (CNPSS 2019; Lozano and Garrido 2015).

Hemophilia offers another example of such an age threshold for treatment. FPGC added treatment coverage in 2011, but only for children under 10 years old. Although its addition represented a positive result for a demand that had been on the agenda for a long time, the way it was defined created concerns about continuity of care for a lifelong disease and patients in need whose age exceeds the threshold.

Both CAUSES and FPGC catalogues remained separate from the provision of public health goods (such as epidemiological surveillance and vector control) and community-based and intersectoral interventions to tackle behavioral risk factors. Although the SP reform included a provision to create a specific fund to protect budgets for nonpersonal interventions from pressures to redistribute additional funding to personal interventions, that fund was never created. These nonpersonal interventions continue to be funded and managed centrally as vertical programs and delivered locally in parallel to the SP.

HBPs IMPLEMENTATION: CHALLENGES AND REPEAL PROCESS

The SP had significant achievements in terms of increased coverage, access to health care, and financial protection for its target population, as documented by Knaul et al. (2023); however, by 2019 it also faced a series of challenges (beyond those outlined in this section, which focuses on implementation of HBPs). Some of those challenges would have merited further policy adjustments or a subsequent reform, especially to consolidate or extrapolate some of the SP results to the overall health system. For example, despite increased coverage and budget allocations to fund the implementation and expansion of SP during its early years, public health spending's share of gross domestic product remained almost equal to the private share from 2016 until the COVID-19 pandemic.[6] In addition, resource pooling for catastrophic interventions was not expanded to the rest of the health system, and mechanisms to enable the cross-delivery between public health care providers had not been fully and effectively put in place. Furthermore, no major steps had been made to explore improvements in resource allocation within the states or to fully incentivize quality assurance through provider payments.

The challenges related to the implementation of HBPs under SP can be framed into three distinct phases. An initial phase related to the launch of the HBPs, with clinics and hospitals racing to deliver the mix of interventions initially listed in the packages. A second phase followed as HBPs matured and new interventions were added without a clear alignment with budgetary space or the human resources needed to deliver more complex and costly interventions. A more recent third phase took place when political and social pressure mounted around a set of excluded interventions that could not be added without significant additional resources and could not be technically justified on the grounds of value for money or significant reductions of the burden of disease. In 2020, by repealing the SP through a congressional reform, the government reverted to implicit rationing of health services, which allowed for less transparency in coverage decisions and more discretionally defined budget allocations to promote political and electoral benefits.

The initial offer of CAUSES and FPGC involved a mix of three groups of health interventions. The first group included interventions already fully offered at the time of the SP launch—for example, antenatal care, HIV services, hypertension and diabetes screening, and basic surgery. The initial HBPs simply recognized those interventions as part of the package, which allowed for a quick acknowledgement of available coverage. The second group consisted of interventions that, although offered, still showed considerable gaps across the continuum of care or inequitable access across geographies. The response was expedient and concentrated on improving the supply of pharmaceuticals and medical devices, and paying for extra time of staff already hired. The third group comprised new interventions requiring high-technology equipment that not only was more expensive to purchase but also challenged existing supply chain logistics and required highly trained personnel to operate. The single most important bottleneck to translating the packages into service delivery involved finding sufficient human resources for health in the form of specialized physicians, nurses, and technicians. Moreover, the supply response lagged across health inputs; for example, the lack of trained personnel to adequately prescribe medication or correctly interpret a mammogram rendered the timely purchase of drugs and imaging equipment ineffective. Poor coordination of care delivery was particularly acute in rural and underserved areas.

As delivery caught up with the scope of the HBPs, the second phase of implementation involved proposal and acceptance of new interventions into the HBPs without the corresponding adjustment in available budgets. The SP's financial rules were fixed by law, including per capita allocations for CAUSES delivery and funds used to directly reimburse certified providers on a cost per case basis in FPGC. Only inflation was used to update annual budget allocations. States' total budgets were set in line with the population enrolled. Inertial additions to both packages fueled by political and social pressures required either funding with additional enrollment targets or improved technical efficiencies in service delivery. As the system matured, it became increasingly difficult to sustain package expansion; reforming the health law again to mobilize additional resources faced sustained opposition from MoF because of limited fiscal space.

Finally, in the third phase of HBP implementation, relatively comprehensive HBPs lost momentum because of the lack of new funds and an insufficient longer-term supply response. HBP dynamics shifted from what to include to how to prevent inclusion of new interventions. Politically less palatable, the focus on exclusions raised concerns of inequality and discrimination. It also made the packages vulnerable to critique for failing to exercise the constitutional human right to health protection enshrined in the 1983 Mexican Constitution. Along populist lines, the new administration attacked the SP and its concomitant HBPs as the main obstacle to comprehensive health care for all. The SP was repealed and purportedly replaced in January 2020 by the National Institute of Health for Well-Being without any clear financial or operational rules or a detailed workplan on how to fulfill its mandate of unfettered UHC. A final challenge thus relates to sheltering HBPs from becoming politized and captured by populist ideology. Dismantling HBPs disempowers citizens, reduces transparency and accountability, and makes the health sector prone to serve political and electoral agendas.

LIMITATIONS AND FUTURE DIRECTIONS

Over the past 30 years, HBPs have not achieved their full potential as the cornerstone to UHC in Mexico. Limitations can be organized across the three subfunctions of health financing: resource mobilization, pooling, and purchasing. HBP expansion lost momentum when increased budget appropriations to fund additional coverage did not match the pressure to include new interventions. HBPs have the capacity to change the narrative when advocating for new resources: framing resource needs in terms of health conditions and the interventions needed to tackle them—rather than as budget line items—can help members of Congress, civil society organizations, and government officials relate more easily to the health sector. That reframing did not happen. Fiscal space for health could have improved if the benefits of excise taxes on sugar sweetened beverages, tobacco, alcohol, or other products deemed harmful for health had been linked to the cost of delivering a set of interventions explicitly listed in the HBP. In fact, new revenues could have been more easily earmarked for health under a properly communicated and functional HBP. Not doing so represents a missed opportunity to mobilize resources.

HBPs greatly improved equity of access at the subnational level only within the SP but failed to improve pooling and equity of access across national subsystems. The other main health insurance schemes, most notably social health insurance institutions and private health care plans, did not adopt the HBPs. In particular, FPGC was a missed opportunity to pool resources to fund risks for expensive health conditions that can be better diversified at the national level across the entire health system.

HBPs failed to make additional improvements to increase value for money. They remained mostly concentrated in facility-based (medical) interventions with no additions into community-based activities and intersectoral policies. Both packages had limited influence to guide long-term resource-generation strategies, basically infrastructure plans and training programs for health professionals. Quality and responsiveness elements of health care were not integrated into the BHP, and quality-assurance efforts were often disconnected from the priority-setting line of work.

LESSONS LEARNED AND OPPORTUNITY AREAS IDENTIFIED FOR FUTURE ANALYSIS

HBPs support country-specific pathways to achieve UHC by introducing an ordered way to make and legitimize decisions on which interventions to cover and for whom. Such decisions also require supporting information and evidence, transparent and rules-based deliberation mechanisms in place, standards of practice, and evaluation. Thus, HBPs are conducive to the development of accompanying information-based tools and decision-making processes, as well as regulations and policies supporting the health system to improve responsive and quality care needed to move forward in the chosen UHC pathway. Implementing an HBP also has implications in terms of guiding an adequately planned and funded human resource formation strategy.

The relevance and role of an HBP depends on which phase the country is in on its path to UHC. A country might choose to transition from positive lists that seek to promote access to negative lists that serve the role of gatekeeping to maintain value for money and allocative efficiency, and sometimes limit abuse of scarce resources. In general, HBP transitions are largely influenced by the stage of HBP implementation and health financing maturity, both in terms of sufficiency and sustainability of HBPs.

In the case of Mexico, dismantling an HBP-based funding scheme after 16 years of implementation entailed the loss of a pivotal element to guide the decision-making process leading to UHC. Eliminating HBPs will most likely not affect services operation in the short term—especially of primary care and general hospitalization interventions, which mostly follow an inertial logic as long as budgets are maintained. What could be missing is a set of rules and a convening platform to discuss the new technologies and interventions to be covered with additional resources. The latter has deeper implications for the high-cost and more complex interventions guided and funded by FPGC.

Just as this chapter analyzes the health system performance benefits derived from HBP implementation, the Mexican experience will generate a natural experiment to understand and document the effects of eliminating HBPs. The evolution along the following three elements that link HBPs with health system performance should be closely watched in the coming years:

1. *The role of HBPs in protecting health budgets and facilitating additional allocations.* HBP packages help bridge the gap between ministries of health advocating for increased funding and ministries of finance and other stakeholders defining fiscal space for health. Discussing health budgets in terms of health interventions, the population benefiting from improved coverage, and measurable access targets should resonate with members of Congress in charge of the budget appropriation process and MoF officials charged with drafting the initial budget proposals and release of allocated budgets. In the absence of CAUSES and FPGC, budget allocation to specific health areas should be affected in directions that remain to be seen (Soucat, González-Pier, and Tandon 2023).
2. *The weakening of MoH stewardship tools that operate in conjunction within HBPs.* HBP implementation tends to be accompanied by a series of measures and tools that feed and are reinforced by HBPs. Those measures and tools include a drug and devices formulary partly guided by health technology assessments, the requirement to provide a need certification to authorize large investments in medical equipment, clinical protocols and practice guidelines, continuous medical education and specialist training, and resource allocation rules. The dismantling of the HBPs might affect or lead to replacement of those elements.
3. *UHC sustainability through HBP-induced patient engagement and empowerment.* The lack of an explicit HBP should result in a loss of accountability and reduced empowerment of citizens to demand rights and access to specific interventions. Not setting explicit limits based on an agreed set of interventions might result in a reversion to rationing of services, which tends to be not only less efficient but also inequitable because wealthier populations and geographies generally have more voice and political influence to leverage health resources in their favor. The absence of HBPs can thus lead to a less vocal and engaged constituency for UHC reforms. Finally, changes in UHC performance indicators in terms of population coverage, access to quality services, and degree of financial protection should reflect the regime shift away from HBPs (box 12.4). The jury is still out.

Box 12.4

Replacement Model and Early Evidence on Its Effect

Mexico's Popular Health Insurance (Seguro Popular, SP) was formally repealed as of January 2020, just as COVID-19 entered the scene. The SP was replaced by the National Institute of Health for Well-Being (Instituto de Salud para el Bienestar, INSABI), with the intention of centralizing resources and functions previously undertaken by the states to provide health services for the population without social security. The new INSABI scheme eliminated previous rules defining federal and state budget allocations along with health benefits packages. The budget is now to be defined annually through the federal government budgeting process and, in principle, should not be less than the amount allocated in the previous year. In practice, states now must negotiate again with the federal government through INSABI and the Ministry of Finance for their annual budgets. Facing pandemic pressure, the government did not immediately enact any secondary rulings to detail further specifics of the new model to replace SP. Concomitantly, under the political leadership of the Mexican Institute of Social Security (Instituto Mexicano del Seguro Social, IMSS), a new proposal emerged to use IMSS-Bienestar as a platform to negotiate with the states regarding the centralization of their financial, human, and physical resources. IMSS-Bienestar—which provides basic primary and secondary care services through its own facilities to 11.6 million people living in marginalized urban and rural areas—receives federal government funding and is run by IMSS in parallel with IMSS's social security medical benefits service platform. In 2022, IMSS-Bienestar was granted an arms-length status to run services for the population without social security in those states that signed a centralization agreement. At present, 18 states have signed such agreements, and IMSS-Bienestar will replace INSABI as the entity responsible for providing services to people without social security. That responsibility includes the centralized procurement of health inputs and management of the Catastrophic Spending Protection Fund (Fondo de Protección para Gastos Catastróficos), which continues as the Wellness Health Fund and is financed through resources retained from budget allocations of states that have signed an agreement with IMSS-Bienestar.

Interestingly, dismantling the SP did not result in widespread rejection by SP beneficiaries. Notwithstanding the rejection to the reform by opposition political parties, approval of the reforms occurred without a major reaction from citizens. Negative reaction from former SP beneficiaries to recent policies changes has come mainly through demonstrations by families of children with cancer because of the widespread lack of medicines after the dismantling of the previous procurement process. The limited public reaction indicates that the intended promotion of entitlement and citizens' empowerment through the SP and health benefits packages did not permeate enough in SP beneficiaries.

So far, little evidence exists on the effect of replacing SP because no formal evaluation has been made to render the new scheme accountable. Some early results, however, can be drawn from national surveys in terms of coverage and financial protection. Notably, some of those results may reflect the combined effect of dismantling the SP and the COVID-19 pandemic, as well as some challenging trends observed in the later years of the SP.

box continues next page

- *Coverage.* The share of the population without access to health services (based on self-reported affiliation or explicit coverage from a public or private institution) increased from 16.2 percent (20.1 million) to 39.1 percent (50.4 million) between 2018 and 2022.
- *Financial protection.* The share of households facing catastrophic expenditures (at a 30 percent threshold of households' disposable income) between 2016 and 2020 showed a slight reduction from 2016 to 2018 (from 2.82 percent to 2.76 percent) and a significant increase from 2018 to 2020 (from 2.76 percent to 3.90 percent) according to a recent World Bank study on health financing sustainability and resilience in Mexico (World Bank 2023). That trend is consistent with recently published estimates by Knaul et al. (2023), which show in addition that excessive spending (that is, catastrophic or impoverishing expenditures) more than doubled between 2018 and 2020 for the uninsured compared with those who have social security.

Sources: CONEVAL 2023; IMSS 2023; IMSS-Bienestar 2022; Knaul et al. 2023; Presidencia de la República 2022, 2023; World Bank 2023.

NOTES

1. Based on data from United Nations Development Programme, Human Development Insights, https://hdr.undp.org/data-center/country-insights#/ranks; World Bank DataBank, World Development Indicators, https://databank.worldbank.org/source/world-development-indicators.
2. The National Development Plan represents the guiding document in each presidential administration; the plan for 2001–06 set five health objectives: ensure fairness in health financing, improve the health conditions of Mexicans, reduce health inequalities, guarantee adequate treatment in public and private health services, and strengthen the health system, particularly its public institutions.
3. States had incentives to register individuals 18 years and older living in the same household as single-person family units. The other argument related to the need to have more accurate enrollment targets. Family size was estimated using a national average that showed variations across states.
4. The package included interventions addressing specific diseases and/or population groups in the following service categories: preventive medicine (immunizations and detection, medical, psychological, diet and exercise counseling services); outpatient consultations (family medicine, community mental health services, reproductive health services); and urgent care, hospitalization, and surgical services (including pregnancy, childbirth, and newborn care).
5. Interventions reflected a combination of diseases covered and specific population groups as well as preventive and community health interventions.
6. Organisation for Economic Co-operation and Development, OECD Data Explorer, Health Expenditure and Financing, https://data-explorer.oecd.org/?fs[0]=Topic%2C1%7CHealth%23HEA%23%7CHealth%20expenditure%20and%20financing%23HEA_EXP%23&pg=0&fc=Topic&bp=true&snb=4.

REFERENCES

53rd World Health Assembly. 2000. *The World Health Report 2000: Health Systems: Improving Performance*. Geneva: World Health Organization.

Basto-Abreu, Ana, Nancy López-Olmedo, Rosalba Rojas-Martínez, Carlos A. Aguilar-Salinas, Vanessa De La Cruz-Góngora, Juan A. Rivera, Teresa Shamah-Levy, et al. 2021. "Prevalence of Diabetes and Glycemic Control in Mexico: National Results from 2018 and 2020." *Salud Publica de Mexico* 63 (6): 725–33.

CNPSS (Comisión Nacional de Protección Social en Salud). 2019. *Informe de Resultados del Sistema de Protección Social en Salud. Enero–Diciembre*. Ciudad de México: Secretaría de Salud.

CONAPO (Consejo Nacional de Población). 2019. "Proyecciones de la Población de los Municipios de México, 2015–2030." https://tabasco.gob.mx/sites/default/files/users /planeacion_spf/6._Proyecciones_de_la_población_de_los_municipios_de_México.pdf.

CONEVAL (Consejo Nacional de Evaluación de la Política de Desarrollo Social). 2023. "El Coneval presenta las estimaciones de pobreza multidimensional 2022." Comunicado No. 7, August 10, 2023, CONEVAL, Ciudad de México. https://www.coneval.org.mx/SalaPrensa /Comunicadosprensa/Documents/2023/Comunicado_07_Medicion_Pobreza_2022.pdf.

Frenk, Julio, ed. 1994. *Economía y Salud: Propuesta para el Avance del Sistema de Salud en México, Informe Final*. Ciudad de México: Fundación Mexicana para la Salud.

Frenk, Julio, Eduardo González-Pier, Octavio Gómez-Dantés, Miguel Angel Lezana, and Felicia Marie Knaul. 2006. "Comprehensive Reform to Improve Health System Performance in Mexico." *The Lancet* 368 (9546): 1524–34. https://doi.org/10.1016/S0140 -6736(06)69564-0.

González-Pier, Eduardo, Cristina Gutiérrez-Delgado, Gretchen A. Stevens, Mariana Barraza-Lloréns, Raúl Porras-Condey, Natalie Carvalho, Kristen Loncich, et al. 2006. "Priority Setting for Health Interventions in Mexico's System of Social Protection in Health." *The Lancet* 368 (9547): 1608–18. https://doi.org/10.1016/S0140-6736(06)69567-6.

IMSS (Instituto Mexicano del Seguro Social). 2023. "IMSS-Bienestar será el modelo de salud más importante a nivel mundial: Zoé Robledo." Press release, June 2023. http://www.imss .gob.mx/prensa/archivo/202306/298.

IMSS-Bienestar. 2022. "Padrón de Población Adscrita 2022: Programa IMSS Bienestar." Government of Mexico. https://www.imss.gob.mx/sites/all/statics/imssBienestar /estadisticas/01-PoblacionAtendida-2022.pdf.

Knaul, Felicia Marie, Hector Arreola-Ornelas, Michael Touchton, Tim McDonald, Merike Blofield, Leticia Avila Burgos, Octavio Gómez-Dantés, et al. 2023. "Setbacks in the Quest for Universal Health Coverage in Mexico: Polarised Politics, Policy Upheaval, and Pandemic Disruption." *The Lancet* 402 (10403): 731–46. https://doi.org/10.1016/S0140 -6736(23)00777-8.

Knaul, Felicia Marie, Eduardo González-Pier, Octavio Gómez-Dantés, David García-Junco, Héctor Arreola-Ornelas, Mariana Barraza-Lloréns, Rosa Hilda Hernández Sandoval, et al. 2012. "The Quest for Universal Health Coverage: Achieving Social Protection for All in Mexico." *The Lancet* 380 (9849): 1259–79. https://doi.org/10.1016/S0140-6736(12)61068-X.

Lozano, Rafael, and Francisco Garrido. 2015. *Improving Health Efficiency—Mexico: Catastrophic Health Expenditure Fund*. Geneva: World Health Organization. https://iris .who.int/handle/10665/186476.

OECD (Organisation for Economic Co-operation and Development). 2021. *Health at a Glance 2021: OECD Indicators*. Paris: OECD Publishing. https://www.oecd-ilibrary.org /social-issues-migration-health/health-at-a-glance-2021_ae3016b9-en.

Presidencia de la República. 2022. "Decreto por el que se crea el organismo público descentralizado denominado Servicios de Salud del Instituto Mexicano del Seguro Social para el Bienestar (IMSS-BIENESTAR)." Diario Oficial de la Federación August 31, 2022. https://www.dof.gob.mx/nota_detalle.php?codigo=5663064&fecha=31/08/2022#gsc.tab=0.

Presidencia de la República. 2023. "Decreto por el que se reforman, adicionan y derogan diversas disposiciones de la Ley General de Salud, para regular el Sistema de Salud para el Bienestar." Diario Oficial de la Federación, May 29, 2023. https://www.dof.gob.mx/nota _detalle.php?codigo=5690282&fecha=29/05/2023#gsc.tab=0.

Secretaría de Salud, Mexico. 2000. Acuerdo por el que la Secretaría de Salud da a conocer las Reglas de Operación Específicas del Programa de Ampliación de Cobertura. Diario Oficial de la Federación, March 14.

Sepúlveda, Jaime, Flavia Bustreo, Roberto Tapia, Juan A. Rivera, Rafael Lozano, Gustavo Olaiz, Virgilio Partida, Lourdes García-García, and José Luis Valdespino. 2006. "Improvement of Child Survival in Mexico: The Diagonal Approach." *The Lancet* 368 (9551): 2017–27. https://doi.org/10.1016/S0140-6736(06)69569-X.

Shamah-Levy, Teresa, Martín Romero-Martínez, Tonatiuh Barrientos-Gutiérrez, Lucía Cuevas-Nasu, Sergio Bautista-Arredondo, M. Arantxa Colchero, Elsa Berenice Gaona Pineda, et al. 2021. *Encuesta Nacional de Salud y Nutrición 2020 sobre Covid-19. Resultados nacionales.* Cuernavaca, México: Instituto Nacional de Salud Pública. https://ensanut.insp.mx/encuestas/ensanutcontinua2020/doctos/informes /ensanutCovid19ResultadosNacionales.pdf.

Soucat, Agnès, Eduardo González-Pier, and Ajay Tandon. 2023. "From Universal Health Coverage Services Packages to Budget Appropriation: The Long Journey to Implementation." *BMJ Global Health* 8 (Suppl 1): e010755. https://doi.org/10.1136/bmjgh -2022-010755.

World Bank. 1993. *World Development Report 1993: Investing in Health.* Washington, DC: World Bank.

World Bank. 2023. "Health Financing Sustainability and Resilience Assessment Report: Mexico Case Study." World Bank, Washington, DC.

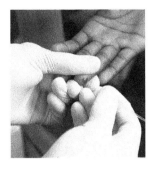

13

Toward Realization of Universal Health Coverage: Designing the Essential Health Benefits Package in Sudan

Jacqueline Mallender, Mohammed Musa, Faihaa Dafalla, Wael Fakiahmed, Mohammed Mustafa, Tayseer Abdelgader, Mark Bassett, Samia Yahia, and Reza Majdzadeh

ABSTRACT

Sudan's transitional government is striving to realize universal health coverage in the context of serious economic, political, and social challenges. To that end, it developed an essential health benefits package, selecting interventions using evidence provided by the World Health Organization Regional Office for the Eastern Mediterranean using evidence sourced from the Disease Control Priorities, among other sources. Health financing for the benefits package remains a challenge, however. The country plans to phase implementation at the state level as funding permits, and to implement institutional arrangements for sustainability. At the time of writing, the armed conflict between the Sudanese Armed Forces and the Rapid Support Forces had halted progress.

INTRODUCTION

Sudan, a vast Northeast African country, shares borders with seven neighboring countries. With a federal structure comprising 18 states, the country has a huge diversity of culture and language across its vast geography. The predominantly young and rural population of Sudan, estimated at about 49 million, is growing by 2.6 percent per annum; life expectancy at birth is 65 years.[1]

Conflict has significantly affected the Sudanese economy. Gross domestic product fell at an estimated rate of 1 percent per annum in 2022, with current gross domestic product per capita estimated at US$1,102 and hyperinflation estimated at 139 percent.[2] The population has also felt the impact of conflict. The United Nations High Commissioner for Refugees reported 1.1 million refugees and asylum seekers and 3.7 million internally displaced people as of December 2022.[3]

In April 2019, Sudan embarked on a transition from the Federal Republic to a new democratic political system, supported by a power-sharing agreement between civilians and the military. That transition was embodied in the establishment of a Sovereign Council and a civilian prime minister. Since October 2021, a military leader has headed the Sovereign Council. Despite ongoing work to agree on the next steps for the transitional government—with facilitation support provided from the the African Union, the Intergovernmental Authority on Development, and the United Nations—the country has experienced armed conflict since April 2023 between the Sudanese Armed Forces and the Rapid Support Forces. As of June 2023, that conflict had resulted in more than 2,000 deaths and internal and overseas displacement of a further 1.9 million people. The ongoing conflict has already caused significant damage to the health system and infrastructure, and a severe economic contraction is expected.[4]

Initially, the transitional government hoped that gaining access to international capital flows would help the country address poverty and the associated poor nutrition, health, and education outcomes that undermine well-being, productivity, and investment. The government made significant progress in the implementation of reforms and policy adjustments agreed with the International Monetary Fund and the World Bank (World Bank 2020). However, the challenging economic situation and the withdrawal of foreign aid following the Sovereign Council's change in leadership have hampered the government's efforts. The World Bank now classifies Sudan as a heavily indebted poor country.

Sudan's Major Health Challenges

Many people in Sudan are at very high risk of exposure to major infectious diseases, including food- or waterborne diseases like typhoid, vector-borne diseases such as malaria, water contact (schistosomiasis), animal contact (rabies), and respiratory diseases. Malnutrition presents a major risk factor issue, and communicable diseases and complications of pregnancy and birth still contribute to the top 10 causes of death and disability.[5] Those figures predate the impact of the COVID-19 pandemic.

COVID-19 and the current armed conflict have made a very challenging situation significantly worse. Sudan currently needs extraordinary aid. According to the mid-May 2023 Humanitarian Response Plan, 24.7 million people need help

(57 percent increase since 2022). The Humanitarian Response Plan targets 18.1 million more people than before the conflict; 11 million people, including 2.4 million people with disabilities, need emergency care for life-threatening physical and mental health concerns. Preconflict Integrated Food Security Phase Classification research in Sudan anticipated that 11.7 million people would be food insecure in 2023 (Phase 3 or worse), including 3.1 million in Phase 4 (emergency) and 8.6 million in Phase 3 (crisis).[6] Currently, their numbers are rising.

Conflict and endemic, waterborne, and vector-borne diseases such as hemorrhagic fevers, vaccine-preventable diseases, and malaria will certainly kill many in the country. The "Measuring the Availability and Affordability of Selected Medicines in Sudan" research concluded that just 31 percent of vital medicines are publicly available, requiring individuals to use private facilities (FMoH 2022a). Hunger and poor coverage of the extended immunization campaign make children under five years vulnerable to vaccine-preventable diseases. Measles vaccination coverage fell to 60 percent in 2022 and varied by region: 56 percent in South Darfur, 54 percent in West Kordofan, 50 percent in Central Darfur, 49 percent in South Kordofan, 46 percent in East Darfur, and 43 percent in Red Sea. Among young people under 15, 3.7 million need measles vaccination, and 700,000 children under five years missed Penta 3 vaccinations. As of September 2022, 10 states had reported 886 measles cases. As many as 50,000 children may also go without sustenance.

A recent report also shows significant challenges related to the health workforce in terms of management, training, funding, and distribution—all of which will have worsened because of the conflict (World Bank 2023). Productivity is down nationwide. Damage to food-manufacturing facilities and markets has disrupted production, so the private sector will need financial and technical help from the international community (particularly from international financial institutions through concessional loans) to restore economic activity and generate employment. Thus, public financing has drastically decreased, public health spending is at a 50-year low, and the country primarily relies on foreign support, estimated at US$1.7 billion in 2023.

Health Financing in Sudan

At the time of writing, the most recent published health accounts reflect data for 2018 (refer to table 13.1 for a summary). In 2018, health expenditure (at about US$60.80 per capita) represented 4.95 percent of gross domestic product. That amount compared with US$132.30 in 2015, a drop largely due to the fall in the exchange rate. General government health expenditure comprises federal and state government expenditure, and social health insurance (the National Health Insurance Fund [NHIF]) was 23.28 percent of current health expenditure; an increase from 14.9 percent in 2015. Out-of-pocket expenditure was relatively high at 66.95 percent of current health expenditure.

Table 13.1 Summary of Health Accounts for Sudan, 2018

Category	
Total population	41,984,512
Exchange rate (SD to US$)	23.8
GDP per capita (SD/US$)	29,270/1,230
CHE as share of GDP (%)	4.95
Per capita health expenditure (SD/US$)	1,448/60.8
GGHE (SD/US$)	337/14.2
GGHE as share of GDP (%)	1.15
GGHE as share of current health expenditure (%)	23.28
Social health insurance (National Health Insurance Fund) as a share of GGHE (%)	27.62
Household OOP expenditure as share of CHE (%)	66.95
Private health expenditure as a share of CHE (%)	70.3
Donor expenditure as a share of CHE (%)	6.42

Source: WHO 2018.

Note: CHE = current health expenditure; GDP = gross domestic product; GGHE = per capita general government health expenditure; OOP = out of pocket; SD = Sudanese pound.

Health System Reform in Sudan

Despite those challenges, for many years, Sudan has aspired to increase coverage of health services and to improve the efficiency and effectiveness of its health system. The universal health effective coverage index increased from 27.5 in 1990 to 51.8 in 2019. Although NHIF has relatively broad coverage, it has relatively low depth of service coverage overall as shown by high levels of out-of-pocket expenditure. Sudan has been part of the Universal Health Coverage Partnership of the World Health Organization (WHO) for the last decade, and the new government has a strong political commitment to improve health care and population health. Currently, the Federal Ministry of Health (FMoH) and NHIF are collaborating to refresh and renew related policies and strategies as part of the newly developed National Health Sector Recovery and Reform Strategic Plan 2022–24 (FMoH 2022b).

As part of that plan, FMOH and NHIF have sought to identify and cost an essential health benefits package (EHBP) to include health care interventions that should ultimately be accessible to the entire population of Sudan. Their work will help inform the development of consistent and standardized clinical protocols and pathways and help identify investment and associated health financing requirements going forward. It will also help inform decisions about revenue contributions from government sources (such as taxation), contributions through the national health insurance, and requirements for risk pooling. This chapter describes the approach taken to designing the EHBP and plans for further development and implementation after the conflict.

DEVELOPING AN ESSENTIAL HEALTH BENEFITS PACKAGE

In 2019, FMoH and NHIF embarked on a joint project to develop an EHBP for citizens of Sudan, with guidance from WHO's Sudan Office and supporting expertise funded by the European Union. The project was governed by a Supervisory Committee chaired jointly by the Undersecretary of FMoH and the NHIF manager and comprising senior representatives of both organizations. A Technical Working Group made up of representatives from both FMoH and NHIF provided day-to-day oversight of the project and its associated tasks. The Supervisory Committee established 13 clinical expert teams comprising senior Sudanese health clinicians, public health experts, and representatives from FMoH programs and departments to provide support and advice on the prioritization process. It set up a core project team to include members of WHO's Sudan office and with the support of experts from Economics by Design Ltd. in collaboration with the University of East Anglia. The project consulted practitioners and stakeholders from state ministries of health and other state government bodies, medical societies, and civil society organizations. The project resulted in a published report (Mallender, Bassett, and Mallender 2020), with results subsequently validated in a large consensus-building workshop involving all stakeholders. The process did not include patient or public representatives, or representatives from industry.

The project ran between December 2019 and September 2020 and included the following steps:

1. *Development of approach.* The development involved a review of international frameworks for designing the EHBP and subsequent agreement on a practical approach with local stakeholders.
2. *Current state assessment.* A current state assessment was undertaken to identify needs, opportunities, challenges, and barriers and to inform priority setting.
3. *Objective setting.* A stakeholder event identified a clear consensus that the EHBP should prioritize financial protection, coverage, quality, and safety and equity.
4. *Categorizing interventions.* A categorizing framework of programs and subprograms for the EHBP list of candidate interventions was developed using draft guidance from the WHO Eastern Mediterranean Regional Office (EMRO) and input from local clinical expert teams.
5. *Priority setting.* Interventions were prioritized on the basis of (1) how well they each addressed need, (2) strong locally relevant supporting evidence, and (3) potential value for money (cost-effectiveness).
6. *Costing.* This step involved the development of local intervention costs to inform an assessment of health financing requirements over time.
7. *Institutionalization.* Proposals were developed for the Institutional and Governance Arrangements for the EHBP going forward, along with an associated road map for implementation.
8. *Capacity building.* This step involved interactive and online training for the ongoing development and implementation of the EHBP.

The original project timeline envisaged completion by April 2020, but the COVID-19 pandemic disrupted that timeline. Work did continue with individuals working remotely and with online delivery of workshops and training. However, the availability of clinical experts was limited because they rightly prioritized the need to respond to the pandemic. FMoH planned to start implementing the EHBP during 2023, funding permitting.

Current Health Benefits Package

The government of Sudan offers its population a minimum health services package that consists mainly of primary care, including medical consultations, routine and laboratory diagnostic tests, and imaging. Although very broad in principle, the current package lacks clarity on selection criteria and specificity. The package includes promotion of child health (immunization against vaccine-preventable diseases, nutrition counseling, growth monitoring, and implementation of integrated management of childhood illnesses package); promotion of reproductive health (safe motherhood and family planning); treatment of common health problems and control of endemic diseases (malaria, tuberculosis, HIV/AIDs, schistosomiasis, and so on); protection and promotion of environmental health and sanitation; treatment of simple diseases, injuries, and mental health; and basic and comprehensive emergency obstetric care. FMoH, in consultation with NHIF, updates a comprehensive list of essential medicines each year. State ministries of health also hold separate lists of medicines at the state level. People covered under health insurance are required to co-pay the cost of medicines (25 percent). Many challenges and issues affect the delivery of the current package, which goes some way in explaining the scale of out-of-pocket expenditure on health. Despite broad coverage, huge geographic variation exists in practice in the quality and availability of many basic health care interventions, and local stakeholders face great challenges in fulfilling commitments to the population.

Selecting Interventions for Inclusion in the EHBP

Designed to cover the entire health system of Sudan, the EHBP encompassed primary health care, secondary care, and specialist tertiary services. Some interventions are already available to citizens (for example, access to malaria nets and to parental advice and support through the essential mother and child health program). Some interventions would require modest expansion (for example, access to meningitis A vaccine for infants) and could be achieved relatively quickly. Others would require significant development in workforce and/or infrastructure (for example, comprehensive antenatal care services). For those reasons, all the candidate interventions for inclusion in the health packages were assessed in terms of current coverage and practical feasibility of coverage expansion over 10 years. Intersectoral and multisectoral interventions were not considered for inclusion in the EHBP because they would be initiated separately as part of a Health-in-All Policies agenda rather than funded directly by health insurance or government health spending.

The WHO EMRO provided draft guidance on the development of priority benefit packages. The draft guide was accompanied by a draft database of interventions classified by program and subprogram. At this stage, the interventions are not consolidated as clinical pathways. It was agreed instead that consolidation would take place once the list of essential interventions had been developed and a first round of prioritization completed. Assessing the interventions as part of clinical pathways is the next stage of development of the EHBP. For each intervention, the WHO EMRO received the following information:

- Package (program and subprogram)
- Intervention description
- Minimum qualification for service provider (health care professional)
- Preferred or minimum level of care (care setting/outlet)—service delivery platform
- Commentary
- Proposed by (source of the evidence base).

Information sources included published guidelines from, for example, WHO and European Union sources, evidence from Cochrane Reviews, and *Disease Control Priorities*, third edition. Interventions were not prioritized at this stage but were instead treated as candidates for Sudan's EHBP. Some health system program interventions were included in the prioritization and costed.

The list was shared with the clinical expert teams, which added and adapted the list of interventions to best match local assessment of need and evidence of effectiveness in context. The result was an expanded list of 740 interventions (the table in annex 13A shows the number of interventions by program and subprogram). For example, in the cardiovascular and respiratory diseases category, selected interventions included the following:

- Anticoagulation for medium- and high-risk nonvalvular atrial fibrillation
- Care of acute stroke and rehabilitation in stroke units, including treatment of acute ischemic stroke with intravenous thrombolytic therapy
- Long-term management of ischemic heart disease, stroke, and peripheral vascular disease with aspirin, beta blockers, angiotensin-converting enzyme inhibitors (ACEi), and statins (as indicated) to reduce risk of further events
- Long-term combination therapy for persons with multiple cardiovascular disease (CVD) risk factors, including screening for CVD in community settings using non-lab-based tools to assess overall CVD risk
- Management of acute coronary syndromes with aspirin, unfractionated heparin, and generic thrombolytics (when indicated)
- Mass media messages concerning healthy eating or physical activity
- Mass media messages concerning use of tobacco and alcohol
- Medical management of acute heart failure
- Medical management of heart failure with diuretics, beta-blockers, ACEi, and mineralocorticoid antagonists

- Opportunistic screening for hypertension for all adults and initiation of treatment among individuals with severe hypertension and/or multiple risk factors
- Primary prevention of rheumatic fever and rheumatic heart diseases by increasing appropriate treatment of streptococcal pharyngitis at the primary care level
- Provision of aspirin for all cases of suspected acute myocardial infarction.

Each intervention was accompanied by an intervention description, an assessment of the minimum qualification for the health care professional providing the service, a preferred care setting (service delivery platform), the target population for the intervention, and any published source for the evidence of effectiveness or guideline recommendations.

Method Used for Priority Setting

The approach for prioritization was based on simple multicriteria decision analysis. Criteria for prioritization were agreed, with each criterion then assigned a weight to reflect its relative importance. Each intervention was then scored on a range of 0–5 to reflect how well it met the criteria. The resulting weighted scores allow for a prioritization assessment.

In two workshops, local stakeholders from FMoH and NHIF agreed on the differentiating criteria to enable comparison of the interventions with each other and prioritization. At the first workshop, stakeholders agreed on a relatively simple structure with only three criteria:

1. *Meets health need (and population impact).* The intervention addresses high-priority needs in terms of the epidemiology of Sudan based on causes of morbidity and mortality, and scale of impact.
2. *Quality of evidence.* The intervention is likely to be effective in the context of Sudan.
3. *Likely value for money.* The intervention is likely to offer good value in the context of Sudan (considering cost-effectiveness with higher priorities given to primary and wider social determinants of health).

At the second workshop, stakeholders agreed that, all other things being equal, interventions meeting health need and having high population impact are to be preferred over interventions with high-quality evidence of effectiveness and good value for money. Importantly, that decision did not mean that the stakeholders felt that quality of evidence and value for money are in themselves less important. Moreover, the draft database of interventions provided by the WHO EMRO came from research showing evidence of effectiveness and value. However, there was concern that the evidence used to score interventions against the effectiveness criteria came mainly from more developed countries and that small relative differences in the source would not be as important in the context of Sudan.

The evidence used to score interventions in terms of their value impact was considered less robust and thus assigned a lower relative weight.

Stakeholders at the second workshop agreed on mean average weights, with quality of evidence and value for money assigned equal importance of 20 percent each, population health need and population impact attracting a weight of 60 percent. Using these weights, interventions that earn high scores for health need and population impact but low scores for quality of evidence and likely value for money will rank higher than interventions that earn high scores for quality of evidence and value for money but low scores for health need and population impact.

Each intervention was assigned a score between 1 (very low) and 5 (very high) against each of the criteria. International expert advisers at the University of East Anglia independently assigned the initial scores using a simple scoring schema for each. Two researchers undertook the scoring independently of each other, with discrepancies referred to a third researcher for resolution. The draft scores went to the clinical expert groups for review and validation, or amendment, as required and to reflect local circumstances. A provisional list of priority interventions was then identified by combining the weights and the scores.

The clinical teams were also asked to assess the extent to which services already existed across Sudan (measured by current population coverage) and the technical feasibility of achieving coverage of more than 75 percent of the target population within three years and seven years. That exercise enabled a high-level strategic assessment of time frames associated with the development at scale, across the country, of each intervention. Finally, stakeholders from different health programs and from national and subnational and relevant agencies reviewed all interventions, defining the most critical, but have not yet finalized medical equipment needed by the level of care.[7]

Sudan is a wide and diverse country with different epidemiological characteristics; therefore, a wide range of defined EHBP interventions might be implemented differently according to the regional context. For that reason, regional workshops will follow to adopt regional interventions and address the local community need.

Using Evidence to Inform Priority Setting

The scoring schema used to prepare the initial scores were based on data and evidence relevant for each of the prioritization criteria. In the absence of comprehensive needs assessments and projections for the population of Sudan, the team used data from the Global Health Data Exchange to estimate levels of need and population impact. Specifically, data were extracted to show the percentage of total disability-adjusted life years (DALYs) attributed to different disease areas for Sudan for 2017. The percentage of DALYs for each disease area was transformed into a quintile distribution of DALYs that could be used to measure need and population impact. Each disease area was mapped into one of five categories based on the percentage of total DALYs accounted for by that disease area. Interventions were then mapped to each disease and assigned a score of 1–5 depending on which disease area they related to. Some risk hazards and public health interventions do not map directly to a specific disease area—for example, COVID-19 and other emerging or reemerging diseases and all hazard risks (such as floods). For such interventions, an attempt was made to match the intervention to the expected health impact of the hazard.

Many of the interventions were proposed because of existing evidence review processes. For those reasons, a more pragmatic approach was adopted to assess the quality of evidence, based on the likely reliability of the source of the evidence included in the database. A scoring schema was developed allowing evidence to be scored on a scale of 1–5. Interventions included in the WHO official guidance attracted the highest score (5), and local anecdotal evidence attracted the lowest score (1).

For value for money, the project team considered using standard databases of cost-effectiveness such as the Tufts Medical Center Global Health Cost-Effectiveness Analysis Registry, to inform the scoring of interventions. For the following reasons, however, the standard databases of cost-effectiveness were not considered suitable at this stage of development of the methodology:

- The databases include a variety of possible definitions of cost-effectiveness, which make them hard to compare. These definitions include
  - Simple cost-efficiency studies (the most efficient way of delivering an outcome measured in natural units—for example, number of deaths);
  - Cost-utility studies (the most efficient way of delivering an outcome measured using standard utility metrics, such as quality-adjusted life years); and
  - Cost-benefit studies (to demonstrate the ratio or value of benefits to costs measured in monetary units).
- For health interventions (pharmacological, devices, or treatment interventions), cost-effectiveness is usually calculated measuring the "marginal" impact of the intervention compared with usual care or a "standard of care." Databases' definitions of usual care and standard of care differ considerably and are also context specific and vary by geography and health system. For the purpose of developing a health benefits package, the usual care is "no care"—rarely the comparator in the economics databases.
- Intervention costs, which are very context specific, vary considerably. Thus, informing local decision-making requires local economic evaluation, which is specific to the intervention in context.
- The value associated with the quality-adjusted life year, often used as the standard utility metric to compare the technical efficiency of different interventions, varies. It is also context specific.

The diversity of study designs and comparators, and the challenges with translating results to a Sudanese context necessitated a more pragmatic approach. As an alternative, the project team developed a simple scoring schema that assigned a score of 1–5 on potential value for money of interventions based on their care setting, disease/risk prevention capability, and stage in the care pathway.

Estimating Intervention Costs

Separately, detailed costing has been prepared for each intervention to show the budget impact of including those services within the EHBP. The international expert led the costing analysis to support the design of the benefits package, and to facilitate the building of a framework and tools to implement it. In a collaborative approach a national team was created to facilitate the costing process, which was composed of the national consultancy and FMoH, with technical and financial support from NHIF and WHO. The costing team was assigned to provide estimates of the potential costs of adopting each intervention at scale in Sudan. The approach taken included a bottom-up costing to include an assessment of

- Protocols and associated activities required for each intervention,
- The population need associated with each intervention,
- Staffing requirements (type and time),
- The care setting and delivery platform,
- Consumables required to support the delivery of the intervention, and
- Overheads associated with the previous items.

The process also used a top-down program budget approach, when appropriate, based on international benchmarks. For the cost of services, the main reference of the interventions' case management was lists of protocols developed by the program technical groups and clinical experts who selected and designed the package mainly using the national program's protocols. If those were not available, then WHO guidelines and standards were used.

Following discussion with the FMoH team, the stakeholders agreed that the OneHealth Tool would be the most appropriate starting point for the costing because it was structured to support the WHO guidance that underpinned many of the selected candidate interventions. The tool also contained default data of potential value in the absence of local information for Sudan. The tool was customized and updated accordingly, and all default data reviewed, edited, and adapted to the country context. Program costs were estimated using a top-down approach. No attempt was made to estimate the health outcomes impact of the interventions because data were not available to support that analysis and because the agreed scope of work for the project did not cover it. Annex 13B provides an overview of the costing methodology.

The cost of current coverage for the initial list of 740 interventions came to an estimated US$1.4 billion based on 2020 prices. Looking solely at the feasibility and time scales of growth and development (driven by infrastructure and staffing requirements), and to achieve target population coverage of 75 percent for each intervention, funding requirements for 2023–24 would increase to an estimated US$2.4 billion. With funding support, the program could achieve full coverage for all interventions by 2030 (notwithstanding growth in demand) at a total cost of US$4.3 billion (2020 prices, 2020 population).

The estimated first-year cost based on current coverage is US$29.3 per capita. Although that first-year cost falls far below per capita health expenditure (US$60), with 67 percent of health spending financed by out-of-pocket payments, financing even the current cost of those services from public funds will be very challenging. Priorities will therefore need to be set according to the availability of health financing, health workforce, and associated infrastructure.

EHBP IMPLEMENTATION PLANS

The National Health Sector Recovery and Reform Strategic Plan 2022–24 sees health services delivery as the main driving instrument for reform of Sudan's health system, and the EHBP as the principal prioritizing tool for effective health interventions and efficient resource use. The EHBP is part of a wider program of reform, including provider payment models and health financing. The health system is also expected to change with a move toward integrated people-centered health systems including primary health care, and intersectoral strategies implemented for localities, provider networks for areas within states, integrated health services for each state, and the development of regionally based tertiary care.

Delivering the Essential Health Benefits

The model of care will be rolled out nationally, together with the technical support for its implementation. Implementation will be phased at the state level. The benefits package will guide the design of the model, which will be adopted and adapted at the local level.

The integrated people-centered health systems at the primary health care level will be implemented through the family health approach. The approach builds upon the identification of the benefits package for each level, identification of the health provider level and skill set, and organizational arrangements (for example, catchment area, referral system, and information system). Subsequently, the benefits package will be enabled by strategies for workforce development, digital health, information technology, supply chain management, and reformed governance arrangements.

The newly designed EHBP is intended to cover Sudan's entire health system and encompass primary health care, secondary care, and specialist tertiary services. Some interventions are already available, some would require modest expansion, and others would require significant development in the workforce and/or infrastructure. The implementation arrangements will keep the package contextualized and adaptable to the future changes in demography and burden of disease. A primary health care mapping survey has taken place in most of Sudan, and information from that survey will address several questions needed to inform the implementation arrangement. Those steps will be taken into consideration during the implementation phase.

With the current war raging since April 2023 and the significant vacuum in health financing, planning for health interventions and successful services delivery funding has required additional emergency prioritization. Consequently, additional prioritization of the EHBP has been undertaken and five criteria agreed upon: illness severity, socioeconomic features, financial protection, disease burden, and practicality and acceptability. Review of all EHBP interventions against those criteria resulted in identification of 280 interventions and 1,818 subactions, which are now being taken forward as emergency priorities.

Health Financing

The health financing strategy combines state and federal tax funding, compulsory insurance premiums collected from those employed in the formal sector, and additional voluntary premiums from citizens as demanded. The intention is to pool state and federal tax funding, combined with funds from international donors, to pay for essential services. Compulsory insurance combined with Zakat will fund a more comprehensive package for the insured population (including the registered poor who will be passported to these services). That package will be combined with a new division of functions into purchasing, provision, and regulation. Purchasers will use new effective provider payment modalities to allocate resources to providers for the delivery of services included in the EHBP. The precise allocation of funding sources to benefits package interventions is yet to be agreed.

Institutionalizing Essential Health Benefits: Ongoing Review and Development

The project team made extensive recommendations for the institutionalization and governance of the program going forward, including proposals for revising the benefits package and for monitoring and evaluation. A document on institutionalization, alongside the development of a service package, was prepared and included as a dedicated chapter in the final technical report (Mallender, Bassett, and Mallender 2020). It proposed a set of governance conventions, management actions, and resources needed to institutionalize the EHBP and related financial mechanisms from 2020 to 2025. The distinctive feature of the document is that the EHBP will ultimately be compatible with the broader governance of Sudan's health system. The document identified all essential functions and activities needed through the five-year period along with the associated governance arrangements. It also defined advisory groups and technical panels, as required, and prepared terms of reference.

Figure 13.1 summarizes the proposed governance structure, showing a national health care board (chaired by the Federal Minister of Health and co-chaired by the Federal Minister of Social Development) for governance and three subordinate boards for delivery, financing, and policy issues. In addition, a dedicated EHBP team will coordinate EHBP activities with input from expert panels. The panels cover various EHBP development areas such as education and training, and monitoring and evaluation. Of the bodies defined as responsible for implementation, NHIF will hold and disburse pooled health care funds, and federal and state ministries of health will cover the sustainable delivery of the EHBP by government-owned health resources and/or in partnership with the private or third sector, meeting standards and targets for efficacy, safety, and values.

Figure 13.1 Proposed Institutional Arrangements for Ongoing Review and Development of Essential Health Benefits

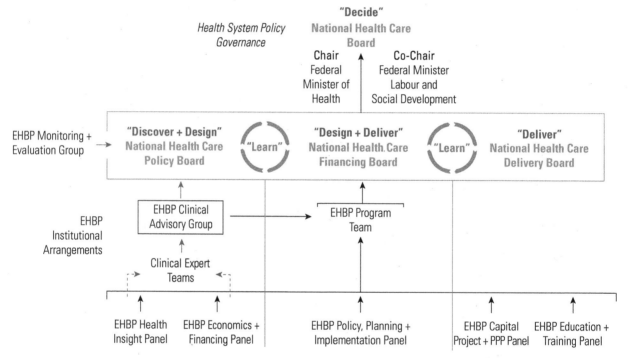

Source: Mallender, Bassett, and Mallender 2020.

Note: EHBP = essential health benefits package; PPP = patient and public participation.

At the time of writing, the final proposals are still under development. However, there is a commitment to ensuring the development of capacity, infrastructure, and governance to oversee the EHBP as a long-term program, maturing into "business as usual." Institutionalization of EHBP development was also considered one of the major milestones in the National Health Sector Recovery and Reform Strategic Plan with distinctive performance indicators to measure the progress toward institutionalization. Since undertaking the work in Sudan, the Joint

Learning Network has also published a guide to health benefits package revision (JLN 2022). That guide features the Sudan case study in relation to the design of the institutionalization of the benefits package.

Wider Health System Reform

The National Health Sector Recovery and Reform Strategic Plan provides a model of care that puts the health services benefits package at the heart of the reform. The plan's vision clearly states, "All people in Sudan enjoy high quality, equitable Access to Essential Health Service and are protected from Emergencies towards a Healthier, Fairer and Safer future" (FMoH 2022b). Thus, it is accompanied by sectorwide reform to be rolled out nationally and demonstrated in a phased manner. The reform includes governance reform, hospital sector reform, emergency care reform, and human resources reform. The governance reform includes revision and updates of health and health-related laws and regulations, such as the Public Health Act, which includes affirmation of primary health care services as a basic right for the people of Sudan.

The National Human Resources for Health Strategy for 2030 aims to provide guidelines for the governance, requirements, hiring, and transfer of human resources based on the identified minimum health services packages. It also states that the criteria and standard working conditions and enabling environment for health workers (such as physical infrastructure, support staff, supplies, and equipment) will be based on the identified services packages at different levels of care.

LIMITATIONS AND FUTURE DIRECTIONS

The COVID-19 pandemic has undoubtedly slowed progress on the project because it diverted attention to addressing the immediate population health need. Notwithstanding the pandemic's impact, several critical success factors and several challenges affected the project (refer to table 13.2 for a summary).

Important things to consider as Sudan moves its health system from the current state toward achieving its long-term goals include the immense transformation involved in the process and how best to ensure continuing improvement and development while the country invests in enabling longer-term changes. Such investment will support workforce training and development; the physical environment (health clinics and hospitals); digital infrastructure and digital health technologies; and equipment, supplies, and supply chains. Parallel investments will be needed in operational and financial management capabilities and capacity. For those reasons, the project team recommended an implementation road map for the near-term tactical transformation required to improve current services, as well as a road map that sets out the steps needed to establish a long-term plan for strategic transformation and associated investment requirements.

Table 13.2 Critical Success Factors and Challenges for Sudan's EHBP

Critical success factors	Challenges
• Ministerial commitment within FMoH despite several political reshuffles	• Gathering timely national and subnational information on population (current and projected), fiscal space, epidemiology of diseases (current and projected), and health system capacity and capabilities (human, built, equipment, consumables) and systems (for example, information, management, financial, logistics)
• Establishment and functioning of ministerially led program Steering Group and TWG (drawn from FMoH and Ministry of Labour NHIF at federal and state levels)	
• Collaboration between top management of FMoH and NHIF (especially within and then beyond the TWG)	• Gathering reliable and detailed historic financial information (at the whole health system level)—despite Sudan's having completed more than five rounds of National Health Accounts
• Engagement of senior clinicians in diverse specialities	• Gathering reliable information about current and planned public expenditure on health in the context of a transitional government
• Pragmatic and timely use of available funds from the European Union to undertake the EHBP development program despite limitations of agreed program scope (preparatory work and implementation both formally out of scope)	• Systematic and sustained engagement with the center of government (one helpful meeting with Deputy Finance Minister)
• An early definition of guiding values and priorities	• Lack of trust that international benchmarks of the cost-effectiveness of interventions have relevance for Sudan (from either utility or costs perspectives)—possibly with some justification
• Identification and adoption of working methods that suited the capacity and developing capabilities of locally employed staff in Sudan—thus aiding skills transfer, program implementation, and sustainability	• Challenges with direct engagement with diverse citizens and communities and associated community engagement given the sensitive political context
• Using the EHBP development program as a "lever" to facilitate political consideration of wider reform of the health system—including capacity building, revisions to the distribution of health care financing roles and responsibilities, and health system governance	• Costing of EHBP conducted from a public sector perspective without considering the health private sector (which is a growing provider for NHIF benefits package)
• Planning for program pilots in two regions, outline planning, and the timeline for wider program implementation	• Lack of available or updated national diseases protocols and management guidelines
• Strong and consistent support from WHO EMRO, and valuable engagement from World Health Organization Geneva.	• Early challenges with involving the TWG and the time needed to increase their commitment and consolidate their support.

Source: Original table compiled for this publication.

Note: EHBP = essential health benefits package; FMoH = Federal Ministry of Health; NHIF = National Health Insurance Fund; TWG = Technical Working Group; WHO = World Health Organization; WHO EMRO = World Health Organization Eastern Mediterranean Regional Office.

LESSONS LEARNED

The value of guidance and support from international bodies cannot be underestimated. Making progress on such complex and challenging programs will require shared learning, knowledge, and expertise. This project offers several important lessons to enhance the value of that guidance still further:

- Distinguish and provide guidance for preparing, designing, implementing, and sustainably embedding a UHC (universal health coverage) EHBP.
- Translate the theory underpinning the development of an EHBP (often well understood) into clear, effective but simple and sustainable practice in highly, and sometimes increasingly, resource-contained contexts.

- Ensure increased sensitivity of guidance to country context—economic, epidemiologic, demographic (for example, urban/rural split), and technical capacity—and to political and institutional context.
- Place greater emphasis (and resources for external support) on the preparatory stage and especially on the implementation and embedding stages of developing a UHC EHBP.
- In the development of future EHBPs, factor in greater emphasis on systemwide resilience and sustainability (disease and events).
- Place greater emphasis on developing UHC EHBPs in the context of wider health system capacity building and/or adjustment and broader institutional development and reform (including governance for performance more than governance of performance).

From the beginning, the newly developed EHBP was seen as a keystone for the ongoing health sector reform because it links so closely with the new strategic directions for health financing, human resources, and service delivery. That strategy will play an important role in strengthening governance and reducing inefficiency due to fragmented pools and contradicted schemes.

The engagement of most of the relevant stakeholders was the key to the project's success. All relevant groups representing clinicians and health systems were invited to add their contributions regarding the proposed EHBP, issues of feasibility, and implementation challenges. The adoption of evidence-informed priority setting to select the most needed and cost-effective interventions was helpful given current data and resource constraints. Despite its difficulty, the task resulted in a very comprehensive and insightful output that facilitated the entire process.

ANNEX 13A. NUMBER OF INTERVENTIONS BY PROGRAM AND SUBPROGRAM (AUGUST 2021)

Communicable diseases	Antimicrobial resistance—infection prevention control	39
	HIV/AIDS	35
	Malaria	19
	Neglected tropical diseases	17
	Pandemic and emergency prep	29
	Sexually transmitted diseases	6
	Tuberculosis	45
	Vaccine-preventable diseases	13
Total		203

(continued)

Noncommunicable diseases	Cancer	26
	Cardiovascular and respiratory diseases	23
	Congenital and genetic disorders	16
	Injury prevention	3
	Poisons	1
	Mental health and drug abuse	35
	Musculoskeletal disorders	6
	Rehabilitation	36
Total		146
Older people and people with disabilities	Elderly	19
Planned procedures	Surgery	147
Women and children	Adolescent health	7
	Child health	11
	Maternal and newborn health	155
	Nutrition	16
	Reproductive health	22
	School age development	14
Total		225
Overall total		740

Source: Based on data provided by the World Health Organization.

ANNEX 13B. METHODOLOGY OF COSTING SUDAN'S EHBP

The OneHealth Tool (OHT) software was the main tool used to estimate recurrent costs of each intervention in five program components across the six delivery sites ranging from community to secondary and tertiary hospital level in the public sector. OHT presents the cost estimates by type of resource and input needed. The costing methodology combined a bottom-up approach to calculate the costs of the medical services at the community, outreach, and facilities levels and a top-down approach to estimate the program management costs.

Bottom-Up Approach

Bottom-up costing, or an engineering approach, is based on a detailed analysis of resources requirements and their costs to estimate the cost of interventions. Interventions costs are classified into direct costs—such as drugs, consumables, investigations, and medical human resources—and indirect costs, which refer to administration and overhead costs. OHT calculates costs by multiplying quantities of resources by their unit cost. Total estimates are built by summing up the percent of estimates in each level, which typically requires close work with relevant technical and clinical experts to obtain and validate detailed resources and inputs used in costing. Sudan's health system delivers health services through six levels: community, outreach, family health unit, family health center, secondary hospital, and tertiary hospital. The bottom-up approach used the following steps.

Assessment of the protocols and associated activities required for each intervention. Data were collected and organized according to the selected intervention and delivery channel, in line with health services and OHT modules. The main reference of the interventions' case management was lists of protocols developed by the program technical groups and clinical experts, who selected and designed the package using mainly the national program's protocols. If those protocols were not available, then WHO guidelines and standards were used. OHT was customized and updated accordingly, and all default data reviewed, edited, and changed to fit the country context. Many consultative meetings with program technical groups and clinical experts were arranged to validate the information used.

Assessment of the population epidemiology associated with each intervention. To compute the annual outputs, the annual number of targets for each intervention in EHBP were calculated as following:

- *Target population.* Refers to the population on which the health intervention focuses, such as pregnant women, under-five children, adults, and so on. Population assumptions for each intervention used Sudan's national census projection 2020.
- *Population in need.* Refers to the percentage of the target population that required the intervention (incidence or prevalence). Data came from the most recent FMoH program reports and studies, such as the 2014 Sudan Multi Indicator Cluster Survey or from global burden studies and estimates when no local data were availble.
- *Coverage.* Reflects the percentage of the population in need that receives the services. Intervention coverages were collected from the FMoH program reports and studies, which represent the baseline coverage for 2020, and then projected up to 2024.

Annual Number of Targets = Target Population × Population in Need × Coverage per Year

Assessment of the average unit cost of interventions. The interventions' costing estimates included the following:

- *Treatment inputs.* The drugs and supplies, medical personnel time requirement, number of outpatient visits, and inpatient days per case. The treatment inputs varied according to the delivery channel, and each delivery channel varied in terms of drugs and supplies, type and time of skilled personnel, and other items required.
- *Unit cost per services.* Calculated using treatment inputs, such as drugs, laboratory tests, human resources type and time, and indirect cost. The project team checked and changed all prices and costs of inputs data to make them more

relevant to the country context. Secondary data collected for input costs included staff salaries and incentives, local prices and costs of laboratory and imaging services, local prices and costs of local visits and inpatient cost, national and international prices of medicines and consumables, and indirect costs including overhead and administrative costs.

Average Unit Cost of Services = Average No. of Drugs, Supplies, and Investigations per Patients per Year × Unit Price of Each Item + Time of Medical Staff Required per Patient per Year × Average Annual Compensation + Average No. of Outpatient Days/Inpatient Day/Patient/Year × Average Outpatient/Inpatient Cost/Patient × Percent of Coverage (Delivery Channels)

EHBP interventions annual cost. The annual intervention cost was calculated by multiplying the annual number of targets with the average total unit cost of services. Finally, the total cost of EHBP was calculated from the annual cost of all interventions and the program cost. All interventions were calculated separately, and the cumulative cost was calculated.

Annual Intervention Cost = No. of Targets × Average Unit Cost of Services

Finally, the total cost of EHBP was calculated by summing up the total annual cost of all interventions and the program's cost.

Top-Down Approach

The management cost estimations of programs were costed with a top-down/ pragmatic approach based on the aggregate programs' budget for the year 2020, according to the programs' plans and strategies. Those plans captured all standardized activities and output conducted by each program at national, state, and local levels, covering detailed information about the program's human resources, training, supervision, advocacy, monitoring, and evaluation.

Data Used for Costing

Figure 13B.1 presents a list of data sources used in the costing exercise. Additionally, in a series of consultative meetings, program managers and clinical experts provided advice on unavailable data.

Figure 13B.1 Data Sources for Sudan's EHBP

Target population and population in need	• Multi-Indicator Cluster Survey 2014 • Population census • Program protocols and reports
Use data	• Program reports and protocols • Sudan Health Statistical Report 2018
Human resources	• Program protocols and reports • FMoH Compensation Chart • Pricing proposal for health services (2020)
Drug and supply costs	• Program protocols and reports • Drug data based on OHT from international drug price list • National Medical Supply Fund price list • International prices (for some locally unavailable drugs and supplies)
Lab and imaging costs	• Program protocols and reports • Pricing proposal for health services (2020) • Program financial report
Overhead and operational costs	• Cost of Hunger in Sudan 2019 • Economic evaluation of vaccines in Sudan (2020)
Health services	• Sudan Statistical Reports 2018 • Program protocols and reports

Source: Original figure developed for this publication.

Note: EHBP = essential health benefits package; FMoH = Federal Ministry of Health; OHT = OneHealth Tool.

OHT contains default data based on standard WHO protocols and expert opinions. The national consultant and the study team checked and modified, when necessary, default data embedded in the tool to fit the country's context. Calculations used the following parameters:

- All EHBP interventions were assumed to be available in the base year (2020).
- The study estimated cost using prices for public sector services.
- All services and interventions were costed using national protocols and procedures, except for some services planned but not currently provided. The costing team built the costs using WHO and international protocols.
- For costing purposes, all needed medicines and laboratory tests were assumed to be available.
- Workers' compensation rates were calculated according to average staff grades and salary scale for the year 2020.
- Allowances and incentives for overtime were calculated using the proposed incentive rates developed by FMoH and NHIF for the year 2020.
- Estimated drug and medical supply prices were calculated using the National Medical Supply Fund list of prices and the international price list, built in OHT software.

- Medical testing estimations were based on the proposed medical services' prices developed by FMoH and NHIF for the year 2020.
- The cost of interventions was estimated using inputs data based on standard protocol and guidelines. For some interventions (mainly injury and surgery interventions) specialists were interviewed regarding their current practices.
- The exchange rate used in the costing study was the official rate estimated by the Central Bank of Sudan for the year 2020 (SD 55 = US$1).

The Costing Team

The exercise was conducted by a team composed of a national consultant and technical team from FMoH. That composition is important to facilitate data collection and adoption of the interventions to the national context. The national consultant was a health economist with experience on OHT.

NOTES

1. World Bank Data, Sudan Overview, https://data.worldbank.org/country/sudan?view =chart.
2. World Bank Data, Sudan Overview.
3. United Nations High Commissioner for Refugees Operational Data Portal, Sudan, https://data.unhcr.org/en/country/sdn.
4. World Health Organization Universal Health Coverage Partnership, Sudan, https://extranet.who.int/uhcpartnership/country-profile/sudan.
5. Institute for Health Metrics and Evaluation, Sudan, https://www.healthdata.org/research -analysis/health-by-location/profiles/sudan.
6. Integrated Food Security Phase Classification, Sudan: Integrated Food Security Phase Classification Snapshot, April 2022–February 2023, https://reliefweb.int/report/sudan /sudan-integrated-food-security-phase-classification-snapshot-april-2022-february-2023.
7. The data presented in this chapter refer to 740 interventions developed to inform the final consensus workshops; however, the final number of interventions has since increased from 740 to 824.

REFERENCES

FMoH (Sudan, Federal Ministry of Health). 2022a. "Measuring the Availability and Affordability of Selected Medicines in Sudan Survey 2022." Government of Sudan, Khartoum.

FMoH (Sudan, Federal Ministry of Health). 2022b. "National Health Sector Recovery and Reform Strategic Plan: Sudan 2022–2024." Sudan Health Observatory.

JLN (Joint Learning Network). 2022. "Making Explicit Choices on the Path to UHC: The JLN Health Benefits Package Revision Guide." World Bank, Washington, DC. https://www .jointlearningnetwork.org/wp-content/uploads/2022/12/Making-Explicit-choices.v4.pdf.

Mallender, Jacqueline Anne, Mark Bassett, and Joe Mallender. 2020. "Health System Benefit Package Design & Provider Payment Mechanisms: Essential Health Benefits Package Technical Report." Economics By Design. https://sudan-ehbp.com/wp-content /uploads/2021/01/WHO_EBD_EHBP-Technical-Report.pdf.

WHO (World Health Organization). 2018. "System of Health Accounts Report 2018." WHO, Geneva. https://extranet.who.int/countryplanningcycles/sites/default/files/country_docs /Sudan/sha_2018_report_v2120201.pdf.

World Bank. 2020. "Sudan Reengagement and Reform Development Policy Financing (P175139)." Report Number PIDA31135, World Bank, Washington, DC. https://documents1.worldbank.org/curated/en/430611615532852121/pdf/Appraisal -Program-Information-Document-PID-Sudan-Reengagement-and-Reform-Development -Policy-Financing-P175139.pdf.

World Bank. 2023. "Sudan's Health Workforce Matters." World Bank, Washington, DC. https://documents.worldbank.org/en/publication/documents-reports/documentdetail /099062823021014007/p175196027650f0c099be0717f6f5ffccf.

Part **2**

Lessons Learned

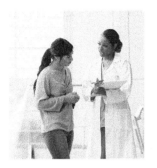

14

From Universal Health Coverage Services Packages to Budget Appropriation: The Long Journey to Implementation

Agnès Soucat, Ajay Tandon, and Eduardo González-Pier

ABSTRACT

Essential packages of health services (EPHSs) contribute to universal health coverage financing through several pathways. Expectations on what an EPHS can achieve for health financing tend to be high, yet stakeholders rarely spell out the pathways to reach desired outcomes. This chapter analyzes how EPHSs relate to the three health financing functions (revenue raising, resource pooling, and purchasing) and to public financial management. The review of country experiences finds that using EPHSs to directly leverage funds for health has rarely been effective. Indirectly, EPHSs can translate into increased revenue through fiscal measures, including health taxes. Through improved dialogue with public finance authorities, health policy makers can refer to specific interventions to connect the value of additional public spending with universal health coverage indicators. However, empirical evidence on EPHSs' contribution to resource mobilization is still pending. EPHS development exercises have had more success in advancing resource pooling across different schemes: EPHSs can help compare the performance of coverage schemes, occasionally leading to harmonization of universal health coverage interventions and identifying gaps between health financing and service delivery. EPHS development and iterative revisions are essential in core strategic purchasing activities as countries develop their health technology assessment capacity. Ultimately, packages must translate into adequate public financing appropriations through country health program design, ensuring that funding flows directly to address obstacles to increased coverage.

INTRODUCTION

Over the past three decades, many countries have invested in developing essential packages of health services (EPHSs), aiming at the progressive realization of universal health coverage (UHC). The focus on both UHC objectives—service coverage and financial risk protection—implies the importance of not only the quantity but also the quality of health finance. High-performing health financing systems for UHC are those in which adequate public funding levels are also predictable and sustainable, prepaid funds are pooled across population groups sharing the financial risk of ill health, and allocations translate into service delivery that both maximizes health outcomes and reduces exposure to catastrophic health expenditures (WHO 2018).

Defining an explicit publicly financed EPHS is a foundational element of UHC reforms across countries (Cotlear et al. 2015; Glassman, Giedion, and Smith 2017). Countries have typically used technical guidelines on what to include based on the burden of disease and cost-effectiveness criteria, sometimes adding considerations such as acceptability, feasibility, equity, and budgetary impact (Glassman et al. 2016). Some countries, including Thailand and Tunisia, have also concentrated on the process using participatory approaches and societal dialogue (Alfers and Lund 2012; Ben Mesmia, Chtioui, and Ben Rejeb 2020). Countries have diverse financing schemes for EPHSs. Armenia's EPHS has taken a pyramid shape, with the poor getting a larger publicly financed package and the well-off co-paying for complementary private health insurance (Chukwuma, Lylozian, and Gong 2021). In Indonesia, contributions are collected from the well-off in exchange for better hoteling amenities and greater provider choice (Tandon and Reddy 2021). In Brazil, Malaysia, and Sri Lanka, publicly financed EPHSs are universal, although the well-off self-select to use private care (Wagstaff 2009).

Clearly defining which services should benefit from public financing is central to achieving UHC. This chapter analyzes how EPHSs relate to the three health financing functions—revenue raising, resource pooling, and purchasing (Kutzin 2001)—and to public financial management. EPHS design, costing (Gaudin et al. 2023), priority setting, and implementation are directly associated with the function of purchasing, indirectly reinforcing resource pooling (through coverage alignment on breadth and depth) but less directly linked to revenue generation. Nevertheless, the process of developing an EPHS contributes to all health financing core functions (figure 14.1).

REVENUE RAISING: THE FISCAL SPACE QUESTION

In most low- and middle-income countries that have undertaken an EPHS exercise, the total cost of the proposed package invariably exceeds the public financing available. Despite great hopes, few of those costing exercises have translated into additional resources, suggesting that the exercise—although useful for health policy

Country-Led Priority Setting for Health | Ala Alwan, Mizan Kiros Mirutse, Pakwanja Desiree Twea, and Ole F. Norheim

Figure 14.1 The Link between EPHS and Health Finance Policy Objectives

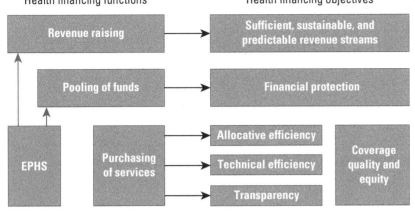

Source: Original figure for this publication.

Note: EPHS = essential package of health services.

makers in identifying priorities—is not the most effective instrument in making the case for additional public resources for UHC. Even when the EPHSs were deemed affordable, resources rarely materialized. Ghana, for example, developed a well-designed EPHS, but no evidence exists that it translated into increased budgets (Blanchet, Fink, and Osei-Akoto 2012). Package development in Kenya did not foster an increase in health resources (Mbau et al. 2020). A review of six countries—Eswatini, Ethiopia, Malawi, Nigeria, Rwanda, and South Africa—shows a systemic disconnect between EPHS processes and health financing policies and frameworks (PMNCH and SIDA 2019). (Refer to box 14.1 for a summary of the role of EPHSs in the health financing dialogue in six additional countries and economies.)

Fiscal space, although not sector specific, has the potential to increase public spending. It depends on macroeconomic growth and stability, how effectively governments can raise revenues, debt sustainability, the capacity to manage overall expenditures, and—in lower-income settings—external financing. In turn, public spending on health is determined by the relative importance assigned to the health sector in the general and subnational budget appropriation processes and by earmarked revenues (such as payroll taxes for social health insurance [SHI] or health taxes). Historically, public spending on health has grown mostly through the impetus of economic growth and improvements in government revenue efforts (Tandon et al. 2020). Few countries have increased public financing through dramatic reprioritization of sectoral allocations to health. Over the first two decades of the twenty-first century, public financing for health in low-income countries more than doubled in real terms from US$5 per capita in 2000 to US$12 in 2019, average real growth of 4.3 percent per year. For lower-middle-income countries, it increased from US$13 to US$30, an average increase of 4.6 percent per year. For upper-middle-income countries, it more than tripled in real terms from US$67 in 2000 to US$286 in 2019—or 7.9 percent per year (figure 14.2).

Financing Essential Packages: Six Case Studies

This chapter reviews the recent experience of Afghanistan, Ethiopia, Pakistan, Somalia, Sudan, and the semiautonomous region of Zanzibar in setting their own essential packages of health services (EPHSs). None conducted a financing dialogue as part of their package discussions. All teams stopped at identifying a theoretical financing gap and estimating its size, comparing a theoretical fiscal space to the cost of the package on a per capita basis. The EPHS literature often refers to that gap analysis approach as the "financing" step, with no evidence provided as to the effectiveness of the simple analysis in improving the health financing framework of a given country. The countries and economy did not see appreciable changes in domestically sourced public financing for health. For example, in Afghanistan and Ethiopia, those expenditures remained largely stagnant in real per capita terms over 2015–19; even others that saw increases had lower growth rates than those among comparators (refer to figure B14.1.1 for information on four of the countries and economy). In Pakistan, the EPHS development process informed the design of a donor-funded joint program. EPHS development aimed at raising externally financed resources to complement some increases in domestic financing for health, although overall numbers remain low and uncertain. Overall, none of the six undertook a dialogue on how to raise revenue, create or consolidate entitlement or pooling mechanisms, identify system inefficiencies to address, establish a new payment provider mechanism, or define a specific program to be included in the multiyear budget.

Figure B14.1.1 Evolution of Public Spending on Health in Selected Countries and Economy 2015–19

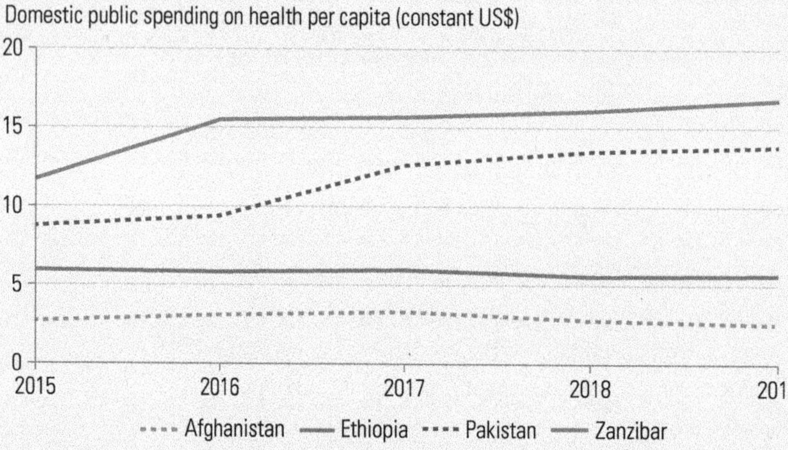

Source: Based on data from World Bank Open Data, https://data.worldbank.org.

Growth in public spending for health can be broken down into three components: economic growth, changes in government spending as a share of gross domestic product (GDP), and changes in health's priority in government budgets. Economic growth—the increase in government revenues due to the increased size of the economy—has contributed most to growth in public spending for health across low- and middle-income countries, followed by overall increases in general spending. Increased priority for health has played a relatively smaller role. In low-income countries, reprioritization can be explained by higher external funding channeled

Figure 14.2 Drivers of Public Financing for Health, 2000–19

a. Drivers, by macro-fiscal determinants

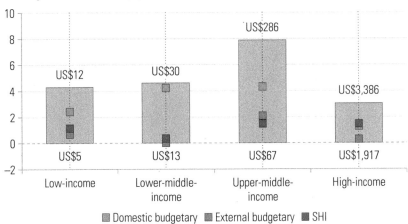

Annual growth rate 2000–19 (%)

☐ Domestic budgetary ☐ External budgetary ■ SHI

b. Drivers, by fiscal source

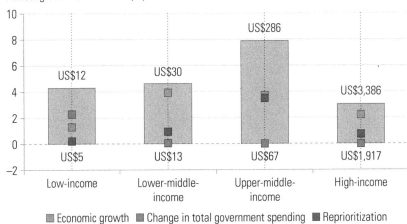

Annual growth rate 2000–19 (%)

☐ Economic growth ☐ Change in total government spending ■ Reprioritization

Source: Based on Soucat, Tandon, and Pier 2023 and data from World Bank Open Data, https://data .worldbank.org.

Note: SHI = social health insurance.

via government budget allocations. Figure 14.3 shows how external sources mostly substituted for domestic funding that declined in aid-dependent countries between 2000 and 2019 (WHO 2019). Most of those countries have not developed UHC financing frameworks to set them on a sustainable trajectory by 2030.

Countries that lack a conducive macro-fiscal environment find it difficult to increase prioritization of health for several reasons. First, governments face competing demands, and other sectors also present well-articulated claims to public funding. Second, many countries do not fully execute health budgets, weakening their case for increased funding. Policy makers may perceive the health sector as inefficient, lacking a clear strategy to optimize available resources and improve service coverage. Sometimes, the inertial increases in public financing for health that derive from

Figure 14.3 External Aid for Health Per Capita and Share of Public Expenditure
Allocated to Health in Aid-Dependent Countries, 2000–19

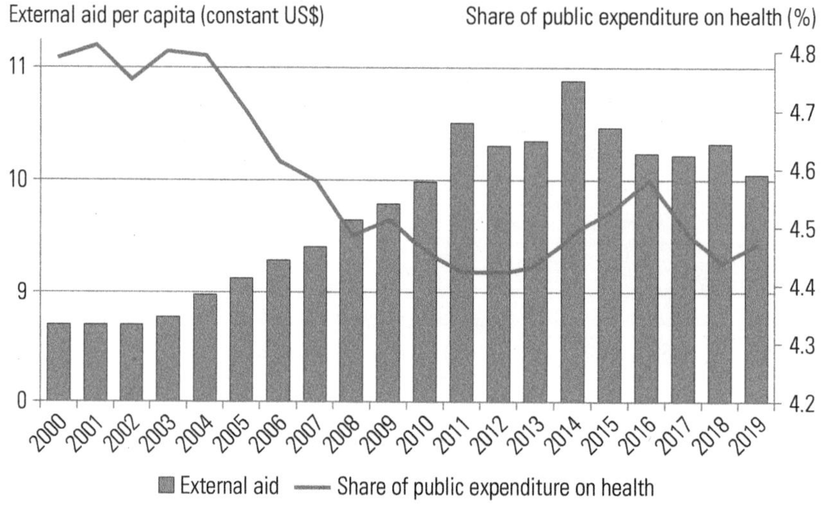

Sources: Based on National Health Accounts data and World Health Organization, Global Health
Expenditure Database, https://apps.who.int/nha/database.

favorable macro-fiscal environments mask relatively low priority for health in
government budgets. Finally, in some countries, identifying a funding gap based on
the cost of an EPHS may lead to calls for more innovative finance (WHO 2019) at
both national and global levels, making the case for more private finance, which can
widen inequalities.

Advocates of expanded service benefits packages often present arguments based
on theoretical economic returns related to improved health outcomes such as lives
saved. That type of argument is not the most convincing for decision-makers when
overall health outcomes and averted premature mortality, in particular, are often the
products of multisectoral action (Caldwell 1979). For example, country evidence
shows a very clear relationship between female education or access to electricity
and child mortality (Shobande 2020). Although the health sector acknowledges
other sectors' health contributions, it is less adept at promoting how investments in
health also contribute to other sectors (for example, poverty alleviation, educational
attainment, and labor productivity), thereby insufficiently leveraging shared
desirable societal benefits to improve budget share.

A more convincing argument would be to connect increases in public financing for
EPHS with improvements in UHC indicators (service coverage and financial risk
protection), which are more easily attributable to government reform efforts within
the health sector. The cost of not implementing reforms should be clearly spelled
out in terms of lost health services benefits and lower associated labor productivity.
Low levels of public financing for health can contribute to inefficiency; for example,
investments in primary health care facilities without health workers or adequate
diagnostics and medicines make wasteful investments in infrastructure.

One clear pathway for benefits packages to increase revenue is the inclusion of behavioral interventions supported by tax policy. Such taxes or subsidies are designed to change the relative prices of commodities and services to promote healthier consumption patterns. Many countries have successfully implemented health taxes on alcohol, tobacco, and sugar-sweetened beverages (Lauer et al. 2023). Removing subsidies for or implementing taxation on fossil fuels can also be considered health taxes, because they reduce the burden of disease related to air pollution and have the potential to raise health budgets. Earmarking is typically not desirable, because it crowds out general taxation; however, earmarking can help increase public support for fiscal reform. For example, France has earmarked the tax on sugar-sweetened beverages for the agriculture worker health scheme (Le Bodo et al. 2022). Additional funding amounts from health taxes may be significant in some countries (for example, Mexico and the Philippines). However, some evidence (for example, from Ghana and Kazakhstan) shows compensating reductions over time in allocations from more discretionary revenues (Cashin, Sparkes, and Bloom 2017).

Introducing local and regional common goods for health into the EPHS (for example, vector control, epidemiological surveillance, public health messaging, and other population-based services) can also constitute a strong argument for additional financing. One of the strongest arguments to justify adequate levels of public finance is that common goods are, by definition, underfunded if left to market forces and can be financed only through general taxation (Soucat 2019). That issue has become particularly salient since the COVID-19 pandemic, which made the high cost of inaction apparent to all finance ministries and treasuries worldwide (Gaudin et al. 2019).

Designing an EPHS may also improve advocacy for resource mobilization by creating a narrative of progress and success on outcomes, as happened in Mexico (Frenk et al. 2006). The capacity of ministry of finance or treasury officials, members of congress or parliament, and other budget decision-makers regarding the health budget improves when dialogue is conducted in terms of health conditions and interventions—and expected health outputs. Without an explicit EPHS, the narrative goes back to staffing, payroll, health commodities and services, and other budget line items, which have a lower potential to resonate with citizens and policy makers. To be credible, the narrative should also build the perception of the sector's effectiveness and efficiency to use the funds well and deliver results.

Using the EPHS to increase revenue for health has limited potential. The disconnect between aspirational health plans and available financial and other resources is identified as the most common failing of existing benefits plans in low-income countries, leading to implicit rationing that is especially harmful to the poor (Glassman and Chalkidou 2012). To be credible, health services packages should be elaborated within the boundaries of likely available fiscal space. Given uncertainties about what will become available—as well as about costs, existing inefficiencies, and levels of service use—it is often preferable not to overly specify the package but rather to incorporate flexibility and adjustment capacity. The Oregon Health Insurance Experiment in the United States started with a tentative fiscal envelope and defined the EPHS within available resources (Finkelstein et al. 2012).

RESOURCE POOLING: FROM VERTICAL STREAMS TO COMPREHENSIVE PACKAGE FUNDING

Pooling is the key health financing function that allows cross-subsidization from the rich to the poor and from the healthy to the sick. From a health financing perspective, a benefits package consists of the services (and conditions for access to them) that the purchaser(s) will pay for from pooled funds. The benefit package definition and implementation processes constitute a critical tool for establishing entitlements for a group of people covered by a health financing pool, supporting a unified framework. A unified benefits framework enables mapping to sources of funding, which can facilitate efforts to either pool them together (for example, combining general revenue transfers and social insurance contributions into one pool) or make them explicitly complementary. It can show how population and cost coverage for those services can be mapped to different funding sources (on the supply side, the insurance/purchaser side, and unfunded parts for which co-payments apply), enabling a depiction of which parts are covered from different pools.

That mapping then enables explicit complementarity among funding sources. Such a framework exists in France (Mutuelles) and the Kyrgyz Republic (contributory SHI). In both cases, a main pool funds a benefits package for the entire population, together with copayments; the framework then has a complementary insurance pool (or more than one pool) for some or all of the copayments (Kutzin et al. 2009). Defining an EPHS can help delineate such a unified national benefits framework for the entire population on the basis of scientific evidence, as done in France (High Authority for Health) and the United Kingdom (National Institute for Care Excellence), as part of health technology assessment.

A specific challenge is to blend supply- and demand-side financing. Indonesia's SHI scheme Jaminan Kesehatan Nasional, which covers about three-fourths of the population, accounts for only one-fourth of total health financing (World Bank Group 2016). The remainder comes from budgetary line-item public financing and user fees to public providers and out-of-pocket fees to private providers. This partial reimbursement SHI model—common in other countries such as India, Kenya, the Philippines, and Viet Nam—is at the same time not adequately leveraged to truly complement other revenue (Cotlear 2018). Similarly, Thailand's public providers have their salaries paid through supply-side budgets whereas the National Health Security Office pays for outputs under the UHC scheme.

Costing a UHC package can help identify potential efficiency gains through service integration and comprehensive planning. In contexts with highly fragmented funding—that is, with multiple public health programs and sources of funding—designing and costing an EPHS creates a level playing field to assess funding needs, harmonizing wage levels, incentives, and service delivery assumptions. An EPHS helps identify economies of scope to be achieved by pooling resources. Identifying an explicit UHC package can consolidate evidence from various service providers and public health programs within a common service delivery framework. Doing so helps reduce overhead levels and better accounts for common costs like human resources and infrastructure, and it reduces overlap. Reducing inefficiencies generates budget space for improved access to other interventions.

Recently, countries have used EPHSs as helpful tools to mainstream externally funded vertical programs into financing schemes funding a broader set of health services. For example, Ghana, Kenya, Nigeria, Tanzania, and Viet Nam successfully integrated their family planning and HIV/AIDS treatment programs into UHC schemes while transitioning away from external funding (Appleford, RamaRao, and Bellows 2020; Regan et al. 2021).

Health services packages may also act as an effective tool for standardizing access criteria across fragmented health insurance schemes. An EPHS can help identify gross inequalities in how governments subsidize different groups through different pools. Defining a national services package establishes a standard to compare current expenditures by different schemes. Assessing an EPHS has flagged unfair access built into segregated insurance pools financed from general taxation. A study conducted in Thailand in 1997 shows how different schemes (low-income, voluntary, social security, and civil service medical benefits schemes) received vastly disparate per capita subsidies and different services packages, highlighting the need to develop an equalized package for all (Khoman 1997). Eventually, that situation led to the merging of most of the schemes with an increasingly harmonized subsidy. Explicit mapping of a UHC package to multiple funding pools allowed for paying providers on the basis of marginal cost: as noted earlier, supply-side budgets pay for Thai public providers' salaries and the National Health Security Office pays for outputs (Tangcharoensathien et al. 2022).

An EPHS can also help estimate the resources required for transferring to a scheme in charge of paying providers and defining how to target subsidies. An open-ended package leads to implicit rationing and inequities because realized benefits are a function of service provider capacity, where richer areas have greater response capacity and the more well-off are more capable of advocating for preferential access. In Indonesia, for example, Jaminan Kesehatan Nasional has an open-ended benefits package. The scheme covers all medically necessary services with no co-payments, no caps, and no limits (other than a negative list of services not covered such as plastic surgery and fertility treatments). Because of the open-ended package and an important part of provider payment (the inpatient part) rewarding the volume of inpatient care, and because of major supply-side imbalances across the country, the national pool results in reverse cross-subsidization—with financing allocations for poorer and rural areas under the single-payer arrangement subsidizing richer and urban areas. Current reforms in Chile aim to address that issue by defining a minimum explicit package of UHC services. Under Chile's Universal Access, an Explicit Guarantees program defines a UHC package to ensure equitable and quality access to benefits.

STRATEGIC PURCHASING: HEALTH SERVICES PACKAGES TO MAXIMIZE EFFICIENCY AND EQUITY

Making the purchasing of health care strategic is probably the most important outcome of a well-designed EPHS. Clarifying which services are to be purchased as a priority—allocative efficiency—is the main role of designing a package. The design and costing of the health services package can even be considered a sub core function of strategic purchasing (Mathauer, Dale, and Meessen 2017).

Translating an EPHS into actual improvements in allocative efficiency requires making investments in developing national institutions. Policy makers need to rely on sound and transparent processes that provide them with high-quality evidence to steer strategic purchasing, including benefits package design and adjustment. Although many discrete country exercises have been conducted, few have led to capacity building or the creation of an agency mandated with health technology assessment or strategic purchasing (Alwan et al. 2023). A key element of institutional construction is to build such an agency and integrate a three-dimensional process—data analysis, dialogue, and decision—whether at the national or at the regional level (WHO 2021). Lebanon, Morocco, and Tunisia have started building such three-dimensional institutions (Dequen-O'Byrne et al. 2020).

Data analysis should take place through autonomous scientific processes under the responsibility of academic institutions. Their conclusions and recommendations should follow transparent procedures, handle the question of conflict of interest, and maintain independence from political processes. Dialogue should be inclusive, elicit the voice of all segments of society, and involve all social and economic groups of society, as happened with the production of the "White Book" in Tunisia (Ben Mesmia, Chtioui, and Ben Rejeb 2020) or during the "Estates General of Health" in France (Caniard and Naiditch 2021). Moreover, decision-making should rest with those responsible for the decision to allocate the proceeds of the collective/public purse, generally parliaments.

EPHSs can help countries improve value for money and maximize the health benefits per financing unit, freeing up resources by identifying cost-saving interventions. Defining a package may also improve technical efficiency. A key difficulty, however, is to translate those potential benefits into actual financing of activities at the point of delivery. For personal, curative care in particular, patients display complaints and symptoms, not specific requests for standard interventions. One critical step to address this issue involves translating the EPHS into a list of essential medicines, diagnostics, and procedures that may be publicly funded, while clarifying in parallel the negative list of those that may not.

A clear EPHS can improve collaboration between public and private delivery systems by leveraging public financing to purchase benefits packages from private providers. Doing so can help expand the delivery capacity of essential services and level the quality of services by linking financing to standardized quality of services. That approach has also been shown to help improve providers' efficiency, creating a level playing field for payments to public and private providers and improving the transparency of providers' activity and management (Or 2014; Trybou et al. 2014). Public providers can benefit from additional budgets for research, training, and more complex care, which are difficult to standardize.

As countries experience a growing burden of chronic conditions, package definitions may also help emphasize integrated financing across levels of care. Such integration can be done by introducing provider payment mechanisms linked to the patient rather than to the illness episode. Case-based or annual per capita payments can then be used for comprehensive follow-up of a patient with chronic care across a provider's network.

Even with explicitly defined benefits, however, challenges arise regarding not just how providers are paid (fee for service, capitation, diagnostic-related groups) but also how much. Inadequate levels of public financing for explicitly and poorly costed benefits are a recipe for misalignment between promises and reality. Reforms targeted to the poor can become weak programs because of inadequate finance. When reforms are implemented and partially funded, do not adequately spell out the EPHS, and/or were not adequately costed and financed, they can spell trouble. The perception of reforms on paper, coupled with implicit rationing and skewed incomplete results, starts a new cycle of problems. A costed package can provide the basis for calculating provider payments, as in the early days of UHC in Thailand (Tangcharoensathien et al. 2020).

FROM FISCAL SPACE TO HEALTH BUDGET SPACE

In countries with conducive macro-fiscal environments, EPHS exercises can be financed even if the government health budget share remains unchanged. In such settings, it is important to be ready to deploy additional health resources, as highlighted by comparing the experiences of China and India (figure 14.4).

Figure 14.4 Public Expenditure on Health, China and India, 2000–19

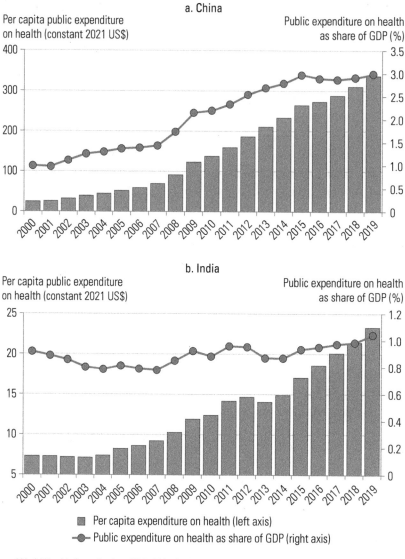

Source: World Health Organization, Global Health Expenditure Database, https://apps.who.int/nha/database.

In 2000, public spending on health represented roughly 1 percent of GDP in both countries, amounting to US$7 in India and US$24 in China. Although India's public spending on health remained at 1 percent of GDP over 20 years, it tripled in real per capita levels, reaching US$23 in 2019, solely because of dramatic GDP growth. New resources enabled a series of reforms, beginning with the rural primary health care expansion (the 2005 National Rural Health Mission expanded reproductive, maternal, newborn, adolescent, and child health). The priority of health in the government budget, however, did not increase over that period. China, by contrast, saw public financing for health increase almost 15-fold from 2000 to 2019, because of a combination of economic growth, increasing government revenue efforts, and higher priority for health in the government budget. Public spending on health in China stands now at 3 percent of GDP, some of the largest growth in fiscal space for health seen in the past decades. China also presents a cautionary tale. Part of expenditure growth was very likely the product of largely unmanaged fee-for-service reimbursement, as well as retaining percentage co-payments (coinsurance), so financial protection did not improve over the period despite the shift in the relative proportion of public and private spending (Meng et al. 2012).

The examples of China and India highlight feasibility as a central concern. A feasible set of UHC EPHSs consists of a set of services that can be realistically financed under existing country circumstances (Escobar, Griffin, and Shaw 2010). Increasing public resources requires identifying strategies to unlock bottlenecks in services package uptake. To be useful, the EPHS must be further translated into a broader program definition as part of the budget cycle. The program should define modalities to fund transfers and provider payments, as well as expected results in terms of direct benefits to the population (access and use).

Linking resources to intended results through program budgeting provides a means to translate EPHS from theory to practice, enabling both alignment of budgets to the promised services and enhanced budget execution (Barroy, Blecher, and Lakin 2022). A key dimension of such linkage involves the loosening of the rigidity of line item budgeting (Piatt-Fünfkirchen et al. 2021). Ultimately, budgets will better match the EPHS and shift from input-based to output-based payment. Examples of such programs include conditional intergovernmental grants, performance-based financing programs, capitation transfers, and health insurance programs, including for specific groups and investment programs. Finally, public financing emanates from taxpayers' and citizens' demand for what the public purse should fund. Services packages need to integrate the broad view of citizens on how best to allocate their taxes. Table 14.1 summarizes pathways by which services packages can generate UHC financing.

Countries with limited public financing would do best to target programs to the poor or for priority services. An important common element across many UHC reforms—for example, in China, Indonesia, Mexico, the Philippines, Thailand, and Viet Nam—is the creation of a publicly subsidized program that expands unremarkable coverage for the poor using general government revenues. The key is to move from scheme to system thinking and differentially support the poor while maintaining a universal vision.

EPHSs differ in how subsidies flow to finance them. Financing can occur directly—with the budget allocated to accredited public and private providers (through subsidies such as line item or global budget or case reimbursement)—or indirectly—with the budget instead flowing to a distinct purchasing agency. India (through Pradhan Mantri Jan Arogya Yojana for private providers—refer to box 14.2), Mexico, and South Africa have direct allocation mechanisms to fund EPHS interventions through decentralized arrangements. By contrast, Argentina, China, Ghana, Indonesia, the Kyrgyz Republic, Rwanda, and Thailand all have important coverage programs in which budget revenues flow to distinct

Table 14.1 Theory of Change: How Health Services Packages Generate UHC Financing

Health financing core function	Pathway	Country cases of resource mobilization, resource pooling, and strategic purchasing
Resource mobilization	(1a) Capacity to advocate for health taxes	(1a) Mexico, Morocco, the Philippines, South Africa
	(1b) Improved dialogue with public finance authorities	(1b) Mexico, Pakistan
	(1c) Identification of cofinancing opportunities	(1c) Armenia
	(1d) Identification of public/common goods for health	
Resource pooling	(2a) Coverage alignment on breadth and depth across funds	(2a) India
	(2b) Equalization of public subsidy between groups	(2b) Thailand
	(2c) Addressing funding gaps of programs	(2c) Indonesia
	(2d) Targeting the poor	(2d) India, South Africa
Strategic purchasing	(3a) Allocative efficiency through priority setting (mostly CEA)	(3a) France, India, Lebanon, Norway, Tunisia, United Kingdom
	• Establishing an HTA agency/practice	(3b) France, Thailand
	(3b) Technical efficiency through levels of care	
	• Improved collaboration between public and private sectors	
	• Integration of financing through levels of care	
	• Identification of provider payment mechanisms	

Source: Based on *BMJ Global Health* 2023.

Note: CEA = cost-effectiveness analysis; HTA = health technology assessment; UHC = universal health coverage.

Box 14.2

The "Long Live India" Ayushman Bharat Program

Ayushman Bharat or "Long Live India"—the umbrella term for health sector reforms in the country—comprises two programmatic components. Health and Wellness Centers rolled out under the National Health Mission's centrally sponsored scheme provide diagnostic tests, free essential medicines, and other comprehensive primary health care services at sub health levels. A new centrally sponsored scheme, the Pradhan Mantri Jan Aarogya Yojana, cofinanced by both the central and state governments, provides government-sponsored noncontributory health insurance coverage for a package of mostly inpatient secondary and tertiary care. The latter serves 100 million poor and near-poor families (an estimated total of 500 million individuals, roughly 40 percent of the country's population) up to a maximum annual limit of 500,000 rupees (approximately US$6,750) per family that can be availed of at government and empaneled private hospitals.

purchasing agencies or subnational entities to include complementary funds and then be allocated to providers. Many countries—including China, the Philippines, and Türkiye—initially expanded per-case reimbursement coverage only for inpatient care, later expanding benefits to include outpatient primary and specialist care. India initiated health reforms aimed at progressively realizing UHC for its population of 1.3 billion.

CONCLUSION

When establishing a dialogue with public finance authorities, health policy makers should translate findings generated during EPHS development into operational approaches and programs to be integrated into the budget cycle. Having explicit evidence-based packages has several advantages, such as defining and implementing program budgeting, assessing costs and whether promised benefits are commensurate with the overall fiscal envelope, absorbing funds that might become available because of conducive macro-fiscal environments, and enabling reforms in risk pooling and strategic purchasing.

On their own, however—except when the services package might include implementation of health taxes—those advantages are not enough to facilitate realization of additional resources from budget-holding authorities. Efforts aimed at connecting increases in public financing for EPHSs with improvements in UHC indicators, identifying and removing absorption-capacity bottlenecks, mainstreaming investments in health for nonhealth and economic outcomes, benchmarking, and demonstrating efficient and equitable improvements in the attainment of health outputs are critical. Such actions fall predominantly in the realm of public financial management reform, from relaxing line-item rigidities to fully moving to program budgets. Defining explicit health services packages offers a useful way to enable that reform, making links between health financing and service delivery explicit and allowing for greater results and accountability.

ACKNOWLEDGMENTS

The Bill & Melinda Gates Foundation sponsored the research underlying this series. The sponsor had no involvement in chapter design; data collection, analysis, and interpretation of the data; or in the writing of the chapter.

This chapter builds on a paper (Soucat, Tandon, and Gonzales Pier 2023) for a series of seven papers coordinated by the Disease Control Priorities 3 Country Translation Project at the London School of Hygiene & Tropical Medicine. The authors thank Dr. Ala Alwan and Dr. Gavin Yamey for their careful review of the paper.

REFERENCES

Alfers, L., and F. Lund. 2012. "Participatory Policy Making: Lessons from Thailand's Universal Coverage Scheme." WIEGO Policy Brief (Social Protection) No. 11, Women in Informal Employment: Globalizing and Organizing, Manchester, UK.

Alwan, A., R. Majdzadeh, G. Yamey, K. Blanchet, A. Hailu, M. Jama, K. A. Johansson, et al. 2023. "Country Readiness and Prerequisites for Successful Design and Transition to Implementation of Essential Packages of Health Services: Experience from Six Countries." *BMJ Global Health* 8 (Suppl 1): e010720.

Appleford, G., S. RamaRao, and B. Bellows. 2020. "The Inclusion of Sexual and Reproductive Health Services within Universal Health Care through Intentional Design." *Sexual and Reproductive Health Matters* 28 (2): 1799589.

Barroy, H., M. Blecher, and J. Lakin, eds. 2022. *How to Make Budgets Work for Health? A Practical Guide to Designing, Managing and Monitoring Programme Budgets in the Health Sector*. Geneva: World Health Organization, https://www.who.int/publications/i/item/9789240049666.

Ben Mesmia, H., R. Chtioui, and M. Ben Rejeb. 2020. "The Tunisian Societal Dialogue for Health Reform (a Qualitative Study)." *European Journal of Public Health* 30 (Supplement 5). https://doi.org/10.1093/eurpub/ckaa166.1393.

Blanchet, N. J., G. Fink, and I. Osei-Akoto. 2012. "The Effect of Ghana's National Health Insurance Scheme on Health Care Utilisation." *Ghana Medical Journal* 46 (2): 76–84.

BMJ Global Health. 2023. "Country Experiences of Developing UHC Packages." Volume 8: Suppl 1, March.

Caldwell, J. C. 1979. "Education as a Factor in Mortality Decline: An Examination of Nigerian Data." *Population Studies* 33 (3): 395–413.

Caniard, E., and M. Naiditch. 2021. "Les États généraux de la santé: un dispositif participatif unique a l'origine de la démocratie sanitaire, histoire et enseignements." *Les Tribunes de la santé* 2021 (67).

Cashin, C., S. Sparkes, and D. Bloom. 2017. "Earmarking for Health: From Theory to Practice." Health Financing Working Paper No. 5, World Health Organization, Geneva. https://iris.who.int/handle/10665/255004.

Chukwuma, A., H. Lylozian, and E. Gong. 2021. "Challenges and Opportunities for Purchasing High-Quality Health Care: Lessons from Armenia." *Health Systems & Reform* 7 (1): e1898186.

Cotlear, D. 2018. "An Anatomy of Progressive Universal Health Coverage Reforms in Low- and Middle-Income Countries." *World Hospitals and Health Services: The Official Journal of the International Hospital Federation* 54 (1): 9–13.

Cotlear, D., S. Nagpal, O. Smith, A. Tandon, and R. Cortez. 2015. *Going Universal: How 24 Developing Countries Are Implementing Universal Health Coverage from the Bottom Up*. Washington, DC: World Bank.

Dequen-O'Byrne, P., M. Sculpher, N. Hawkins, J. C. Thompson, and K. Abrams. 2020. "PCN255 Health Technology Assessment in Low- and Middle-Income Countries: Where to Begin? A Case Study of Tunisia's First Assessment of Trastuzumab in Early and Locally Advanced HER-2 Positive Breast Cancer." *Value in Health* 23 (Supplement 20): S468.

Escobar, M. L., C. C. Griffin, and R. P. Shaw. 2010. *Impact of Health Insurance in Low- and Middle-Income Countries*. Washington, DC: Brookings Institution Press.

Finkelstein, A., S. Taubman, B. Wright, M. Bernstein, J. Gruber, J. P. Newhouse, H. Allen, et al. 2012. "The Oregon Health Insurance Experiment: Evidence from the First Year." *Quarterly Journal of Economics* 127 (3): 1057–106.

Frenk, J., E. González-Pier, O. Gómez-Dantés, M. A. Lezana, and F. M. Knaul. 2006. "Comprehensive Reform to Improve Health System Performance in Mexico." *The Lancet* 368 (9546): 1524–34.

Gaudin, S., W. Raza, J. Skordis, A. Soucat, K. Stenberg, and A. Alwan. 2023. "Using Costing to Facilitate Policy Making towards Universal Health Coverage: Findings and Recommendations from Country-Level Experiences." *BMJ Global Health* 8 (Supplement 1): e010735.

Gaudin, S., P. C. Smith, A. Soucat, and A. S. Yazbeck. 2019. "Common Goods for Health: Economic Rationale and Tools for Prioritization." *Health Systems & Reform* 5 (4): 280–92.

Glassman, A., and K. Chalkidou. 2012. *Priority-Setting in Health: Building Institutions for Smarter Public Spending*. Washington, DC: Center for Global Development.

Glassman, A., U. Giedion, Y. Sakuma, and P. C. Smith. 2016. "Defining a Health Benefits Package: What Are the Necessary Processes?" *Health Systems & Reform* 2 (1): 39–50.

Glassman, A., U. Giedion, and P. C. Smith. 2017. *What's In, What's Out? Designing Benefits for Universal Health Coverage*. Washington, DC: Center for Global Development. https://www.cgdev.org/publication/whats-in-whats-out-designing-benefits-universal-health-coverage.

Khoman, S. 1997. "Rural Health Care Financing in Thailand: Innovations in Health Care Financing." Discussion Paper 365, World Bank, Washington, DC.

Kutzin, J. 2001. "A Descriptive Framework for Country-Level Analysis of Health Care Financing Arrangements." *Health Policy* 56 (3): 171–204.

Kutzin, J., A. Ibraimova, M. Jakab, and S. O'Dougherty. 2009. "Bismarck Meets Beveridge on the Silk Road: Coordinating Funding Sources to Create a Universal Health Financing System in Kyrgyzstan." *Bulletin of the World Health Organization* 87: 549–54.

Lauer, J. A., F. Sassi, A. Soucat, and A. Vigo, eds. 2023. *Health Taxes: Policy and Practice*. World Health Organization.

Le Bodo, Y., F. Etilé, C. Julia, M. Friant-Perrot, E. Breton, S. Lecocq, C. Boizot-Szantai, et al. 2022. "Public Health Lessons from the French 2012 Soda Tax and Insights on the Modifications Enacted in 2018." *Health Policy* 126 (7): 585–91.

Mathauer, I., E. Dale, and B. Meessen. 2017. *Strategic Purchasing for Universal Health Coverage: Key Policy Issues and Questions: A Summary from Expert and Practitioners' Discussions*. Geneva: World Health Organization.

Mbau, R., E. Kabia, A. Honda, K. Hanson, and E. Barasa. 2020. "Examining Purchasing Reforms towards Universal Health Coverage by the National Hospital Insurance Fund in Kenya." *International Journal for Equity in Health*, February 3, 2020. https://equityhealthj.biomedcentral.com/articles/10.1186/s12939-019-1116-x.

Meng, Q., L. Xu, Y. Zhang, J. Qian, M. Cai, Y. Xin, J. Gao, et al. 2012. "Trends in Access to Health Services and Financial Protection in China between 2003 and 2011: A Cross-Sectional Study." *The Lancet* 379 (9818): 805–14.

Or, Z. 2014. "Implementation of DRG Payment in France: Issues and Recent Developments." *Health Policy* 117 (2): 146–50.

PMNCH (Partnership for Maternal, Newborn & Child Health) and SIDA (Swedish International Development Cooperation Agency). 2019. "Prioritizing Essential Packages of Health Services in Six Countries in Sub-Saharan Africa: Implications and Lessons for SRHR." SIDA, Stockholm. https://evidentdesign.dk/wp-content/uploads/2020/06/53306-WHO-One- PMNCH-report-web.pdf.

Piatti-Fünfkirchen, M., H. Barroy, F. Pivodic, and F. Margini. 2021. "Budget Execution in Health: Concepts, Trends and Policy Issues." World Bank, Washington, DC. https://openknowledge.worldbank.org/entities/publication/ad0715ec-3f5d-5418-96f0-7db475fff5bf.

Regan, L., D. Wilson, K. Chalkidou, and Y.-L. Chi. 2021. "The Journey to UHC: How Well Are Vertical Programmes Integrated in the Health Benefits Package? A Scoping Review." *BMJ Global Health* 6 (8): e005842.

Shobande, O. A. 2020. "The Effects of Energy Use on Infant Mortality Rates in Africa." *Environmental and Sustainability Indicators* 5 (2):100015.

Soucat, A. 2019. "Financing Common Goods for Health: Fundamental for Health, the Foundation for UHC." *Health Systems & Reform* 5 (4): 263–67.

Soucat, A., A. Tandon, and E. Gonzales Pier. 2023. "From Universal Health Coverage Services Packages to Budget Appropriation: The Long Journey to Implementation." *BMJ Global Health* 8 (Suppl 1): e010755. https://gh.bmj.com/content/8/Suppl_1/e010755.

Tandon, A., J. Cain, C. Kurowski, A. Dozol, and I. Postolovska. 2020. "From Slippery Slopes to Steep Hills: Contrasting Landscapes of Economic Growth and Public Spending for Health." *Social Science & Medicine* 259 (August): 113171.

Tandon, A., and K. S. Reddy. 2021. "Redistribution and the Health Financing Transition." *Journal of Global Health* 11: 16001.

Tangcharoensathien, V., W. Patcharanarumol, W. Suwanwela, S. Supangul, W. Panichkriangkrai, H. Kosiyaporn, and W. Witthayapipopsakul. 2020. "Defining the Benefit Package of Thailand Universal Coverage Scheme: From Pragmatism to Sophistication." *International Journal of Health Policy Management* 9 (4): 133–37.

Tangcharoensathien, V., S. Sachdev, S. Viriyathorn, K. Sriprasert, L. Kongkam, K. Srichomphu, and W. Patcharanarumol. 2022. "Universal Access to Comprehensive COVID-19 Services for Everyone in Thailand." *BMJ Global Health* 7 (6): e009281.

Trybou, J., M. De Regge, P. Gemmel, P. Duyck, and L. Annemans. 2014. "Effects of Physician-Owned Specialized Facilities in Health Care: A Systematic Review." *Health Policy* 118 (3): 316–40.

Wagstaff, A. 2009. "Social Health Insurance Reexamined." *Health Economics* 19 (5): 503–17.

WHO (World Health Organization). 2018. *Public Spending on Health: A Closer Look at Global Trends*. Geneva: WHO.

WHO (World Health Organization). 2019. *Global Spending on Health: A World in Transition*. Geneva: WHO.

WHO (World Health Organization). 2021. *From Value for Money to Value-Based Services: A Twenty-First Century Shift*. Geneva: WHO.

World Bank Group. 2016. "Indonesia: Health Financing System Assessment." World Bank, Washington, DC. https://openknowledge.worldbank.org/entities/publication/411630a0 -64e8-58ce-8132-e89a0c180f23.

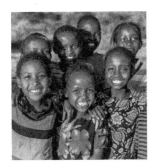

15

Decision-Making Processes for Essential Packages of Health Services: Experiences from Six Countries and Economies

Rob Baltussen, Omar Mwalim, Karl Blanchet, Manuel Carballo,
Getachew Teshome Eregata, Alemayehu Hailu, Maryam Huda, Mohamed A.
Jama, Kjell Arne Johansson, Teri Reynolds, Wajeeha Raza, Jacqueline Mallender,
and Reza Majdzadeh

ABSTRACT

Many countries and economies around the world strive for universal health coverage, and an essential package of health services (EPHS) offers a central policy instrument to achieve that aim. An EPHS defines the coverage of services the country or economy makes available, the proportion of costs covered by different financial schemes, and who can receive the services. This chapter reports on the development of an analytical decision-making framework for EPHS revision and a review of practices of six economies presented in this volume (Afghanistan; Ethiopia; Pakistan; Somalia; Sudan; and Zanzibar, a semiautonomous part of Tanzania), as well as lessons from India.

The analytical framework distinguishes the practical organization, fairness, and institutionalization of decision-making processes. The review shows that these economies (1) largely follow a similar practical stepwise process but differ in their implementation of some steps, such as the choice of decision-making criteria; (2) promote fairness in their EPHS process by involving a range of stakeholders, which in the case of Zanzibar included patients and community members; (3) act transparently in at least some of the steps of their decision-making process; and (4) in terms of institutionalization, express a high degree of political will for ongoing EPHS revision, with almost all having a designated governing institute for EPHS revision.

The lessons in this chapter indicate that countries and economies should organize meaningful stakeholder involvement and foster the transparency of the decision-making process, because those approaches are key to fairness in decision-making. Countries and economies should also take steps toward the institutionalization of their EPHS revision processes.

INTRODUCTION

Many countries and economies around the world strive for universal health coverage (UHC), to provide the health services their populations need without causing financial hardship. An essential package of health services (EPHS) offers a central policy instrument to achieve that goal, because an EPHS defines the coverage of services available, the proportion of costs covered under different financial schemes, and who can receive the services. Such an EPHS can guide both the delivery of care and the associated resource allocation, including human resources, provider payment, procurement, and budgeting (Baltussen et al. 2016; Chalkidou et al. 2016; Glassman, Giedion, and Smith 2017).

Traditionally, analytical work to support EPHS revision has emphasized evidence and analysis of themes such as effectiveness, safety, cost, cost-effectiveness, burden of disease, and budget impact of health services (Baltussen et al. 2016). Only recently has attention been paid to the process of EPHS revision. The way a country or economy organizes its decision-making process can have far-reaching consequences for the content, fairness, and impact of its EPHS (Bertram, Dhaene, and Tan-Torres Edejer 2021; Castro, Suharlim, and Kumar 2020; Glassman, Giedion, and Smith 2017; iDSI 2018; Ottersen et al. 2014; Terwindt, Rajan, and Soucat 2016; Verguet et al. 2021).

This chapter reviews the experience of six economies (Afghanistan; Ethiopia; Pakistan; Somalia; Sudan; and Zanzibar, in organizing their EPHS decision-making processes and substantiates that experience with lessons from India. The selection was based on their use of evidence from the third edition of *Disease Control Priorities (DCP3)*[1] in EPHS revision, and subsequent involvement in the DCP3 Country Translation Review Initiative. The review team included persons leading and involved in the management of EPHS development and revision in the six countries and economies during the period 2019–22, and all of whom are listed as authors of this chapter. For the review, the team developed an analytical framework including a country or economy information template (annex 15A) on the decision-making process for EPHS revision. That framework was based on intensive discussions using several review rounds among all authors, with reference to guides relevant to EPHS revision (Bertram, Dhaene, and Tan-Torres Edejer 2021; Castro, Suharlim, and Kumar 2020; Glassman, Giedion, and Smith 2017; Ottersen et al. 2014; Terwindt, Rajan, and Soucat 2016). The team also developed general recommendations on how countries and economies can improve their current EPHS revision process, on the basis of review results, discussions among authors, and available sources on EPHS revision. Recognizing, however, that countries and economies will have their own decision-making processes, this chapter does not provide a blueprint for EPHS revision.

Because countries differ in their institutional arrangements regarding EPHS revision, this chapter uses the term "governing body" when referring to the principal agency governing the EPHS—often the Ministry of Health or an agency external to it. It also refers interchangeably to "countries," using the term also to relate to governing bodies in countries. Whenever the chapter uses "EPHS revision," that term may also refer to EPHS design if a country has yet to establish its EPHS.

ANALYTICAL FRAMEWORK

The analytical framework distinguishes three interrelated topics of a country's decision-making process: practical organization, fairness, and institutionalization (figure 15.1). To address practical organization, the team developed a seven-step EPHS revision process, informed by several sources and the six economies' experience on questions such as what evidence must be collected and for which services, who should decide which services to include and on what basis, and how to take the current health system into account (Bertram, Dhaene, and Tan-Torres Edejer 2021; Castro, Suharlim, and Kumar 2020; Glassman, Giedion, and Smith 2017; Oortwijn and Baltussen 2021; Ottersen et al. 2014; Terwindt, Rajan, and Soucat 2016).

Figure 15.1 The Stepwise EPHS Revision Process

A. Install an advisory committee
B. Map and select services for evaluation
C. Define decision criteria for prioritization of services
D. Collect evidence on decision criteria for each service
E. Prioritize services
F. Integrate implementation planning into EPHS revision
G. Communicate decisions and establish an appeal mechanism

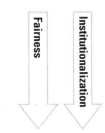

Fairness | Institutionalization

Source: Original figure developed for this publication.
Note: EPHS = essential package of health services.

The fairness of EPHS revision refers to the reasonableness of decisions as perceived by domestic stakeholders, an important requisite for societal support for the final EPHS (Daniels 2000; Ottersen et al. 2014). There is growing acknowledgement of the need for decision-makers to organize fair processes and to do so in a pragmatic manner (Daniels 2000; Ottersen et al. 2014). The team used the evidence-informed deliberative processes framework, which distinguishes four elements that countries can use in each step of their decision-making process to foster the fairness of their process: meaningful stakeholder involvement, ideally operationalized through deliberation; evidence-informed evaluation; transparency; and appeal (Oortwijn, Jansen, and Baltussen 2022).

Institutionalization refers to how a set of activities becomes an integral part of a planning system and becomes embedded in ongoing practices (Bertram, Dhaene, and Tan-Torres Edejer 2021; Machado-da-Silva, Fonseca, and Crubellate 2005). Countries and economies may want to institutionalize the decision-making process to facilitate any ongoing EPHS revision and realize a lasting impact on the EPHS. The institutionalization of EPHS revision relates to issues such as legal framework, governance, and capacity.

The following sections describe the seven steps of the EPHS decision-making process. For each step, the sections provide review results of how the six economies implemented the steps. The subsequent section provides review results on the topic of institutionalization. Refer to table 15.1 for a list of the general recommendations.

Table 15.1 Recommendations for Implementing an EPHS Decision-Making Process

Step A. Install an advisory committee

1. Have a governance structure in place that clearly describes the roles and mandates of the various institutions and stakeholders involved.

2. Install an advisory committee whose main task is to prepare recommendations on EPHS revision to the final decision-maker.

3. Install technical task forces that can support the advisory committee.

4. Compose the advisory committee so that it reflects the diversity of social values present in the population and involves nonhealth professionals as well as health experts.

5. Describe the membership and recruitment process of the advisory committee in a publicly available document.

6. Actively involve all relevant stakeholders in the decision-making process—for example, through participation, consultation, or communication.

Step B. Map and select services for evaluation

1. Assess which model package (such as the DCP3 HPP or EUHC) is most relevant to the decision-making context.

2. Assess the relevance of included services relative to the sociocultural and epidemiological context, and compare the resulting list of services with the existing package.

3. Decide whether to evaluate all services in detail or to concentrate evaluation activities on a selected set of services.

4. Involve stakeholders in the selection of services, and describe the process in a publicly available document.

Step C. Define decision criteria for prioritization of services

1. Define decision criteria in consultation with stakeholders and consider their values.

2. Describe the decision criteria and their selection process in a publicly available document.

table continues next page

Table 15.1 Recommendations for Implementing an EPHS Decision-Making Process
(continued)

Step D. Collect evidence on decision criteria for each service

1. Organize an independent review of quality of evidence by stakeholders and experts.

2. Make the used evidence available publicly.

Step E. Prioritize services

1. Present evidence in a way that is easily accessible and understandable by the advisory committee.

2. Use a structured approach to interpret the evidence and to trade off decision criteria, such as qualitative, quantitative, or decision rules analysis.

3. Always include a deliberative component in this structured approach to secure the quality of the decision.

4. Involve stakeholders in the prioritization of services.

5. Describe the prioritization process in a publicly available document and report on the deliberations and the underlying argumentation for specific decisions.

Step F. Integrate implementation planning into EPHS revision

1. Establish a plan that describes how services are implemented in terms of various health system aspects such as co-payments, delivery platform, health system barriers, and required investments.

2. Secure an integrated service delivery—that is, include foundational services for undifferentiated conditions in the package and coordinate services across different levels of the health system to foster continuity of care.

3. Develop the implementation plan in conjunction with stakeholders and make it publicly available.

Step G. Communicate decisions and establish an appeal mechanism

1. Ensure that EPHS coverage decisions are communicated to all relevant stakeholders, using a variety of channels.

2. Establish a protocol for appeal, including the requirements regarding provision of new evidence and clear revision rules.

Institutionalization

1. Institutionalize the decision-making process for ongoing EPHS revision.

2. Establish an explicit requirement—such as a legal framework—that ensures ongoing EPHS revision.

3. Designate an institution for governing ongoing EPHS revision.

4. Describe the EPHS revision process in a formal document.

5. Secure sufficient funds for EPHS revision.

6. Secure sufficient technical capacity for EPHS revision and make plans to improve capacity when insufficient.

Source: Original table developed for this publication.

Note: DCP3 = Disease Control Priorities, third edition; EPHS = essential package of health services; EUHC = essential universal health coverage; HPP = high-priority package.

STEP A. INSTALL AN ADVISORY COMMITTEE

Advisory committee. Countries and economies can install an advisory committee—that is, a central decision-making committee that prepares recommendations on EPHS revision for consideration by the final decision-maker, typically the Ministry of Health (Bertram, Dhaene, and Tan-Torres Edejer 2021). In developing its recommendations, the committee makes scientific and social judgments on the coverage of services, costs, and populations in the health benefits package (Oortwijn and Baltussen 2021). To avoid cognitive overload, the advisory committee can receive support from subcommittees that develop preparatory recommendations on specific disease programs. The governing body may also wish to install technical task forces that can assist the advisory committee, for example, in terms of evidence collection (Oortwijn and Baltussen 2021). Analysis shows that all six focus economies had an advisory committee in place, often assisted by subcommittees and receiving some form of technical support (table 15B.1 in annex 15B).

Stakeholder involvement. Given that the advisory committee informs public decision-making, its members should ideally reflect the needs and interests of the broader public (Bertram, Dhaene, and Tan-Torres Edejer 2021). The composition of the committee should mirror the demographic and social diversity of the population and its social values, needs, and preferences; the committee can involve both health experts (such as clinicians, public health professionals, program managers, and patient organizations) and nonhealth professionals (such as community members, policy makers, politicians, researchers, development partners, and civil society) (Kunz et al. 2012). Countries and economies often neglect the critical and valuable practice of involving community representatives in advisory committees.

Decision-making processes can involve such stakeholders in three different ways (Abelson et al. 2016). First, stakeholders can *participate* in meetings and engage in deliberations with or without voting. Second, they can be *consulted*—that is, involved in nondeliberative ways, such as through the provision of verbal comments at meetings. Finally, stakeholders can receive *communication* informing them about the processes and/or decisions. The review for this chapter shows that, in four of the focus economies (Afghanistan, Ethiopia, Pakistan, and Zanzibar), advisory committees and subcommittees involved stakeholders such as health professionals, provincial representatives, and development partners. In Zanzibar, the committee also involved patient representatives and people from within the community. Stakeholders actively participated in deliberations in all countries, with stakeholders in Pakistan also having voting rights.

Conflict of interest and transparency. Because the advisory committee is ideally independent and free of undue external influences, it should not include stakeholders with interests in specific services (Oortwijn and Baltussen 2021). If potential conflicts of interests do exist, they can be openly declared (as occurred in Pakistan), with appropriate steps taken to resolve any conflicts identified (NICE 2019). Countries and economies can describe the membership and recruitment process in publicly available documents, as four of the six did (Afghanistan, Pakistan, Sudan, and Zanzibar), and typically in a written report. In Somalia, that information was proactively sent to stakeholders.

STEP B. MAP AND SELECT SERVICES FOR EVALUATION

Countries and economies can use model packages as a starting point for their EPHS revision to describe a set of services typically included in an EPHS. Central to DCP3 are (1) the high-priority package, which includes 108 services and is most relevant for low-income countries, and (2) the essential universal health coverage package, which includes 218 services and is most applicable to lower-middle-income countries (Oortwijn and Baltussen 2021). However, countries and economies may wish to combine the DCP3 packages with other recommended packages or listings of services, such as the UHC Compendium,[2] in order to have a more comprehensive starting point for analysis. The review for this chapter shows that the economies used various packages as the starting point of analysis (table 15B.2 in annex 15B). Three countries (Pakistan, Somalia, and Sudan) used the DCP3 essential universal health coverage package, Somalia added services from the UHC Compendium reflecting the need to cover services for common symptomatic presentations, and Sudan added services from the World Health Organization Eastern Mediterranean Region UHC Priority Benefit Package. Afghanistan used the DCP3 high-priority package as a starting point for its analysis.

Countries and economies can involve stakeholders in the selection of services for evaluation and describe the process in a publicly available document.[3] In most cases, stakeholder involvement occurred through membership in subcommittees. Two countries (Afghanistan and Somalia) made information on the selection of services public.

STEP C. DEFINE DECISION CRITERIA FOR PRIORITIZATION OF SERVICES

Decision criteria reflect the broad goals of a country's or economy's health system (for example, maximization of population health, fair distribution of health, and financial protection) and underlying values (for example, equity, solidarity, and access to good quality care) (Bertram, Dhaene, and Tan-Torres Edejer 2021; Tromp and Baltussen 2012). The advisory committee can use decision criteria for the assessment and subsequent appraisal of services; in this way, recommendations on the inclusion or exclusion of services in the package of essential health services are based on social preferences. Countries and economies are generally advised to define such decision criteria in consultation with stakeholders and to consider their different needs, interests, and values (Bertram, Dhaene, and Tan-Torres Edejer 2021). Such a consultation can be organized in various ways, for example, through a policy document review, survey, or workshop. Countries and economies can publish decision criteria in a publicly available document.

Analysis for this chapter shows that economies most frequently used cost-effectiveness as a criterion (Ethiopia, Pakistan, Somalia, Sudan, and Zanzibar), followed by financial risk protection and equity (Afghanistan, Ethiopia, Pakistan, and Zanzibar) and budget impact (Ethiopia, Pakistan, Somalia, and Sudan) (table 15B.3 in annex 15B). Less commonly used decision criteria concerned feasibility/ health system capacity (Afghanistan, Pakistan, Somalia, and Sudan), economic impact (Pakistan), and social and cultural acceptability (Ethiopia and Zanzibar). Both Somalia and Sudan used integrated service delivery as a criterion. In five economies, stakeholders were involved in the definition of decision criteria (Ethiopia, Pakistan, Somalia, Sudan, and Zanzibar). In Pakistan, decision criteria were based on a policy document review, followed by a survey among stakeholders and consultation in a workshop (annex 15C). Several economies reported on decision criteria in publicly available documents (table 15B.3).

STEP D. COLLECT EVIDENCE ON DECISION CRITERIA FOR EACH SERVICE

Developing an EPHS should ideally be based on explicit criteria and the most updated local evidence available (Bertram, Dhaene, and Tan-Torres Edejer 2021; Glassman, Giedion, and Smith 2017). As noted earlier, some of the most commonly used criteria included burden of disease, equity, financial risk protection, and cost-effectiveness. For illustrative purposes, annex 15D describes the use of local evidence in Afghanistan (Blanchet et al. 2019), and annex 15E describes the use of cost-effectiveness in the countries.

The governing body can organize a review of the quality of evidence by experts and/or stakeholders before using that evidence to prioritize services—all six countries and economies have such a mechanism in place. Countries and economies are generally advised to make public the evidence used in defining the EPHS (Bertram, Dhaene, and Tan-Torres Edejer 2021). Most in the review shared that evidence either on a website, in a report, or in a document sent to stakeholders (table 15B.4).

STEP E. PRIORITIZE SERVICES

In the appraisal step, the advisory committee interprets the results of the assessment in a broad perspective and then formulates recommendations for decision-makers. Governing bodies can best present evidence to make it easily accessible and understandable by the advisory committee (Oortwijn and Baltussen 2021). Subsequent deliberation or discussion can offer a way of interpreting the evidence and developing social and scientific judgments. The central challenge in such deliberations involves trading off the different decision criteria.

A performance matrix can be a useful starting point; it simply presents the performance of a service against the decision criteria (Baltussen et al. 2019). Advisory committees have different options for interpreting the matrix. First, they can undertake a *qualitative approach,* which simply involves deliberating on the performance matrix using explicitly defined criteria. Second, they can adopt a *quantitative approach,* typically referred to as a multicriteria decision analysis, using scoring and weighting techniques. In practice, however, the multicriteria decision analysis has important methodological challenges such as the neglect of the principle of opportunity costs (Baltussen et al. 2019). Third, they can use an *approach with decision rules,* interpreting the performance matrix using a set of simple rules—for example, first ranking services by cost-effectiveness and then using deliberations to assess whether other criteria may affect the ranking. Irrespective of the approach, countries and economies may always want to include a deliberative component in their appraisal process and to report on decisions, including argumentation, in a publicly available document (Baltussen et al. 2019). Five economies (Afghanistan, Ethiopia, Pakistan, Somalia, and Zanzibar) used a qualitative approach, and one (Sudan) used a combined qualitative and quantitative approach (table 15B.5). All reviewed economies used deliberation in their approaches.

Other Aspects of Prioritization

Stakeholders involved in the prioritization of services need to have the necessary capacity and sufficient training for the task at hand (Surgey, Mori, and Baltussen 2022). All six focus economies involved a wide range of stakeholders in prioritizing services. In addition, it is generally recommended that countries and economies consider the available fiscal space in the prioritization of services (Glassman, Giedion, and Smith 2017).

Although, for the sake of fairness, reimbursement decisions are ideally reached by consensus, in some cases stakeholders may, for a variety of reasons, continue to disagree. The advisory committee can also reach a decision by majority voting when consensus is not otherwise achievable (Oortwijn and Baltussen 2021). All six reviewed economies aimed to reach consensus, and Pakistan used majority voting when stakeholders could not reach consensus.

No economy conducted its committee meetings in public. Only Afghanistan made the recordings/proceedings of the committee meetings available to the public. In all countries, publicly available documents described the prioritization process.

STEP F. INTEGRATE IMPLEMENTATION PLANNING INTO EPHS REVISION

Countries and economies can establish a plan that describes implementation of services in terms of various health system aspects, such as co-payments, delivery platform, health system barriers, and required investments. They may want to make special efforts to secure integrated service delivery—that is, to include foundational services in the package for undifferentiated conditions such as cough or fever, and to coordinate services across different levels of the health system to foster continuity of care. Such a plan can be developed in conjunction with stakeholders and described in a publicly available document. Four reviewed economies (Ethiopia, Pakistan, Somalia, and Zanzibar) established an implementation plan as an integral part of their EPHS revision (table 15B.6 and annex 15F). Most considered co-payments, delivery platforms, health systems barriers, and investments; and five also involved stakeholders. Five economies made the implementation plan publicly available.

STEP G. COMMUNICATE DECISIONS AND ESTABLISH AN APPEAL MECHANISM

Communication and appeal are important features that enhance the legitimacy of decision-making by making the decision and underlying argumentation public. Countries and economies should strive to ensure that they communicate EPHS coverage decisions to all relevant stakeholders, using a variety of channels (Bertram, Dhaene, and Tan-Torres Edejer 2021). All reviewed economies had communication strategies in place to inform stakeholders.

Appeal refers to the need for a mechanism that gives stakeholders the possibility to apply for a revision of a decision, or to provide (new) arguments or evidence and receive a reasoned response (Daniels 2000). Countries and economies can establish a protocol for appeal, including the requirements regarding provision of new evidence and clear revision rules. Various focus countries had appeal mechanisms in place (table 15B.7).

INSTITUTIONALIZATION

The economies had varying experiences regarding institutionalization of their decision-making process (refer to table 15B.8 and annex 15G for an example on Sudan). Although most demonstrated a high political will for ongoing EPHS revision, only Ethiopia established that will through regulation. Most economies designated a governing institute for EPHS revision. In addition, countries had recently revised their EPHSs, and most countries therefore had a good description of the decision-making process. That process nevertheless needs to be endorsed as an established procedure in the health system and described in a formal document.

CONCLUSION

This chapter reviews the experiences of six economies in terms of their decision-making processes for EPHS revision. The analytical framework on the *practical organization* distinguished several distinct steps, finding that all the economies appear to have applied those steps. This finding confirms the relevance and validity of the framework: economies embarking on a similar exercise should follow the same stepwise approach in shaping their decision-making process.

The steps, however, should not be considered as prescriptive or formulaic. Countries and economies are encouraged to adapt the number, order, and contents of steps to fit their own decision-making context. The reviewed economies indeed differed in their implementation of various steps—for example, on the use of subcommittees to support the central advisory committee. Countries and economies can learn from each other and select best practices accordingly. Not all countries and economies necessarily design or revise their health benefits package following the stepwise decision-making process described in this chapter. For example, box 15.1 illustrates the case of India.

Box 15.1

The Process of Health Benefits Package Revision in India

India has in recent years designed its benefits package for two flagship federal programs under the Ayushman Bharat reforms. One program expands the package of comprehensive primary care services to include noncommunicable diseases; ophthalmic and ear, nose, and throat care; oral health care; elderly and palliative care; emergency care; and mental health services at frontline public facilities across India through upgrading existing frontline primary health infrastructure into health and wellness centers. The other program, Pradhan Mantri Jan Arogya Yojana, provides tax-financed health insurance coverage for a package of inpatient secondary and tertiary hospital care to 100 million poor and near-poor families at both public and empaneled private facilities. In both programs, specialist committees were established to determine the inclusion of services, considering evidence on burden of disease, comprehensiveness, financial risk protection, equity, and cost-effectiveness. On the latter, the government also commissioned studies to assess the cost-effectiveness of some of the interventions including screening for cervical cancer, diabetes, and hypertension under the health and wellness center reforms.

Source: Refer to chapter 10 in this volume.

As with their practical organization, the economies shared many characteristics on how they promoted the *fairness* of their decision-making process. For example, all organized some form of stakeholder involvement, although its implementation differed in terms of (1) number of stakeholders involved (Ethiopia involved no fewer than 80 stakeholders), (2) type of stakeholders involved (Zanzibar sets a nice example on patient and community involvement), and (3) mode of involvement (Pakistan allowed all stakeholders to fully participate in meetings, with voting power). Meaningful stakeholder involvement is key to fair decision-making processes, and countries and economies are advised to prioritize it when revising their EPHS development or revision process. In addition, all were transparent in terms of at least some of the steps of their decision-making process, for example, on the governance structure or on the decision criteria. Countries and economies should be attentive to the need for transparency in all steps and describe those steps in publicly available documents. When necessary, informing stakeholders on the decision-making process may require proactive efforts.

The review on *institutionalization* shows that all six economies had a high degree of political will, an institution to pursue the work, the required capacity, and an explicit prioritization process. In addition, the economies secured financial resources, either from domestic sources or development aid. In most cases, however, the work was considered a project and not an ongoing activity embedded in the respective health systems. Countries and economies are strongly advised to foster the institutionalization of their EPHS development/revision process (Verguet et al. 2021).

All six economies provide successful examples of EPHS development and revision. In other countries, despite initial intentions, the process of defining or revising the EPHS has not yet started or, if it has begun, has not led to the final list of services as a package. This chapter reviews only successful experiences and does not cover lessons learned from possible failures.

ANNEX 15A. COUNTRY AND ECONOMY INFORMATION TEMPLATE

A. Install an advisory committee.
   1. Have advisory committees, program area advisory committees, and/or Technical Working Groups been established? Describe membership in terms of number and affiliation.
   2. How were members selected?
   3. Do members need to sign a conflict-of-interest form before they are installed?
   4. How were stakeholders involved? Describe their involvement in terms of communication/consultation, participation without voting, participation with voting, and how the process was organized in practice.
   5. Did committee members and stakeholders receive training on the EPHS process? Describe.
   6. Is the membership and recruitment process described in a publicly available document?
   7. Has a link been established with the Ministry of Health and Ministry of Finance? Describe.

B. Map and select services for evaluation.
   1. How did the country select services for evaluation—that is, for detailed evidence-based assessment (for example, compare existing package to DCP high-priority package)? Describe.
   2. How many services were evaluated? Describe if evaluation was limited to certain DCP program areas and/or delivery platforms.
   3. Were stakeholders involved in selecting services for evaluation? If so, describe which stakeholder groups and how.
   4. Is the selection of services for evaluation described in a publicly available document?

C. Define decision criteria for prioritization of services.
   1. How were decision criteria defined? Please describe if definition was based on a survey, identification of social values through document analysis, or a combination.
   2. Were stakeholders involved in the definition of decision criteria? If so, describe which stakeholder groups and how.
   3. Which decision criteria were identified?
   4. Were decision criteria operationalized in a way that allows evidence collection on these criteria?
   5. Are defined decision criteria described in a publicly available document?

D. Collect evidence on decision criteria for each service (note that, following the scope of the chapter, this step does not make an inventory of sources and methods of data collection, except for cost-effectiveness).

1. How was evidence on cost-effectiveness collected? Describe, for example, review and contextualization processes.

2. Was the quality of evidence reviewed by experts and/or stakeholders? If so, describe which experts/stakeholder groups and how.

3. Is the collected evidence available in a public document?

E. Prioritize services.

1. How was evidence presented to the advisory committee or Technical Working Groups (for example, through color-coded evidence briefs and/or summary tables)?

2. Did committee members deliberate on the prioritization of services? If so, describe whether they followed a structured process to interpret the evidence and trade-off criteria (for example, weighing and scoring, or first ranking on cost-effectiveness and then modifying rankings in deliberations).

3. How was reference made to the overall available fiscal space? (Were costs of prioritized services added up to a total budget, and was an explicit budget constraint used?)

4. Were feasibility concerns included in the prioritization of services?

5. Were stakeholders involved in the prioritization of services? If so, which stakeholder groups and how? (communication/consultation/participation without voting/participation with voting)

6. What is the mandate of the committee—to develop recommendations or to make decisions? If it is to develop recommendations, to whom was it presented for endorsement?

7. How did the committee come to a decision/recommendation? (for example, consensus or voting)

8. Are the committee meetings public, and/or are recordings/proceedings available to the public?

9. Is the prioritization process described in a publicly available document?

F. Integrate implementation planning into benefit package design

1. Was an implementation plan established in terms of, for example, co-payments (user fees), delivery platform, health system barriers, and required health system investments? Describe which health systems aspects were taken into account.

2. Were stakeholders involved in the development of the implementation plan? If so, which stakeholder groups and how?

3. Is the implementation plan described in a publicly available document?

G. Communication and appeal

1. What mode of communication was used to inform stakeholders (including the broad public) of the outcomes of the EPHS decision-making, if any?

2. Are appeal options available for stakeholders wishing to revise decisions, and are these options proactively communicated to stakeholders?

Table 15B.1 Summary of Country and Economy Experiences in Installing an Advisory Committee (Step A)

Indicator	Afghanistan	Ethiopia	Pakistan	Somalia	Sudan	Zanzibar
What is the composition of the advisory committee?	National advisory group with four members: MoPH, deputy Minister; Director of Information and Evaluation, and Director of Health Financing and Economics with support from a group of international experts	National advisory group with 30 members; regional advisory group with 36 members (3 from each region)	NAC[b] with 90 members: health professionals, development partners, provincial representation	Intergovernmental committee of 7 members: Federal Minister of Health, State Ministries of Health, advisers, academics, the private sector, and international experts from international health partners	Supervisory committee (5 representatives from National Health Insurance Fund and FMoH)	National advisory team with 15 members from MoH, MoF, tertiary hospital representative, and Office of Chief Government Statistician
Was the advisory committee supported by subcommittees that developed preparatory recommendations on specific disease programs?	Yes, 9 working groups constituted in Afghanistan, including representatives from MoPH, development partners, and provincial directors	Yes, 9 working groups including 80 representatives (subject matter experts from primary, secondary, and tertiary level; academia; MoH; regional health bureau; and development partners)	Yes, 4 TWGs including a total of 183 members	No	Yes, 1 TWG, consisting of 9 representatives from the National Health Insurance Fund and FMoH and 2 representatives from WHO	Yes, 6 TWGs including health professionals (50), program managers (45), and representatives from civil society organizations including patient organizations (55), local government authorities (45), development partners (15), and MoH (15)
Was technical support provided?	By MoPH staff, international experts, WHO, international academic institutes, and international development partners	By international academic institutes, WHO, Harvard School of Public Health, and Addis Ababa University	By project team (UHC-BP secretariat), including staff from MoH and (inter) national academic institutes	By MoH TWGs, and a task force including national and international development partners	By a project team comprising international experts in health economics and UHC development and 13 clinical expert teams comprising Sudanese health professionals	By international academic institutes and project team (core team) of 12 members from MoH, MoF, and Office of Chief Government Statistician
Did the (sub)committee involve patients or patient representatives?	No	No[a]	No	No	No	Yes
Did the (sub)committee involve public representatives?	No	No	No	No	No	Yes

table continues next page

Table 15B.1 Summary of Country and Economy Experiences in Installing an Advisory Committee (Step A) (continued)

Indicator	Afghanistan	Ethiopia	Pakistan	Somalia	Sudan	Zanzibar
How were stakeholders involved in the (sub) committee?	Consultation and participation in deliberations but without voting rights	Participation in deliberations	Participation in deliberations, with voting power	Stakeholders (representatives from service providers, policy makers, purchasers, financiers, academia, and private sector) were involved in the service package development through a steering committee (voting mechanism not part of the process)	Consultation and participation in deliberations but without voting rights	Consultation and participation in deliberations
Did members declare conflict of interest?	No	No	Yes	No	No	No
Are the membership and recruitment process described in a publicly available document? If yes, how (report, website)?	Yes	Yes, direct email communication and an official letter from the Office of the Minister sent to stakeholders	Yes, in a report	Yes, through a letter sent to all stakeholders	Yes, in a report (only in summary and not including the recruitment process)	Yes, in a report
Were stakeholders involved in still other ways—that is, outside the mentioned subcommittees?	Yes, consulted to review the final version of the IPEHS	Yes	No	Yes, stakeholders review of service package before it was endorsed by the MoH	No	Yes

Source: Original table prepared for this publication.

Note: FMoH = Federal Ministry of Health; IPEHS = Integrated Package of Essential Health Services; MoF = Ministry of Finance; MoH = Ministry of Health; MoPH = Ministry of Public Health; NAC = National Advisory Committee; TWG = Technical Working Group; UHC-BP = Universal Health Coverage–Benefit Package; WHO = World Health Organization.

a. Patient representatives (for cancer, chronic kidney disease, diabetes mellites) were involved in steps B (map and select services for evaluation) and C (define decision criteria for prioritization of services).

b. In addition, a steering committee was established involving stakeholders who reported to the Minister of Health. The National Advisory Committee reported to the steering committee.

Table 15B.2 Summary of Country and Economy Experiences in Mapping and Selecting Services for Evaluation (Step B)

Indicator	Afghanistan	Ethiopia	Pakistan	Somalia	Sudan	Zanzibar
Which model package was used as a starting point?	DCP3 HPP	DCP3, WHO-CHOICE	DCP3 EUHC	DCP3 EUHC expanded with service listing in UHC Compendium	DCP3 EUHC expanded with WHO-EMRO UHC-Priority Benefit Package	DCP3 EUHC
Was this model package compared to the existing package?	—	Yes, to the 2005 EHSP	Yes, it was compared to the existing packages	Yes	Yes	EHCP
Were all services evaluated or only a selection?	All services	All services	All services	All services	All services	All services
Were services assessed on their relevance?	Yes, based on BoD	Yes, based on BoD	Yes	Yes, based on the common undifferentiated problems and BoD	Yes	Yes
Were stakeholders involved in the selection of services?	Yes, national advisory group and Expert Committee members involved	Yes, committees involved	Yes, TWGs involved	Yes, experts, donors, and providers from the public and private sectors involved	Yes, 13 expert clinical committees involved	Yes, 6 TWGs involved
Is information on selection of services publicly available? If yes, how (report, website)?	Yes	Yes	Yes, publicly available on website	Not publicly accessible	Yes[a]	Report

Source: Original table developed for this publication.

Note: BoD = Burden of Disease; *DCP3 = Disease Control Priorities*, third edition; HPP = highest-priority package; EHCP = Essential Health Care Package; EMRO = Eastern Mediterranean Regional Office; EHSP = essential health services package; EUHC = Essential Universal Health Coverage package; TWG = Technical Working Group; WHO = World Health Organization; — = not available.

a. Refer to Sudan, "Essential Health Benefits Package," https://sudan-ehbp.com/essential-health-benefits-package.

Table 15B.3 Summary of Country and Economy Experiences in Defining Decision Criteria for Prioritization of Services (Step C)

Indicator		Afghanistan	Ethiopia	Pakistan	Somalia	Sudan	Zanzibar
Selected criterion[a]	Burden of disease		✓		✓	✓ (Meets health need)	✓
	Effectiveness	✓		✓ (Avoidable burden)		✓	
	Quality of evidence			✓		✓	
	Financial risk protection	✓ (Affordability)	✓	✓			✓
	Equity	✓	✓	✓			✓
	Cost-effectiveness		✓	✓ (Health gain for money spent)	✓ (Likely value for money)	✓ (Likely value for money)	✓
	Budget impact		✓	✓	✓ (Affordability)	✓	✓
	Integrated service delivery				✓	✓	
	Feasibility	✓		✓	✓	✓ (To inform potential timing)	
	Socioeconomic impact			✓			
	Public and political acceptability		✓		✓ (Political acceptability)		✓
How were decision criteria defined and by whom?		National advisory group and international expert group	Literature review, followed by deliberation among MoH leadership and all stakeholders (final list of criteria based on decision by MoH)	Policy document review, followed by survey among stakeholders and consultation in workshop	Proposed by expert group followed by stakeholder consultation (MoH staff, program managers and service providers, international partners)	Decision process, criteria and weighting selected in a workshop with the TWG and other ministry stakeholders	Proposal from deliberative meetings discussed and final list decided by the executive committee of the MoH
Were stakeholders involved in this step?		No	Yes	Yes	Yes	Yes	Yes
Is information on process and criteria definitions publicly available? If yes, how (report, website)?		Yes (how?)	Yes, in report	Yes, in report	The process of work published and endorsed by the MoH	Yes[b]	—

Source: Original table developed for this publication.

Note: MoH = Ministry of Health; TWG = Technical Working Group; — = not available.

a. The names of the criteria used by the countries were interpreted in terms of common criteria definitions. The countries' original naming of the criterion is provided in parentheses.

b. Refer to Sudan, "Essential Health Benefits Package," https://sudan-ehbp.com/essential-health-benefits-package.

Table 15B.4 Summary of Country and Economy Experiences in Evidence Collection (Step D)

Indicator	Afghanistan	Ethiopia	Pakistan	Somalia	Sudan	Zanzibar
Was evidence reviewed before it was used for decision-making?	Yes	Yes	Yes	Evidence collected from trusted global sources so considered reliable	Yes	Yes
Were stakeholders involved in the collection and review of evidence?	Yes, international expert group and national working groups involved	Yes, committees and TWGs established at different levels involved	Yes, TWG members engaged in review of service descriptions and evidence collection	Yes, all relevant stakeholders including MoH and partners/donors involved	Yes, 13 expert groups engaged to review all services	Yes, all TWGs engaged in reviewing the evidence
Is information on this step publicly available? If yes, how (report, website)?	Yes, on MoPH website	Yes, report	No	Document shared with stakeholders elaborates data sources and criteria used	Not yet, but to be published upon completion of the final selection	Yes, report

Source: Original table developed for this publication.

Note: MoH = Ministry of Health; MoPH = Ministry of Public Health; TWG = Technical Working Group.

Table 15B.5 Summary of Country and Economy Experiences in Prioritization of Services (Step E)

Indicator	Afghanistan	Ethiopia	Pakistan	Somalia	Sudan	Zanzibar
Did the committee use a structured approach to prioritize services?	Qualitative approach using deliberations based on explicit criteria	Qualitative approach using deliberations based on explicit scored criteria	Qualitative approach using deliberations based on explicit scored criteria	Qualitative approach using deliberations based on explicit criteria	Combined qualitative and quantitative approach, including scoring and weighing as starting point for deliberation	Qualitative approach using deliberations based on explicit criteria
Did the committee deliberate to prioritize services?	Yes	Yes	Yes	Yes	Yes	Yes
Did the committee consider the required budget and available budget (fiscal space) when prioritizing services?	The required budget estimated but not the fiscal space	Yes, in fiscal space	Yes, both required budget and available fiscal space	The required budget estimated but not the fiscal space	The required budget estimated but not the fiscal space	Projection for the coming 10 years made and fiscal space to be done using the FairChoices tool
Did the committee consider feasibility concerns when prioritizing services?	Yes	Yes	Yes	Yes	Yes, in relation to timing	Yes
Were stakeholders involved in prioritizing services?	Yes, through all committees as mentioned in table 15B.1	Yes	Yes, through all committees as mentioned in table 15B.1	Yes, through all committees as mentioned in table 15B.1	Yes, through all committees as mentioned in table 15B.1	Yes, through all committees as mentioned in table 15B.1

table continues next page

Table 15B.5 Summary of Country and Economy Experiences in Prioritization of Services (Step E) (continued)

Indicator	Afghanistan	Ethiopia	Pakistan	Somalia	Sudan	Zanzibar
How did the committee come to a decision?	Consensus	Consensus	TWG members voted on classification of services as low, medium, or high priority. If consensus was not achieved, majority vote was used. In NAC and SC consensus was used.	Consensus	Consensus	Consensus
How was evidence presented to the committee?	Analysis reports with summaries and Excel sheet	Draft report and interactive Excel sheet	Evidence sheets with color-coded evidence on the criteria burden of disease, budget impact, and cost-effectiveness	Results from the Somalia Health and Demographic Survey 2020, color-coded matrix of the burden of disease analysis, and resources mapping and expenditure tracking analysis	Excel sheet	FairChoices model used to present evidence on cost-effectiveness, budget impact, and health benefit gains in low, moderate, and high performance for each delivery platform
Are the committee meetings public?	No	No	No	No	No	No
Are recordings and/or proceedings of the committee meetings available to the public?	Yes	No	No	No	No	No
Is the prioritization process described in a publicly available document? If yes, how (report, website)?	Yes	Yes, on a website	Yes, in a report	Yes, in a report available online (prioritization not yet finalized)	Yes[a]	Yes, well described in the report

Source: Original table developed for this publication.

Note: NAC = National Advisory Committee; SC = steering committee; TWG = Technical Working Group.

a. Refer to Sudan, "Essential Health Benefits Package," https://sudan-ehbp.com/essential-health-benefits-package.

Table 15B.6 Summary of Country and Economy Experiences in Development of Implementation Planning (Step F)

Indicator	Afghanistan	Ethiopia	Pakistan	Somalia	Sudan	Zanzibar
Was an implementation plan developed?	No, due to the arrival of Taliban	Yes	Yes	Yes, developed as part of the EPHS	No clear implementation plan (though recommendations are in place)	Yes
Were levels of co-payment considered?	Yes	Yes	No	The rollout of the package to be done incrementally depending on the available resources and capacity	Not yet	Currently Zanzibar offers health care services free of charge
Were delivery platforms considered?	Yes	Yes	Yes	Yes, package targeted to offer services at all levels	Yes, package explicitly includes delivery platform	Yes
Were health system barriers considered?	Yes	Yes	Yes	Yes, including consideration of nomadic populations, IDPs, and insecure areas of the country	Yes, in terms of current coverage	Yes
Were health system investments considered?	Were supposed to be calculated	Yes	Yes, as a percentage of costs of the package	Yes, and the investment case for the health sector was developed to focus mainly on service delivery and prioritized health system strengthening provisions.	Not yet	Yes
Were stakeholders involved in developing the implementation plan?	Yes	Yes	Yes, through their membership in the TWGs	Yes, through their membership in the task force	Not yet	Yes, plan developed by the core team and shared with experts and program managers for their input
Is the implementation plan (becoming) available in a public document? If yes, how (report, website)?	No	Yes, in report	Yes, on website	Yes, in report	Yes[a]	Yes, in report

Source: Original table developed for this publication.

Note: EPHS = Essential Package of Health Services; IDPs = internally displaced persons; TWG = Technical Working Group.

a. Refer to Sudan, "Essential Health Benefits Package," https://sudan-ehbp.com/essential-health-benefits-package.

Table 15B.7 Summary of Country and Economy Experiences in Communication and Appeal (Step G)

Indicator	Afghanistan	Ethiopia	Pakistan	Somalia	Sudan	Zanzibar
What mode of communication was used to inform stakeholders on the outcomes of the EPHS decision-making?	Consultation	Official letter, email, public launching, media release, and press release	Official letter, email, steering committee meeting/inter-ministerial forum, public report, press release	Through health sector coordination meetings, formal launching with stakeholders and media participation, emails and reports shared directly and through MoH website	EHBP not yet finalized or approved	Through consultative meetings
Were appeal options available for stakeholders wishing to revise decisions?	Through two consultation rounds in 2021	Yes, appeal can be made to the Executive Committee of the MoH	Yes, provinces were given opportunity to revise the decisions at the national level	Was not part of the process	Not yet	No
Were appeal options proactively communicated to stakeholders?	Yes	Yes	Yes	No	Not yet	No

Source: Original table developed for this publication.

Note: EHBP = Essential Health Benefits Package; EPHS = essential package of health services; MoH = Ministry of Health.

Table 15B.8 Summary of Country and Economy Experiences in Institutionalization

Indicator	Afghanistan	Ethiopia	Pakistan	Somalia	Sudan	Zanzibar
Is there an explicit requirement (for example, legal framework) in place that ensures the use of ongoing EPHS revision in the country?	The political will existed, evident from a president's letter, but revision not enforced as an explicit obligation.	Yes, there is a resolution and legal framework in place.	The concept is elaborated in upstream documents as policy but not as an explicit requirement.	Yes, although it is a decision by the Minister of Health, it is still not a written requirement.	This is stated by directorates of the MoH, but not yet translated into a formal requirement.	There is no specific explicit requirement for the package.
Is an institution designated for governing ongoing EPHS revision in the country?	Yes	Yes, the FMoH is solely designated.	Responsibilities were clear at the federal level. At the provincial level, local institutions will be designated.	The MoH is responsible for guiding and overseeing the revision through a participatory process.	A governing structure has been proposed but is not yet established.	The process is led by the MoH with technical support. Strengthening of existing bodies has already started, such as establishing a financing unit in the MoH.
Is the ongoing EPHS revision process described in a formal document?	No	Yes, the process is described in a national document.	The process is well defined but not described in a formal document.	The MoH developed a concept note describing the revision process.	The process is well defined but not described in a formal document.	Yes, the process is described in a report.

table continues next page

Table 15B.8 Summary of Country and Economy Experiences in Institutionalization (continued)

Indicator	Afghanistan	Ethiopia	Pakistan	Somalia	Sudan	Zanzibar
Does this institution have sufficient funds for ongoing EPHS revision activities?	No	The FMoH allocates some funding, but that funding is not sufficient.	No	No	It is stated as an activity in the upcoming plan that can guarantee sufficient resources.	It relies on development partners.
Are there plans to build the required technical capacity?	No	Yes, training on health economics at the master and PhD level is ongoing.	The federal ministry envisages the provinces; however, further technical capacity is needed at the federal level.	There is no plan yet.	It is proposed in the plan.	Yes, a team of 12 members has been established and trained, and PhD opportunities obtained.

Source: Original table prepared for this publication.

Note: EPHS = essential package of health services; FMoH = Federal Ministry of Health; MoH = Ministry of Health.

ANNEX 15C. IN THE SPOTLIGHT: DEFINING DECISION CRITERIA IN PAKISTAN

The selection and definition of decision criteria involved several steps.

1. The project team, with representatives from the Ministry of National Health Services Regulations and Coordination and academic institutes, carried out a review of national health policy documents to identify relevant criteria.
2. The team matched identified criteria to the criteria proposed in the international literature, taken from a recent published review.
3. The team further specified the criteria and their definitions for feedback and approval by members of the Technical Working Groups, which led to the preselection of eight criteria (effectiveness, health gain for money spent, avoidable burden of disease by the intervention, budget impact, feasibility, equity, financial risk protection, and social and economic impact).
4. The Ministry of National Health Services Regulations and Coordination conducted a Likert scale survey that asked members of the Technical Working Groups to indicate the importance they attached to these criteria, whether they believed any criteria were missing, and to provide any additional comments or suggestions. A total of 52 Technical Working Group members responded (a response rate of 52 percent).

Using the survey results, and feedback following the first appraisal workshop, several of the criteria were redefined (mainly phrased more in less technical language). Because the cost-effectiveness criterion proved difficult for participants to grasp, it was rephrased as "health gain for money spent." No additional criteria were suggested.

Although effectiveness was one of the eight original criteria, it was not used during the prioritization exercise because the services subjected to deliberation and prioritization were all considered effective, a requirement for their inclusion in the DCP3 list of recommended interventions.

ANNEX 15D. IN THE SPOTLIGHT: VERNACULAR EVIDENCE IN AFGHANISTAN

The revision of Afghanistan's health priority package in 2018–21 generated a particular mix of knowledge sharing and information use, creating a bank of evidence in a way unique to this particular development process. Contexts and processes really shape "vernacular evidence" produced in a specific place and at a specific time.[4] Analysis, interpretation, and discussion of evidence lead to debates bringing new understandings and parameters to light. Experts applied keen and careful judgment, taking the micro and macro levels of the health system into account, guided by their experience and the dynamics within the group. In humanitarian response in particular, decision-makers will have to use their professional judgment "amidst the uncertainty of whether the existing research evidence can be applied to their unique setting" (Khalid et al. 2020). The Integrated Package of Essential Health Services development is a good illustration of production of vernacular evidence, with decision-making surrounding available evidence often coming down to discussions and experience, rather than published material. At times vernacular evidence was a compromise considering absence of specific evidence and shaped by consensus building, shared ethics, and morality. It is not less robust than other evidence; in fact, one could suggest that through its adaptations it is more explicit and tailored to the situation at hand. However, despite the "social" vetting of vernacular evidence, it is still at the mercy of the authority of those at the table with the most power.

ANNEX 15E. USING COST-EFFECTIVENESS ANALYSES FOR PRIORITIZATION AND BENEFIT PACKAGE DESIGN

Cost-effectiveness analysis (CEA) is a popular approach because it provides a useful way of health gains within a budget constraint; however, generating local CEA data can be extremely resource-intensive, especially for low- and middle-income countries (Glassman et al. 2016). Review of the experiences of six low- and middle-income countries in developing evidence for CEA using a short questionnaire finds that, given the lack of context-specific CEA studies, countries used one of three approaches to estimate CEA: (1) using existing tools and software to generate CEA estimates, (2) transferring existing evidence on CEA from similar health systems or global databases, and (3) using expert opinion to estimate value for money. For the first approach, some of the tools used predominantly in Ethiopia, Somalia, and Zanzibar include the WHO-CHOICE tool, the UHC Compendium, and the FairChoices tool, respectively (Eregata et al. 2021). Other countries such as Afghanistan and Pakistan used the second approach, transferring evidence on incremental cost-effectiveness ratios from global databases like DCP3, or evidence from countries with the most similar health systems. Expert opinion and contextualization of published CEA evidence applied in the Ethiopian case (Hailu et al. 2021). Sudan employed the third approach, with local and international experts providing a rating for each intervention based on its expected value for money.

Overall, all countries clearly considered CEA an important criterion, but none had an institutionalized process for generating local CEA data. Of the different approaches countries used to incorporate CEA, each approach has its own strengths and limitations; for instance, using tools to generate local values for CEA helped provide local and updated estimates, but developing these estimates still involved a resource-intensive process, made more challenging by the limited availability of primary data. Although potentially less time consuming, the second approach to transfer evidence on CEA raises questions about the generalizability of the incremental cost-effectiveness ratios used. The third approach using expert opinion, although likely the quickest, has the obvious limitation of relying on the judgment of individuals. Given the variation of approaches, further work comparing these methodologies and tools to generate local evidence on CEA will provide useful guidance for low- and middle-income countries and economies looking to incorporate CEA in their prioritization process.

ANNEX 15F. IN THE SPOTLIGHT: INTEGRATED SERVICE DELIVERY APPROACH IN THE REVISION OF SOMALIA'S HEALTH SERVICE PACKAGE

Frontline health workers deliver care across a range of conditions according to the demand of people. People seek health care for undifferentiated conditions, such as cough or fever, rather than complaining about a specific disease like pneumonia or tuberculosis. Therefore, listing interventions based on diseases (even if they have a high burden) might lead to a discrete package that is not responsive to demand. On the contrary, the health system should clearly specify what it does for each common demand, such as a simple intervention providing analgesics to relieve pain due to a particular cancer. Moreover, services should be coordinated across different levels of the health care system and lower- and higher-level services aligned. For example, mechanisms should be in place to refer patients from peripheral health centers to hospitals in case of complications.

These two elements (health system responsiveness to common demands and continuity of care across levels of service) constitute the main components of the integrated service delivery approach used in the revision of the health service package in Somalia. The country's approach provides a foundation for providing people-centered services and has the following characteristics: it addresses the way people present, includes all high-burden conditions, makes it easier for the user to understand what services are covered and where they are delivered, and ensures people's movement across the health system and the coordination of referral with higher-level services.

ANNEX 15G. IN THE SPOTLIGHT: ARRANGEMENTS FOR INSTITUTIONALIZATION OF SUDAN'S SERVICE PACKAGE

In Sudan, a specific document was prepared for institutionalization alongside the development of the Essential Health Benefits Package (EHBP). The document suggested a set of governance conventions, management actions, and resources needed to "institutionalize" the EHBP and related financial mechanisms from 2020 to 2025. The distinctive feature of the document is that it will ultimately make the EHBP compatible with the broader governance of Sudan's health system.

In developing this document, (1) all essential functions and activities needed through the five-year period were identified, (2) the governance arrangements required for those functions and activities were mapped, and (3) advisory groups and technical panels were defined, as required. The result was a board of national health care (chaired by the Federal Minister of Health and cochaired by the Federal Minister of Labour and Social Development) for governance and three subordinate boards for delivery, financing, and policy issues. In addition, a dedicated EHBP program team will coordinate EHBP activities using inputs from expert panels. The panels cover various EHBP development areas such as education and training or monitoring and evaluation.

The process also defined the bodies responsible for implementation. The National Health Insurance Fund will hold and disburse pooled health care funds. Federal and state Ministries of Health will cover the sustainable delivery of the EHBP by government-owned health resources, and/or in partnership with the private or third sector, and meeting standards and targets for efficacy, safety and values.

FUNDING SOURCES

Funding was made available through a grant from the Bill & Melinda Gates Foundation, number OPP1201812. This chapter builds on a paper (Baltussen et al. 2023), part of a series of papers coordinated by the DCP3 Country Translation Project at the London School of Hygiene & Tropical Medicine. The sponsor had no involvement in chapter design; collection, analysis, and interpretation of the data; or the writing of the chapter.

NOTES

All authors were involved in the study development and data collection and interpretation. Rob Baltussen, Omar Mwalim, and Reza Majdzadeh analyzed the data and wrote the first version. All authors contributed to writing the final version. Rob Baltussen is responsible for the overall content as guarantor.

1. For more on DCP3, refer to University of Washington, Department of Global Health, DCP3, Economic Evaluation Methods, https://www.dcp-3.org/economic-evaluations.
2. University of Washington, Department of Global Health, "DCP3 Country Translation Project," https://www.dcp-3.org/translation.
3. World Health Organization, UHC Compendium: Health Interventions for Universal health Coverage, https://www.who.int/universal-health-coverage/compendium.
4. Annex 15D is adapted from Lange et al. (2022).

REFERENCES

Abelson, J., F. Wagner, D. DeJean, S. Boesveld, F.-P. Gauvin, S. Bean, R. Axler, et al. 2016. "Public and Patient Involvement in Health Technology Assessment: A Framework for Action." *International Journal of Technology Assessment in Health Care* 32 (4): 256–64. https://doi.org/10.1017/S0266462316000362.

Baltussen, R., M. P. Jansen, E. Mikkelsen, N. Tromp, J. Hontelez, L. Bijlmakers, and G. J. Van der Wilt. 2016. "Priority Setting for Universal Health Coverage: We Need Evidence-Informed Deliberative Processes, Not Just More Evidence on Cost-Effectiveness." *International Journal of Health Policy and Management* 5 (11): 615–18. https://doi.org/10.15171/ijhpm.2016.83.

Baltussen, R., K. Marsh, P. Thokala, V. Diaby, H. Castro, I. Cleemput, M. Garau, et al. 2019. "Multicriteria Decision Analysis to Support Health Technology Assessment Agencies: Benefits, Limitations, and the Way Forward." *Value in Health: The Journal of the International Society for Pharmacoeconomics and Outcomes Research* 22 (11): 1283–88. https://doi.org/10.1016/j.jval.2019.06.014.

Baltussen, R., O. Mwalim, K. Blanchet, M. Carballo, G. T. Eregata, A. Hailu, M. Huda, et al. 2023. "Decision-Making Processes for Essential Packages of Health Services: Experience from Six Countries." *BMJ Global Health* 8: e10704. https://doi.org/10.1136/bmjgh-2022-010704.

Bertram, M., G. Dhaene, and T. Tan-Torres Edejer, eds. 2021. *Institutionalizing Health Technology Assessment Mechanisms: A How to Guide.* Geneva: World Health Organization. https://www.who.int/publications/i/item/9789240020665.

Blanchet, K., F. Ferozuddin, A. J. J. Naeem, F. Farewar, S. A. Saeedzai, and S. Simmonds. 2019. "Priority Setting in a Context of Insecurity, Epidemiological Transition and Low Financial Risk Protection, Afghanistan." *Bulletin of the World Health Organization* 97 (5): 374–76. https://doi.org/10.2471/BLT.18.218941.

Castro, H., C. Suharlim, and R. Kumar R. 2020. "Moving LMICs toward Self-Reliance: A Roadmap for Systematic Priority Setting for Resource Allocation." *The Medicines, Technologies, and Pharmaceutical Services (MTaPS) Program* (blog), September 14, 2020. https://www.mtapsprogram.org/news-blog/moving-lmics-toward-self-reliance-a-roadmap-for-systematic-priority-setting-for-resource-allocation/#:~:text=Home%20%3E%20News%20%3E%20Blogs-,Moving%20LMICs%20Toward%20Self%2Dreliance%3A%20A%20Roadmap%20for%20Systema.

Chalkidou, K., A. Glassman, R. Marten, J. Vega, Y. Teerawattananon, N. Tritasavit, M. Gyansa-Lutterodt, et al. 2016. "Priority-Setting for Achieving Universal Health Coverage." *Bulletin of the World Health Organization* 94 (6): 462–67. https://pmc.ncbi.nlm.nih.gov/articles/PMC4890204/pdf/BLT.15.155721.

Daniels, N. 2000. "Accountability for Reasonableness." *BMJ* 321 (7272): 1300–01.

Eregata, G. T., A. Hailu, K. Stenberg, K. A. Johansson, O. F. Norheim, and M. Y. Bertram. 2021. "Generalised Cost-Effectiveness Analysis of 159 Health Interventions for the Ethiopian Essential Health Service Package." *Cost Effectiveness and Resource Allocation* 19 (1): 2.

Glassman, A., U. Giedion, Y. Sakuma, and P. C. Smith. 2016. "Defining a Health Benefits Package: What Are the Necessary Processes?" *Health Systems & Reform* 2 (1): 39–50.

Glassman, A., U. Giedion, and P. C. Smith. 2017. *What's In, What's Out? Designing Benefits for Universal Health Coverage*. Washington, DC: Center for Global Development. https://www .cgdev.org/publication/whats-in-whats-out-designing-benefits-universal-health-coverage.

Hailu, A., G. T. Eregata, A. Yigezu, M. Y. Bertram, K. A. Johansson, and O. F. Norheim. 2021. "Contextualization of Cost-Effectiveness Evidence from Literature for 382 Health Interventions for the Ethiopian Essential Health Services Package Revision." *Cost Effectiveness and Resource Allocation* 19 (1): 58.

iDSI (International Decisions Support Initiative). 2018. "Health Technology Assessment Toolkit." iDSI Secretariat, London, https://idsihealth.org/HTATOOLKIT.

Khalid, A. F., Lavis, J. N., El-Jardali, F., and Vanstone, M. (2020). "Supporting the Use of Research Evidence in Decision-Making in Crisis Zones in Low- and Middle-Income Countries: A Critical Interpretive Synthesis." *Health Research Policy and Systems* 18 (1): 1–12.

Kunz, R., A. Fretheim, F. Cluzeau, T. J. Wilt, A. Qaseem, M. Lelgemann, M. Kelson, et al. 2012. "Guideline Group Composition and Group Processes: Article 3 in Integrating and Coordinating Efforts in COPD Guideline Development. An Official ATS/ERS Workshop Report." *Proceedings of the American Thoracic Society* 9 (5): 229–33. https://doi .org/10.1513/pats.201208-056ST.

Lange I., F. Feroz, A. J. Naeem, S. A. Saeedzai, F. Arifi, N. Singh, and K. Blanchet. 2022. "The Development of Afghanistan's Integrated Package of Essential Health Services (IPEHS): Vernacular Evidence, Expertise and Ethics in a Priority Setting Process." *Health Policy and Planning* 305 (July): 115010.

Machado-da-Silva, C. L., V. S. Fonseca, and J. M. Crubellate. 2005. "Unlocking the Institutionalization Process: Insights for an Institutionalizing Approach." *Brazilian Administration Review* 2 (1): 1–20.

NICE (National Institute for Health and Care Excellence). 2019. *Policy on Declaring and Managing Interests for NICE Advisory Committees*. London: National Institute for Health and Care Excellence.

Oortwijn, W., M. Jansen, and R. Baltussen. 2022. "Evidence-Informed Deliberative Processes for Health Benefit Package Design—Part II: A Practical Guide." *International Journal of Health Policy and Management* 11 (10): 2327–36. https://www.ijhpm.com/article_4166.html.

Ottersen, T., O. F. Norheim, B. M. Chitah, on behalf of the World Health Organization Consultative Group on Equity and Universal Health Coverage. 2014. "Making Fair Choices on the Path to Universal Health Coverage." *Bulletin of the World Health Organization* 92 (6): 389.

Surgey, G., A. T. Mori, and R. Baltussen. 2022. "Health Technology Assessment in Tanzania: Capacity and Experience of HTA Committee Members." *Journal of Global Health Economics and Policy* 2: e2022004. https://doi.org/10.52872/001c.33116.

Terwindt, F., D. Rajan, and A. Soucat. 2016. "Priority Setting for National Health Policies, Stratgeies and Plans." Chapter 4 in *Strategizing National Health in the 21st Century: A Handbook*. Geneva: World Health Organization.

Tromp, N., and R. Baltussen. 2012. "Mapping of Multiple Criteria for Priority Setting of Health Interventions: An Aid for Decision Makers." *BMC Health Services Research* 12: 454. https://bmchealthservres.biomedcentral.com/articles/10.1186/1472-6963-12-454.

Verguet, S., A. Hailu, G. T. Eregata, S. T. Memirie, K. A. Johansson, and O. F. Norheim. 2021. "Toward Universal Health Coverage in the Post-COVID-19 Era." *Nature Medicine* 27 (3): 380–87. https://www.nature.com/articles/s41591-021-01268-y.

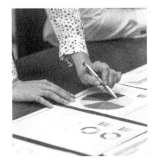

16

Analytical Methods and Tools Used for Priority Setting and Costing for Health Benefits Packages in Low- and Lower-Middle-Income Countries and Economies: Current Approaches

David A. Watkins, Pakwanja Desiree Twea, Sylvestre Gaudin, and Karin Stenberg

ABSTRACT

The design of health benefits packages requires a range of data on the characteristics of candidate interventions, such as their cost-effectiveness and budget impact. This chapter reviews the analytical processes that eight country and economy teams undertook to appraise interventions for their health benefits packages. It summarizes the methods and tools used, including their limitations, and challenges that teams faced. The chapter provides recommendations for future work in this area, with an emphasis on standardization of methods and ongoing support from the international community to build and strengthen analytical capacity among country and economy teams.

INTRODUCTION

Over the past two decades, ever-increasing numbers of countries have committed to universal health coverage (UHC) through political processes such as Sustainable Development Goal target 3.8 ("Achieve universal health coverage") and through World Health Assembly resolutions including WHA58.33 (58th World Health Assembly 2005). To advance the UHC agenda, low- and lower-middle-income countries have undertaken a range of reforms, including the establishment and revision of explicit health benefits packages (HBPs), defined here as prespecified sets of health interventions to which beneficiaries are entitled, usually via public finance and/or publicly mandated benefits.

A 2021 report by the World Health Organization (WHO) outlined eight principles for the design of HBPs (WHO 2021). Although most of the principles relate to processes covered elsewhere in this volume (for example, in chapter 15), principle 4 stresses the need for data-driven, evidence-based approaches that are revised considering new evidence, and principle 6 stresses the need to link HBPs explicitly to domestic health financing strategies. To follow those principles, analysts working on HBP reform benefit greatly from having local data, using consistent analytical methods (for example, on costing), and employing modeling tools that can generate summary estimates of intervention- and package-level costs and impacts.

The Disease Control Priorities (DCP) project was established in part to provide guidance on the sorts of interventions that are likely to provide very good value for money in low-resource settings. The first *DCP* publication proposed the idea of essential packages of interventions designed primarily using cost-effectiveness evidence (World Bank 1993). The third edition of *DCP* (*DCP3*) built on that concept and responded to growing global interest in UHC and HBPs by identifying a core set of interventions that, taken together, represented a model HBP addressing common health needs and constraints across low- and lower-middle-income countries. It called that list "essential universal health coverage" (EUHC).

EUHC was intended as a starting point for country-level deliberation, rather than a prescription for all countries. It was constructed around 218 interventions that had compelling evidence for cost-effectiveness, feasibility, and relevance in low- and lower-middle-income countries. The interventions were identified through systematic literature reviews (emphasizing cost-effectiveness studies) appraised by a network of over 500 international experts, supported by 230 peer reviewers in a process overseen by the US National Academies of Medicine (Jamison et al. 2018). The 218 interventions were identified through a process of harmonizing, de-duplicating, and standardizing all of the interventions recommended across the nine volumes of *DCP3* (Watkins et al. 2017).

In general, *DCP3* did not produce and report de novo estimates of intervention cost-effectiveness in different settings; it presented data from the literature for selected contexts. The exception, a paper released after *DCP3* was published, reported the potential costs of EUHC in stylized low- and lower-middle-income countries settings (Watkins et al. 2020). The expectation was that local technical experts would do additional analyses to contextualize DCP3's qualitative recommendations. As reported herein, several countries did conduct such analyses, using existing tools and guidance.

Upon the release of *DCP3* in 2018, several "country translation" initiatives were undertaken to adapt the recommendations into policy and practice. (Of course, those initiatives also drew on several other evidence repositories, each with its own unique value.) Part 2 of this volume explains those country initiatives in detail. This chapter focuses on the analyses done to generate cost-effectiveness evidence, financial costs, and other parameters that would inform the processes for selecting which interventions to include in the HBP.

The motivation for this chapter is the observation that countries have used a range of data, methods, and tools for those sorts of analysis. Although acknowledging that no "one-method-fits-all" approach exists for HBP design, the chapter notes that countries have struggled to find the methods and tools that fit the data they have available for use. A major focus of the fourth edition of the *DCP* series *(DCP4)* will be to develop new mechanisms and tools for priority setting that add value to existing tools and better meet the needs of users.

To inform the future efforts of DCP4 and partner institutions that support technical work on HBPs, this chapter summarizes the analytical tools, methods, and types of evidence used in intervention prioritization and costing exercises in eight countries and economies where DCP3 recommendations played a key role in HBP development: Afghanistan (chapter 4), Ethiopia (chapter 2), Malawi (chapter 7), Nigeria (chapter 9),[1] Pakistan (chapter 3), Somalia (chapter 6), Sudan (chapter 13), and the semiautonomous region of Zanzibar (chapter 5). The source material for this chapter largely comes from the case study chapters in part 1 of this volume. (This chapter does not include DCP4 case studies from Colombia, India, the Islamic Republic of Iran, and Mexico because of data limitations and differences in the scope of those chapters.) This chapter also summarizes the findings of an in-depth survey of costing methods done for the related DCP3 country translation review process (Gaudin et al. 2023). In reviewing those experiences, the chapter outlines an agenda for research and development of new tools for priority setting for UHC.

IDENTIFYING CANDIDATE INTERVENTIONS AND ASSESSING COST-EFFECTIVENESS

As mentioned, the EUHC list provided an important starting point for identifying HBP candidate interventions in the eight countries and economies, but most made use of other data sources that complemented DCP3 recommendations. For example, they frequently considered interventions included in the WHO-CHOICE (CHOosing Interventions that are Cost-Effective) project or in the OneHealth Tool, along with the contents of the WHO UHC Compendium, a comprehensive database of health services that was developed around the same time the eight country and economy HBP initiatives were being undertaken.[2] Finally, local experts—for example, clinicians participating in technical working groups—were an important source of interventions in some countries, especially for specialist and tertiary interventions that were not the focus of DCP3 (Eregata et al. 2020).

Processes for identifying and appraising interventions vary widely across countries, leading to divergent definitions of interventions at different levels of granularity. For example, the total reported number of interventions analyzed ranges from 97 interventions in Malawi to 1,018 in Ethiopia. Because both countries were looking at a comprehensive HBP that covered the entire health care system, this difference in the number of interventions did not reveal differences in HBP scope or quality; indeed, much of the difference can be attributed to the level of granularity at which country and economy teams defined and understood the term "intervention." What is clear is that appraising a larger number of interventions places more burden on the assessment process, extending the time and effort required (and potentially requiring new or improved tools). One implication is that the community of experts in HBP design would benefit from developing a common definition/delimitation of an "intervention" for the purpose of cost-effectiveness analysis and costing, regardless of the level of granularity required for informing service delivery arrangements during the HBP implementation phase. Standardization would also help make tools and recommendations more transferable across settings.

Cost-effectiveness is widely accepted as a core criterion for designing HBPs and is highlighted in WHO guidance (WHO 2014). Nearly all countries and economies reviewed in this chapter used cost-effectiveness as a criterion in their priority-setting processes. Because of limited local data, most countries used cost-effectiveness estimates from the literature to guide their selection. That approach has three main challenges.

The first challenge relates to topical relevance. Most cost-effectiveness analyses that appear in the literature are done as part of health technology assessment processes for newer drugs, diagnostics, or procedures, with the explicit objective of determining whether they will be covered by purchasers. For example, a published cost-utility analysis of trastuzumab as an add-on to current breast cancer treatment protocols may be relevant to a range of countries with a similar burden of breast cancer and similar drug prices, but it will not yield any useful insights into whether conventional breast cancer treatment (that is, without trastuzumab) is cost-effective in a low-income country where conventional treatment is not widely available. Using a trastuzumab study as a rough indicator of overall breast cancer cost-effectiveness could lead to incorrect conclusions.

The second challenge relates to the limitations of common analytical approaches. Most published estimates focus on the incremental cost-effectiveness of new technologies in comparison to the current service mix provided in that setting ("incremental approach"). However, an HBP might seek to improve allocative efficiency, in which case the appropriate comparison might be a "do nothing" scenario ("sectoral approach") instead of the current service mix (Baltussen et al. 2023). The approach should be tailored to the policy question at hand.

The third challenge relates to the transferability of cost-effectiveness estimates to very different contexts. For example, the cost-effectiveness of malaria prevention and treatment interventions varies greatly depending on the drug regimens used and seasonality and transmissibility (Conteh et al. 2021). Extrapolating cost-effectiveness estimates from a study done in a high-transmission setting to a low-transmission setting may result in a false positive—that is, the analyst might determine the intervention is cost-effective when it in fact is not. Conversely, the cost-effectiveness of sickle-cell disease interventions varies by an order of magnitude depending on the incidence of this genetic disorder (Kuznik et al. 2016). Extrapolating cost-effectiveness estimates from a study done in a low-incidence setting to a high-incidence setting may result in a false negative—that is, the analyst might determine the intervention is not cost-effective when it in fact is. A variant of the false negative risk is that many interventions do not have robust evidence for effectiveness, mostly because they have been in use since before the era of randomized clinical trials (and therefore would be unethical to trial nowadays), yet they are core to any health system. Many surgical interventions fit into this category of being recommended despite lack of gold-standard trial evidence (McCulloch et al. 2002).

Despite the limitations of using cost-effectiveness estimates from the literature, it was the most common approach in the eight country and economy case studies. Local experts reviewed the literature (which was in many cases skewed toward high-income and upper-middle-income countries) for cost-effectiveness estimates. In the Ethiopia initiative, the team translated those estimates to local values using a standardized process (Hailu et al. 2021). International cost-effectiveness evidence has been used in other HBP initiatives, such as in Ghana (Vellekoop, Odame, and Ochalek 2022). Table 16.1 provides information on the data and tools that fed into each assessment of intervention cost-effectiveness. Countries and economies used the cost-effectiveness literature semi-quantitatively to rank most interventions, and some countries analyzed some of the interventions using quantitative approaches (GCEA, Health Interventions Prioritization Tool, FairChoices Tool, or in the case of Malawi a locally developed tool). Ethiopia went further than the other initiatives by conducting de novo analyses to generate locally contextualized GCEA estimates; doing so required a great amount of work but likely enhanced the credibility and accuracy of the priority-setting process (Eregata et al. 2021).

Table 16.1 Cost-Effectiveness Data and Tools Used in Country and Economy Case Studies

	Source(s) of cost-effectiveness information on different interventions	Tools used to analyze intervention cost-effectiveness, if applicable	Number of interventions considered[a] (final number of interventions in the package[b])	Other comments
Afghanistan	DCP3	Health Interventions Prioritization Tool (http://hiptool.org)	149	n.a.
Ethiopia	Locally generated estimates, DCP3, Tufts CEA Registry, WHO-CHOICE peer-reviewed articles	WHO-CHOICE GCEA Tool	Originally considered 1,442 unique interventions; 1,018 included (549 high priority)	n.a.
Malawi	Tufts CEA Registry, DCP2, WHO-CHOICE, systematic reviews	EHP Tool[e]	258 (97)	n.a.
Nigeria	—	—	—	Process done separately from the formal government health benefits package design process
Pakistan	DCP3,[c] Tufts CEA Registry[d]	n.a.	193 (88)	Transferability of global data was done through an explicit process that included matching of the intervention and comparator and a quality assessment
Somalia	DCP3, locally generated estimates	—	412 (412)	Interventions identified and prioritized through a deliberative process
Sudan	Did not use cost-effectiveness per se for ranking; used the following criteria: health need, population impact, quality of evidence, value for money	—	740 (The number of interventions later increased to 824)	Ranking criteria decided through deliberation; interventions scoring by two experts, adjudicated by a third expert; draft scores validated by clinical expert groups
Zanzibar	FairChoices Tool, peer-reviewed articles	FairChoices Tool	302	n.a.

Source: DCP4 chapters 2, 3, 4, 5, 6, 7, 9, and 13.

Note: CEA = cost-effectiveness analysis; *DCP2 = Disease Control Priorities*, second edition; *DCP3 = Disease Control Priorities*, third edition; *DCP4 = Disease Control Priorities*, fourth edition; EHP = essential health package; GCEA = generalized cost-effectiveness analysis; WHO-CHOICE = World Health Organization CHOosing Interventions that are Cost-Effective; n.a. = not applicable; — = not available.

a. Total initial number of interventions considered prior to prioritization.

b. Number of interventions included in the package.

c. University of Washington, Department of Global Health, DCP3, Economic Evaluation Methods, https://www.dcp-3.org/economic-evaluations.

d. Tufts Medical Center, Center for the Evaluation of Value and Risk in Health, "GH CEA Registry," https://cevr.tuftsmedicalcenter.org/databases/gh-cea-registry.

e. The EHP Tool is an Excel-based, locally developed tool designed for the collection, collation, and analysis of disease burden and cost data associated with interventions under consideration for inclusion in the HBP.

METHODS AND TOOLS FOR COSTING AND BUDGETING

Costing is acknowledged as a critical component of any HBP reform process (Cashin and Özaltın 2017). Costing is required both to inform the ranking of interventions for priority setting—presuming it includes criteria like cost-effectiveness and budget impact—and to inform the overall budget envelope/resource needs to implement the HBP. It is important to stress that the approach to costing differs depending on how the cost estimate will be used. Economic costs used for analyzing the long-run cost-effectiveness of an intervention will be numerically different from financial costs used for short-run budgeting and will have a different interpretation. Clarifying the purpose of a cost analysis is therefore essential to the conduct of the costing. A 2021 systematic review of 29 HBP costing studies (2000–20) from 19 countries summarized the approaches and data typically used (Jeet et al. 2021). Those 29 estimates used a range of different costing methods and tools, and study quality (assessed by external criteria) varied considerably. Most studies conducted financial costing using a predominately bottom-up approach.

The Global Health Cost Consortium reference case on cost analyses laid out several principles that could be relevant to HBP costing (Vassall et al. 2017). Those principles include, importantly, the following:

- *Purpose of the analysis*. Is it for doing cost-effectiveness analysis? For medium- to long-term financial planning? For annual budgeting? (The previous section of this chapter covers cost-effectiveness analysis; this section covers the costing done for assessing affordability and medium-term financial planning.)
- *Type of costs*. Are they economic or financial costs (refer to the earlier discussion)? Are they based on norms (for example, provided in best-practice guidelines) or real-world observations (for example, using on-site data collection approaches and/or expenditure data)?
- *Costing dynamics*. What is the time horizon of the analysis? Are the estimates net of any future savings (for example, from preventive interventions)? Do they include the costs of supporting system change and/or improving implementation?

All eight country and economy HBP initiatives featured in this chapter performed a cost analysis of their candidate HBP package. The initiatives most frequently used the OneHealth Tool (OHT)[3] for modeling financial costs for a three- to five-year implementation plan. Country and economy analyses made use of OHT default data on prices and quantities, and incorporated local data. Table 16.2 provides an overview. As mentioned in the related paper from Gaudin et al. (2023), most of the cost analyses were heavily supported by international consultants. The main purpose of the HBP costing was to assess affordability and raise resources. None of the eight countries and economies linked the HBP cost estimates explicitly to budgeting and purchasing arrangements, raising concerns about the translation of those estimates into practice and highlighting an important area for future efforts (Soucat, Tandon, and Gonzales Pier 2023). Linking costing to budgeting and purchasing thus needs to be an important feature of HBP tools in the future and is a priority for the new Integrated Health Tool intended to supersede OHT (box 16.1).

Table 16.2 Costing Tools Used to Generate Full Package Costs in Country and Economy Case Studies

	Source(s) of cost information on different interventions (for example, ingredients and cost drivers)	Tools used to generate local estimates of package costs, if applicable	Time horizon of costing of the final package	Final package cost per capita (% of GDP)
Afghanistan	Local data collection	Cost Revenue Analysis Tool Plus	3 years	US$6.9 (1.3%)
Ethiopia	OneHealth Tool default data, supplemented by local data collection	OneHealth Tool	10 years	US$34 for 2020 under low-cost scenario (3.7%)
Malawi	Local data collection based on standard treatment guidelines	OneHealth Tool	5 years	US$30 for 2021/22 (4.8%)
Nigeria	—	OneHealth Tool	9 years	—
Pakistan	Local data collection	Excel; each intervention was costed separately using a normative, ingredients-based "rapid" approach	Primary analysis: 1 year; secondary analysis of projected costs by province: 7 years	US$12.98 for district-based package (0.98%)
Somalia	—	OneHealth Tool	10 years	US$33 by 2030 (5.9%)
Sudan	OneHealth Tool default data, reviewed and updated to fit the country context	OneHealth Tool	7 years	US$29.3 for first-year cost (4.8%)
Zanzibar	OneHealth Tool default data, supplemented by local data collection	OneHealth Tool	10 years	—

Source: DCP4 chapters 2, 3, 4, 5, 6, 7, 9, and 13. For additional details, please refer to Gaudin et al. (2023).

Note: DCP4 = Disease Control Priorities, fourth edition; GDP = gross domestic product; HBP = health benefits package; — = not available.

Box 16.1

The OneHealth Tool: Status and Future Directions

The OneHealth Tool (OHT)[a] is a tool supported by various United Nations entities (Joint United Nations Programme on HIV/AIDS, United Nations Children's Fund, United Nations Development Programme, United Nations Population Fund, and the World Health Organization) that, since its launch in 2012, has been applied in over 80 countries to support cost and impact modeling for health interventions and strategies. OHT allows users to select interventions, set targets, produce multiyear projections of cost and health impact, and map costs to budget areas and funding sources. Governance mechanisms for OHT include a Country Reference Group, ensuring that user feedback is a guiding principle for the tool design and functionalities.

box continues next page

As shown in table 16.2, most countries and economies covered in this chapter use OHT during their package costing process. The OHT is currently being reprogrammed as an online Integrated Health Tool for Costing, designed to bring standard methods into a modern, online interface.

a. WHO, OneHealth Tool, https://www.who.int/tools/onehealth

OTHER CRITERIA, METHODS, AND TOOLS USED

In addition to cost-effectiveness and budget impact, other highly relevant criteria when prioritizing interventions for HBPs include disease burden addressed, risks versus benefits of an intervention, equity, financial risk protection, feasibility, economic and social impact, and political acceptability (WHO 2021), as well as locally developed criteria. For example, development of Ethiopia's HBP focused on seven criteria: burden of disease, cost-effectiveness, equity impact, financial protection, budget impact, acceptability to the public, and political acceptability (Eregata et al. 2020). Those criteria mirror the ones most commonly used for health technology assessment in high-income countries, including cost-effectiveness, clinical effectiveness, and budget impact (Paris, Deveaux, and Wei 2010).

Although each of the eight country and economy teams used different criteria with different implications for analytical needs, some criteria were used in multiple countries. Examples include health impact, equity impact, and impact on financial protection. Additionally, several conducted an analysis of the potential fiscal space available for health, which they could then compare against the cost of the HBP, helping them determine whether they could afford the HBP as designed.

Six of the eight countries and economies analyzed the overall health impact of the HBP—that is, the anticipated health gains at the population level, with four using OHT (or the related Lives Saved Tool) and two using the Health Interventions Prioritization Tool. The Zanzibar team used a prototype version of the FairChoices Tool, a tool currently under development for DCP4 to support HBP design with a focus on including equity and financial protection alongside cost-effectiveness. Most teams conducted an assessment of potential fiscal space available for health, though as noted in a related paper, those analyses were not done in collaboration

Table 16.3 Other Criteria and Analytics Used to Assess HBPs in Country and Economy Case Studies

	Health impact analysis?	Fiscal space for health analysis?	Consideration of equity?	Consideration of financial protection?	Other comments
Afghanistan	Yes, as an output from the HIP Tool	Yes (HIP Tool)	—	—	n.a.
Ethiopia	—	Yes	Yes (Delphi process)	Yes (Delphi process)	Additional criteria included cost-effectiveness, disease burden, public acceptability, and political acceptability
Malawi	Yes, as an output of the OneHealth Tool	Yes	Yes (qualitative assessment via dialogue)	Yes (specified EHP as free at point of access)	n.a.
Nigeria	Yes, as an output of the Lives Saved Tool	—	Yes (Delphi process)	—	n.a.
Pakistan	Yes, derived from the cost-effectiveness literature	Yes (standard World Bank methods)	Yes, qualitatively	Yes	n.a.
Somalia	Yes, as an output of the OneHealth Tool	Yes (ad hoc method)	—	—	n.a.
Sudan	—	—	Yes, through weighting process	—	Does not explicitly indicate equity but implied in the meet health needs criteria
Zanzibar	Yes, as an output from the FairChoices Tool	Yes (FairChoices Tool)	—	—	n.a.

Source: DCP4 chapters 2, 3, 4, 5, 6, 7, 9, and 13.

Note: Assessments for health impact analysis, equity, and financial risk protection are based on whether the countries addressed these considerations quantitatively through modeling approaches or qualitatively through discussions and incorporating explicit criteria. *DCP4 = Disease Control Priorities,* fourth edition; EHP = essential health package; HIP = Health Interventions Prioritization; n.a. = not applicable; — = not available.

with ministries of finance, limiting their validity and usability (Soucat, Tandon, and Gonzales Pier 2023). Most countries and economies assessed equity impact, but did not use quantitative approaches. Only Ethiopia did a structured assessment of the financial protection properties of the candidate interventions. The range of tools and methods used throughout these initiatives suggests considerable room for methodological innovation and standardization, including quantitative approaches to modeling equity and financial protection alongside cost-effectiveness (WHO 2014). Table 16.3 summarizes the criteria retained in each of the eight countries and the tools used in each case.

LESSONS LEARNED AND FUTURE DIRECTIONS

This chapter summarizes the use of various analytical tools and approaches to support review of interventions for inclusion in HBPs in Afghanistan, Ethiopia, Malawi, Nigeria, Pakistan, Somalia, Sudan, and Zanzibar. Despite some commonalities—for example, all country and economy initiatives made some attempt to appraise intervention cost-effectiveness, and all costed their entire HBP—the depth and scope of the analyses conducted varied widely across countries. Several lessons can be gleaned from their experiences that point to directions for DCP4 and related work.

Given the challenging fiscal environments of many low- and lower-middle-income countries, accurate estimates of HBP costs continue to be an important part of any HBP reform process. As noted by Gaudin et al. (2023), however, several methodological, data, and technical capacity limitations threaten the success of HBP costing exercises. Box 16.2 summarizes those limitations and the way forward.

Another observation involves the substantial amount of time required for the HBP costing exercises (usually 6–20 months) (Gaudin et al. 2023). This could be partly explained by the diverse range of interventions that need to be considered to deal with the health care system holistically. An alternative approach would be to

---

Box 16.2

Key Messages on Health Benefits Package Costing Exercises

Message 1. Health benefits package (HBP) costing exercises to date have used different costing approaches, and it is not clear that analysts in different settings have a shared understanding of the various use cases for costs and why certain methods are appropriate (or not) to a specific use case. There appears to be confusion around cost estimation for cost-effectiveness/cost-efficiency assessments versus costing for financial planning and budgeting. Interpretation of costing terminology also varied, especially around the shared health system–related costs and constraints to scale up. A "reference case" for HBP-related costing that accounts for the different use cases could be developed to improve the quality of future costing studies.

Message 2. Health economists agree that there is no such thing as one "true" cost estimate. All costs are based on a range of assumptions and are only as good as the underlying data. Costing studies need to incorporate a standard set of sensitivity analyses (for example, as recommended by a future reference case, refer to message 1), acknowledge the range of uncertainty in cost estimates, and update their findings regularly as new data are collected.

Message 3. Most costing exercises for HBPs are still being done by international consultants rather than local experts. Health economics capacity-building projects can be an excellent target for future development assistance to countries and regions. Still, short-term trainings that address one-off policy problems are insufficient: training programs need to focus on building institutional capacity over the long term.

Message 4. Most countries make HBP costing and budgeting separate processes, which severely hinders the implementation of the HBP. Tools for HBP costing need to link to budgeting and medium-term financial planning processes, for example, by using a common set of data inputs and assumptions. Future directions for HBP analytics might also include an explicit linkage to provider payment mechanisms and other dimensions of strategic purchasing.

Source: Adapted from Gaudin et al. 2023.

consider a set of distinct "compartments" or "modules" within the health care system (Norheim and Watkins 2023) that can be analyzed separately and at different times, making better use of limited local capacity. For example, a child health program is conceptually distinct enough from an adult mental health program (for example, workforce implications, health outcomes addressed, and financing sources) that the two programs could undergo separate revisions—that is, as "subpackages" of the broader HBP, perhaps on a rolling basis. A system of rolling updates can reflect political priorities and new evidence. For example, many countries are currently examining priority setting for primary health care interventions and/or noncommunicable disease interventions. It should also be recognized that countries usually have more than one HBP, and each HBP would have a defined scope of services, a unique governance mechanism, and a specific budget. For example, some countries have separate packages for community or primary care versus hospital or referral care. Country mechanisms should be set up to inform local institutions and local processes. Another approach is to further development processes of "adaptive health technology assessment." Adaptive health technology assessment explicitly considers the time, data, and resource needs of different methods to generate and synthesize evidence for different decision criteria and has been applied in India and Rwanda, shortening the assessment time. Further work is ongoing to better understand the risks of using simplified analytical methods to inform decision-making (Nemzoff et al., n.d.).

As noted in box 16.2, many low- and lower-middle-income countries lack robust institutions with locally built and sustained technical expertise to inform HBP analysis without relying heavily on external support. In this era of decolonizing global health, the international community needs to pay close attention to the ways it perpetuates dependency and exacerbates an unequal distribution of technical capacity between the global North and the global South (Kwete et al. 2022). Addressing this issue requires three types of changes. First, countries and economies need to institutionalize HBP (and where applicable, health technology assessment) processes to create a permanent system/structure for this sort of work to ensure it has an influence on policy implementation. Second, the development assistance community needs to support investments in technical capacity within these institutional structures so that HBPs can, over time, be completely locally driven and not reliant on external partners. Third, greater investment is needed in guidance and tools that are truly global public goods, along with international financial support for local institutions and programs that have a track record of successful skills and knowledge transfer. Such tools can aid in capacity building and help fast-track HBP-related analyses. At a minimum, country teams need to be empowered to expect more of international consultants, including built-in efforts to strengthen local capacity and greater local ownership of data and outputs from their analyses.

It remains to be seen whether a wide range of countries will prioritize equity and financial protection and whether they can successfully integrate those outcomes alongside cost-effectiveness data. Few examples exist of how to use extended cost-effectiveness analysis to estimate the consequences of multiple interventions in these dimensions (Verguet et al. 2015). Since DCP3 was published, some progress has been made on quantifying equity outcomes (Johansson et al. 2020) and on optimizing health and financial protection within HBPs (Lofgren et al. 2021). The latter is especially important in countries where out-of-pocket payments for essential services are still very high. In those environments, planners face a trade-off between spending available resources on financial protection and spending available resources to expand the population coverage of the HBP or the range of interventions included. Still, additional work is needed to fully bring those criteria into health and population modeling frameworks. The aforementioned FairChoices Tool seeks to do so.

Finally, in addition to the challenges in linking HBP costs to financing arrangements, there are challenges in linking HBP interventions (and their properties) to health system arrangements and constraints. Without explicitly considering shared human resources (for example, primary care nurses) or physical resources (for example, general hospital wards) and the sorts of services that such "multivalent" resources can provide, a purely technocratic analysis focusing on the most cost-effective interventions may lead to an incoherent health care system. Such issues, which form a critical part of the research agenda for new HBP tools, are discussed in detail elsewhere (Reynolds et al. 2023). Ideally, HBP analytics will also inform—and be informed by—a set of core service delivery indicators that can be used to monitor implementation (Danforth et al. 2023) and identify the next set of reforms needed to continue making progress along the path to universal health coverage.

NOTES

1. The Nigeria case study describes the review and selection of high-value interventions for investment done as part of the Lancet Nigeria Commission.
2. World Health Organization, UHC Compendium: Health Interventions for Universal Health Coverage, https://www.who.int/universal-health-coverage/compendium.
3. Avenir Health, "OneHealth Tool," https://www.avenirhealth.org/software-onehealth.

REFERENCES

58th World Health Assembly. 2005. "Sustainable Health Financing, Universal Coverage, and Social Health Insurance." World Health Organization, Geneva. https://iris.who.int/handle/10665/20383.

Baltussen, R., G. Surgey, A. Vassall, O. F. Norheim, K. Chalkidou, S. Siddiqi, M. Nouhi, et al. 2023. "The Use of Cost-Effectiveness Analysis for Health Benefit Package Design—Should Countries Follow a Sectoral, Incremental or Hybrid Approach?" *Cost Effectiveness and Resource Allocation* 21 (1): 75.

Bertram, M. Y., J. A. Lauer, K. Stenberg, T. Tan-Torres Edejer. 2021. "Methods for the Economic Evaluation of Health Care Interventions for Priority Setting in the Health System: An Update from WHO CHOICE." *International Journal of Health Policy and Management* 10 (11): 673–77.

Cashin, C., and A. Özaltın. 2017. *At What Price? Costing the Health Benefits Package.* Washington, DC: Center for Global Development.

Conteh, L., K. Shuford, E. Agboraw, M. Kont, J. Kolaczinski, and E. Patouillard. 2021. "Costs and Cost-Effectiveness of Malaria Control Interventions: A Systematic Literature Review." *Value in Health* 24 (8): 1213–22.

Danforth, K., A. M. Ahmad, K. Blanchet, M. Khalid, A. R. Means, S. T. Memirie, A. Alwan, and D. Watkins. 2023. "Monitoring and Evaluating the Implementation of Essential Packages of Health Services." *BMJ Global Health* 8 (Suppl 1).

Eregata, G. T., A. Hailu, Z. A. Geletu, S. T. Memirie, K. A. Johansson, K. Stenberg, M. Y. Bertram, A. Aman, and O. F. Norheim. 2020. "Revision of the Ethiopian Essential Health Service Package: An Explication of the Process and Methods Used." *Health Systems & Reform* 6 (1): e1829313.

Eregata, G. T., A. Hailu, K. Stenberg, K. A. Johansson, O. F. Norheim, and M. Y. Bertram. 2021. "Generalised Cost-Effectiveness Analysis of 159 Health Interventions for the Ethiopian Essential Health Service Package." *Cost Effectiveness and Resource Allocation* 19 (1): 2.

Gaudin, S., W. Raza, J. Skordis, A. Soucat, K. Stenberg, and A. Alwan. 2023. "Using Costing to Facilitate Policy Making towards Universal Health Coverage: Findings and Recommendations from Country-Level Experiences." *BMJ Global Health* 8 (Suppl 1).

Hailu, A., G. T. Eregata, A. Yigezu, M. Y. Bertram, K. A. Johansson, and O. F. Norheim. 2021. "Contextualization of Cost-Effectiveness Evidence from Literature for 382 Health Interventions for the Ethiopian Essential Health Services Package Revision." *Cost Effectiveness and Resource Allocation* 19 (1): 58.

Jamison, D. T., A. Alwan, C. N. Mock, R. Nugent, D. Watkins, O. Adeyi, S. Anand, et al. 2018. "Universal Health Coverage and Intersectoral Action for Health: Key Messages from *Disease Control Priorities*, 3rd Edition." *The Lancet* 391 (10125): 1108–20.

Jeet, G., E. Masaki, A. Vassall, and S. Prinja. 2021. "Costing of Essential Health Service Packages: A Systematic Review of Methods from Developing Economies." *Value in Health* 24 (11): 1700–13.

Johansson, K. A., J. M. Okland, E. K. Skaftun, G. Bukhman, O. F. Norheim, M. M. Coates, and Ø. A. Haaland. 2020. "Estimating Health Adjusted Age at Death (HAAD)." *PLoS One* 15 (7): e0235955.

Kuznik, A., A. G. Habib, D. Munube, and M. Lamorde. 2016. "Newborn Screening and Prophylactic Interventions for Sickle Cell Disease in 47 Countries in Sub-Saharan Africa: A Cost-Effectiveness Analysis." *BMC Health Services Research* 16: 304.

Kwete, X., K. Tang, L. Chen, R. Ren, Q. Chen, Z. Wu, Y. Cai, and H. Li. 2022. "Decolonizing Global Health: What Should Be the Target of This Movement and Where Does It Lead Us?" *Global Health Research and Policy* 7 (1): 3.

Lofgren, K. T., D. A. Watkins, S. T. Memirie, J. A. Salomon, and S. Verguet. 2021. "Balancing Health and Financial Protection in Health Benefit Package Design." *Health Economics* 30 (12): 3236–47.

McCulloch, P., I. Taylor, M. Sasako, B. Lovett, and D. Griffin. 2002. "Randomised Trials in Surgery: Problems and Possible Solutions." *BMJ* 324 (7351): 1448–51.

Nemzoff, Cassandra, Francis Ruiz, Kalipso Chalkidou, Abha Mehndiratta, Lorna Guinness, Francoise Cluzeau, and Hiral Shah. n.d. "Adaptive Health Technology Assessment to Facilitate Priority Setting in Low- and Middle-Income Countries." *BMJ Global Health* 6 (4). http://orcid.org/0000-0003-2735-0644.

Norheim, O. F., and D. A. Watkins. 2023. "The Role of HTA for Essential Health Benefit Package Design in Low or Middle-Income Countries." *Health Systems & Reform* 9 (3): 2273051.

Paris, V., M. Deveaux, and L. Wei. 2010. *Health Systems Institutional Characteristics: A Survey of 29 OECD Countries*. OECD Health Working Papers, No 50. Paris: OECD Publishing.

Reynolds, T., T. Wilkinson, M. Y. Bertram, M. Jowett, R. Baltussen, A. Mataria, F. Feroz, and M. Jama. 2023. "Building Implementable Packages for Universal Health Coverage." *BMJ Global Health* 8 (Suppl 1).

Soucat, A., A. Tandon, and E. Gonzales Pier. 2023. "From Universal Health Coverage Services Packages to Budget Appropriation: The Long Journey to Implementation." *BMJ Global Health* 8 (Suppl 1).

Vassall, A., S. Sweeney, J. G. Kahn, G. Gomez, L. Bollinger, E. Marseille, B. Herzel, et al. 2017. "Reference Case for Estimating the Costs of Global Health Services and Interventions." Global Health Cost Consortium. https://ghcosting.org/pages/standards/reference_case.

Vellekoop, H., E. Odame, and J. Ochalek. 2022. "Supporting a Review of the Benefits Package of the National Health Insurance Scheme in Ghana." *Cost Effectiveness and Resource Allocation* 20 (1): 32.

Verguet, S., Z. D. Olson, J. B. Babigumira, D. Desalegn, K. A. Johansson, M. E. Kruk, C. E. Levin, et al. 2015. "Health Gains and Financial Risk Protection Afforded by Public Financing of Selected Interventions in Ethiopia: An Extended Cost-Effectiveness Analysis." *The Lancet Global Health* 3 (5): e288–96.

Watkins, D. A., D. T. Jamison, A. Mills, R. Atun, K. Danforth, A. Glassman, S. Horton, et al. 2018. "Universal Health Coverage and Essential Packages of Care." In *Disease Control Priorities* (third edition), Volume 9, *Disease Control Priorities: Improving Health and Reducing Poverty*, edited by D. T. Jamison, H. Gelband, S. Horton, P. Jha, R. Laxminarayan, C. N. Mock, and Rachel Nugent. Washington, DC: World Bank.

Watkins, D. A., J. Qi, Y. Kawakatsu, S. J. Pickersgill, S. E. Horton, and D. T. Jamison. 2020. "Resource Requirements for Essential Universal Health Coverage: A Modelling Study Based on Findings from *Disease Control Priorities*, 3rd Edition." *The Lancet Global Health* 8 (6): e829–39.

WHO (World Health Organization). 2014. *Making Fair Choices on the Path to Universal Health Coverage*. Final Report of the WHO Consultative Group on Equity and Universal Health Coverage. Geneva: WHO.

WHO (World Health Organization). 2021. *Principles of Health Benefit Packages.* Geneva: WHO.

World Bank. 1993. *World Development Report 1993: Investing in Health*. New York: Oxford University Press. https://openknowledge.worldbank.org/handle/10986/5976.

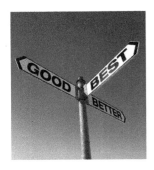

17

Building Implementable Packages for Universal Health Coverage

Teri A. Reynolds, Thomas Wilkinson, Melanie Y. Bertram, Matthew Jowett, John Fogarty, Rob Baltussen, Awad Mataria, Ferrozudin Ferroz, and Mohammad Jama

ABSTRACT

Because no country or health system can provide every possible health service to everyone who might benefit, the prioritization of a defined subset of services for universal availability is intrinsic to universal health coverage. Creating a package of priority services for universal health coverage, however, does not in itself benefit a population: packages have impact only through implementation. There are inherent tensions between the way services are formulated to facilitate criteria-driven prioritization and the formulations that facilitate implementation, and service delivery considerations are rarely well incorporated into package development. Countries face substantial challenges bridging from a list of services in a package to the elements needed to get services to people. The failure to incorporate delivery considerations already at the prioritization and design stage can result in packages that undermine the goals that countries have for service delivery. Based on a range of country experiences, this chapter discusses specific choices about package structure and content and summarizes some ideas on how to build more implementable packages of services for universal health coverage, arguing that well-designed packages can support countries to bridge effectively from intent to implementation.

INTRODUCTION

The central tenet of universal health coverage (UHC) is that all people should have the high-quality care they need without suffering financial hardship.[1]

Because no country or health system can provide every possible health service to everyone who might benefit, the process of prioritizing a defined subset of services for universal availability is intrinsic to UHC. Strongly, though not inevitably, linked to the UHC agenda is the idea that the process should be executed according to certain principles. The World Health Organization (WHO) recommends that prioritization be based on explicit criteria and that it should incorporate consideration of service delivery realities (WHO 2021). Given limited individual resources in most contexts, the UHC requirement for financial protection usually carries with it an implication that public funds will be preferentially directed toward prioritized services (Soucat, Tandon, and Gonzales Pier 2023); in some contexts the explicit goal is to make those services free at the point of care. In general, population access to services intended for UHC may be protected through a variety of government assurance mechanisms, including but not limited to direct financing or direct provision for some groups, mandatory contribution and prepayment schemes, and regulatory structures that constrain what public and private entities pay for or deliver. There are, of course, many other kinds of health service packages and subpackages, designed for a range of uses. This chapter focuses exclusively on packages of priority services intended for UHC (UHC packages, often called essential packages of health services). The component services of a UHC package, sometimes also referred to more generically as *interventions*, span a wide scope of health care activities that depend in turn on specific health system *inputs*, such as health workforce, medications, devices, protocols, and other resources.

The elaboration of a UHC package, however, even when done in perfect accordance with the principles stated earlier, does not in itself benefit a population—packages have impact only through implementation. Despite increasing country interest in (and improving processes for) UHC package development and revision in recent years, a vast implementation gap remains, with coverage of many essential services remaining low even when they are included in a package (Mohamed et al. 2022; Sohail, Wajid, and Chaudhry 2021; Verguet et al. 2021).

Failures of implementation are often attributed to financial resource limitations, but not all barriers are economic. There are inherent tensions between the way services are formulated to facilitate criteria-driven prioritization and the formulations that facilitate implementation, and service delivery considerations are rarely well incorporated into package development. As described later in this chapter, when burden of disease is used as a criterion for inclusion in a UHC package, high-burden health *conditions*, for example, must be "translated" or mapped to the *services* that address those conditions. Interventions taken from a series of independent cost-effectiveness studies (which may span from single drugs or procedures to entire programs), for example, may be too heterogenous to support a consistent delivery approach.

Countries face substantial challenges bridging from a UHC package list to the capacity-building, human, and material resources, and the organizational and financing elements, needed to get services to people. They struggle to account for the interdependence of services and platforms, and to bridge from disease- or population-specific services to integrated service delivery. Finally, they struggle to create a coherent approach to people's health needs from lists of individual interventions that often leave out the foundational demand-driven health services for common conditions that make up much of primary care.

The premise of this chapter is that UHC packages are powerful mechanisms for influencing service delivery (for better or worse), and that there are key strategic choices that countries can make in package design and implementation approaches to facilitate successful delivery of the included health services. Well-designed packages can support countries in bridging effectively from prioritization to implementation; at the same time, the failure to incorporate delivery considerations at the prioritization and design stage can result in packages that undermine the goals that countries have for service delivery, particularly regarding integration and people-centeredness. Of course, well-designed packages are not sufficient in themselves to ensure successful implementation, but they are a necessary foundation and can help ensure that countries' package development processes support their goals for service delivery.

Technical support for package implementation is increasingly identified as a high priority for countries, and this chapter aims to capture ideas on package design based on experiences across many countries—including but not limited to those addressed by other papers in this series (Alwan et al. 2023; Baltussen et al. 2023; Danforth et al. 2023; Gaudin et al. 2023; Siddiqi et al. 2023; Soucat, Tandon, and Gonzales Pier 2023). Recognizing that package implementation is highly context-dependent, this chapter focuses on how considerations related to service delivery can be incorporated into package structure and content to design more implementable packages.

THE USES AND ABUSES OF PACKAGES FOR UHC

Even in highly constrained environments, a complex range of services is provided to different population groups. A UHC package does not seek to encompass all possible services offered by a given health system but explicitly outlines a subset of interventions to be offered universally at a defined level of quality based on need and protected by government assurance mechanisms. A UHC package may be quite small to begin with, containing a limited set of interventions, and its contents progressively expanded over time. Or a UHC package may be larger from the beginning, containing a broad range of services beyond those widely available, and its implementation progressive. In the former case, the package can be operationalized in the near term; in the latter, it sets a horizon of policy intent as resources and capacities expand over time.

Packages that start small have a different relationship to implementation mechanisms than packages that start large (including services that stretch or exceed the current capacity of the system for service delivery). A smaller UHC package is more immediately "operational" and is usually intended to be provided universally in the near term (in such a case, the health system as a whole may deliver much of its care outside the package and its associated UHC guarantees, such as through private sector services paid for by users). An expansive UHC package containing services that exceed current delivery capacity, by contrast, aims to set goals (which are ideally feasible) for what the health system should achieve over time. Fundamentally, UHC packages aim to bridge a gap between people's health needs and the services available to them, but they do so in different ways in different policy contexts. Many countries' packages are a blend of operational and aspirational.

Country experiences show that, whatever the initial intent for package development (and that intent varies among stakeholders), defined packages of services are ultimately used for many purposes (Eregata et al. 2020; Lange et al. 2022; Mallender, Bassett, and Mallender 2020; MoHHS 2021; MoPH 2020; Wright and Holtz 2017). Those purposes include the more traditional use for defining entitlements, but packages are also used to define contracting responsibilities for service providers, and for budgeting purposes. They are widely used to support service planning, including as a foundation for health workforce competencies and training, and for material resource (and supply chain) planning. Finally, they may be used for program reporting, to communicate to donors and partners what is being done for particular diseases or subpopulations. Taken together, those uses confer the power of a UHC package to transform health care delivery, and each of those use cases has implications for the way packages should be designed to best meet country needs.

The most basic presentation of a package is a simple static list of services, perhaps organized by platform of care, health area, or life course stage. Although the exercise of collating such a list should be based on available evidence and accountable deliberative processes, the failure to consider major implementation mechanisms while constructing the package at best limits the power of the package to drive improvements in health outcomes and at worst undermines countries' values and goals for service delivery.

Delivering against a UHC package means bridging the gap from development to implementation, and that delivery process starts with the package itself. There is critical translational work to be done between traditional steps of package development and successful implementation. To that end, approaches to service prioritization, and the package documents that result, should not be driven primarily by what makes prioritization most convenient, or by a theoretical construct of what "ought" to inform relative trade-offs between competing investments, but by the goal of getting care to people and people to care. UHC packages should already incorporate the terminology, content, and structure that will best support implementation. Otherwise, countries risk uncoupling robust package development processes from the service delivery that gives them meaning.

BUILDING IMPLEMENTABLE PACKAGES

The purpose of a UHC package is to influence the care and services that people receive (in that sense, a package is also a plan), and that purpose has substantial implications for how a package should be formulated. The process of implementation-oriented package design is a deliberate adjustment from a historical pattern of service delivery to a model based on available evidence, deliberative processes, and strategic policy direction.

The criteria commonly used for prioritization, particularly burden of disease and cost-effectiveness, strongly shape package terminology and granularity and create interdependence among services. Criteria should be considered together and alone: equity may lead in a different direction than cost-effectiveness, cost-effectiveness formulations may not align with integrated service delivery, and political priorities may conflict with protection of the vulnerable or addressing the local burden of disease. Moreover, each criterion leads to interventions that are formulated in different ways. Movement from criteria-based formulations to implementation, therefore, has many pitfalls and must be actively managed. For example, identifying which services address what part of the burden of disease requires substantial interpretation and often results in services formulated as diseases ("management of asthma" or simply "asthma") that lack the specificity to support implementation (or costing, for that matter). A service described as "initial evaluation and referral for X" (a formulation that appears in several sources) may be effective and cost-effective only when the complementary referral service is available, but such complementary services are rarely considered as a linked prioritization choice.

The reality of service delivery, including information about where services will be delivered and the interdependence among local service delivery platforms, must be considered and the terminology that derives from different selection criteria rationalized to create an implementable package. Formulations from burden of disease lists, for example, are not the same as those from cost-effectiveness analysis (CEA) studies, and neither is optimal for successful implementation (refer to the examples in the following subsections). The structure of packages should support decision-making that incorporates relational health system aspects (for example, referral across platforms), and the content of packages should include foundational services and be expressed in terminology that reduces ambiguity and supports implementation.

Package Structure and Content

Package terminology and structure affect the ability to implement and cost a UHC package. Formulations that lack detail, for example, can be interpreted in many ways and correspond to different resource requirements. For a given reference source to be applicable, the service implemented should be broadly the same as the service studied. Experience in many countries shows that they rarely have any mechanism to ensure that the intervention studied in a reference source is the one included in an implementation plan (for example, a country might have studied "management of ectopic pregnancy," and deemed it cost-effective as a bundle including medical and surgical management, when only surgical management is available in a given context). Interventions are often modified or adapted, and rarely are original evidence sources available or accessed during consultations, nor would such use of such sources always be practical. If that limitation is not made explicit and managed, it can uncouple selection criteria and service delivery in ways that fundamentally affect the legitimacy of the package development and delivery processes.

Often because they aggregate formulations from heterogenous scholarly literature, standard references formulate lists of services that include single drugs or procedures, microprograms, diseases, and subpopulations (Jamison et al. 2018). That approach creates many challenges for implementation. It is difficult to articulate a stepwise implementation strategy that will work for both a single medication (for example, "provision of cotrimoxazole to children born to HIV-positive mothers") and a complex bundle comprising many services (for example, "adolescent-friendly health services including provision of condoms to prevent sexually transmitted infections (STIs), provision of reversible contraception, treatment of injury in general and abuse in particular, and screening and treatment for STIs") (Jamison et al. 2018, annex 3C). It would be even more challenging to develop distinct implementation strategies for each of a list of highly variable package entries.

Package design elements that support implementation considerations, and that can be included in a simple spreadsheet, include the following:

- *Use of a rationalized architecture of interventions with consistent granularity* and nested levels of granularity for different needs. This approach allows choices at the relevant level for different stages of prioritization and assessment, and working groups can view or hide detail as needed (figure 17.1).
- *Use of an architecture of interventions that includes the foundations of care*, such as services for people presenting with undifferentiated syndromes and services associated with the core continuity and coordination functions of primary care (for example, longitudinal care planning, medication review, management of referral, and counter-referral). This practice ensures that the bulk of primary care activities can be represented in the package (figure 17.2).
- *Entries expressed as services rather than diseases*, which supports translation to the delivery context, including assignment to service delivery platforms,

monitoring, mapping of health worker competencies, and other uses such as coverage estimation. Examples include "external hemorrhage control with tourniquet" or "internal fracture fixation" rather than "treatment of injury in general."

- *Specification of local delivery platforms and assignment of services to platforms.* Adding local information on platform names and staffing norms, for example, can guide decisions and foreground feasibility considerations to ensure that the total list of services assigned to a given platform is appropriate. Refer to figures 17.1–17.4 for examples from WHO, Afghanistan, and Somalia.
- *Use of a structure that visually represents relationships among platforms* (for example, by aligning related interventions across rows) to ensure that interdependent interventions (such as lower-level services that depend on higher-level services for their effectiveness and cost-effectiveness) are always seen, reviewed, and prioritized together (figures 17.1–17.3).
- *Creating a mechanism that visually represents current service delivery* and highlights the gaps that must be overcome to deliver the intended package. This type of mechansim helps ensure that feasibility and implementation considerations are foregrounded.

Figure 17.1 WHO UHC SPDI Platform: Mapping Services to Context-Relevant Delivery Platforms to Support Package Implementation

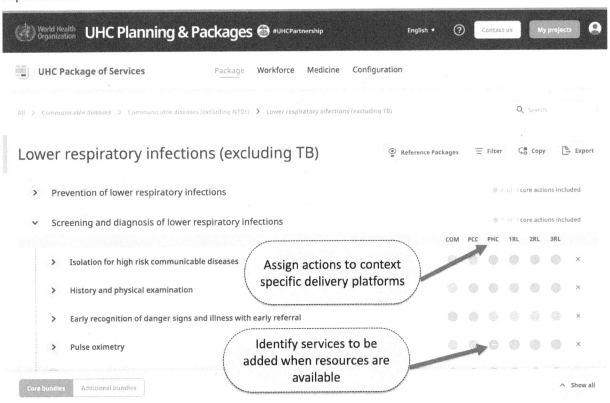

Source: WHO Universal Health Coverage Service Planning, Delivery and Implementation platform (UHC SPDI), https://uhcc.who.int/uhcpackages/ (accessed November 15, 2024).

Note: SPDI = Service Planning, Delivery, and Implementation; TB = tuberculosis; UHC = universal health coverage; WHO = World Health Organization.

Figure 17.2 WHO UHC SPDI Platform: Use of Structured Architecture to Support Explicit Inclusion of Primary and Emergency Care Services

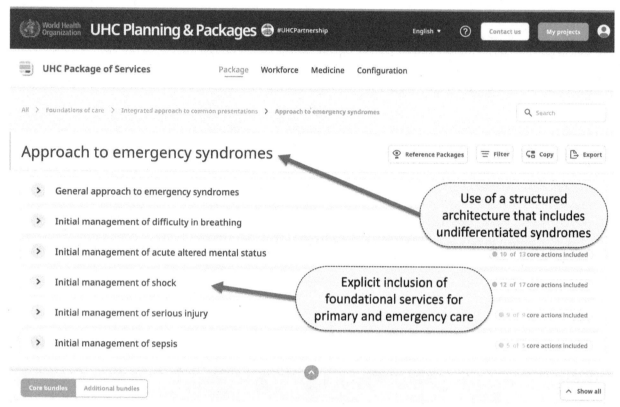

Source: WHO Universal Health Coverage Service Planning, Delivery and Implementation platform (UHC SPDI), https://uhcc.who.int/uhcpackages/ (accessed November 15, 2024).

Note: SPDI = Service Planning, Delivery, and Implementation; UHC = universal health coverage; WHO = World Health Organization.

- *Visualizing linkage to burden of disease, prior packages, and regional or global reference packages.* This process might include, for example, color coding for services addressing top causes of death and disability. It allows simultaneous consideration of this criterion and others and supports prioritization of services and designation of delivery platforms that match the country's health needs. Refer to figures 17.2 and 17.3 for examples from WHO and Somalia.
- *Using symbols or colors that indicate a progressive horizon for implementation,* such as arrows to indicate a shift from the initial platform on which a new service might be introduced to the optimal platform for delivery once capacity or funding is available. Refer to figures 17.1 and 17.3 for examples from WHO and Somalia.
- *Using formulations that have adequate detail* and are organized to support mapping to the human and material resources required for implementation (figure 17.4). This process may also include the use of bundles of services and visits to support costing and cost-effectiveness analyses.

Figure 17.3 Somalia Essential Package of Health Services, 2020: Visual Representation of Services across Platforms to Ensure Prioritization of Interdependent Interventions

Community	Primary health unit (PHU)	Health Centre (Show the Inspector)	District Hospital (DH)	Regional Hospital/ National Hospital	*Additional services
Mental health and substance use disorders					
★ Education on mental health	◉ Support for families	← ★ Detection and referral for depressive disorders with validated interview based tools [WHO-UHC]	◉ Provide psychological interventions for depression [WHO-UHC]	◉ Provide psychological interventions for depression [WHO-UHC]	X-HC Medications for maintenance treatment of bipolar disorder (WHO-UHC)
★ Referral of people needing care		← ◉ Monitor oral regimen for depression [DCP-H]	◉ Initiate oral agents for depression [DCP-H]	◉ Initiate oral agents for depressive disorders [DCP-H]	
			◉ Provide outpatient psychiatric treatment by mental health nurses	◉ Inpatient psychiatric care for depression	
		← ★ Detection and referral for anxiety disorders for all age groups using validated interview based tools [WHO-UHC]	★ Provide psychological interventions for anxiety [WHO-UHC]	★ Provide psychological interventions for anxiety [WHO-UHC]	X-PHU Cognitive behavioural therapy for persons with subthreshold symptoms of mood and anxiety disorders [DCP-P]
		← ★ Monitor oral therapy for anxiety disorders [DCP-H]	★ Initiate oral agents for anxiety [DCP-H]	★ Initiate oral agents for anxiety [DCP-H]	
		← ★ Monitor oral therapy of psychotic disorders [DCP-H]	★ Initiate oral agents for psychotic disorders [DCP-H]	★ Manage refractory psychosis with advanced oral agents [DCP-P]	
			← ★ Administer IM and IV antipsychotic therapies [DCP-P]		
			◉ Provide inpatient psychiatric care for psychotic disorders		
	★ Provide harm reduction services such as safe injection equipment [DCP-H]	★ Provide screening and brief interventions for alcohol use disorders [DCP-E]		← ★ Manage alcohol withdrawal [WHO-UHC]	
		◉ Provide tobacco and khat cessation counselling and nicotine replacement therapy when relevant		← ★ Manage opiate withdrawal [WHO-UHC]	
◉ Promotion of avoidance of FGM	◉ Promotion of avoidance of FGM	◉ Psychosocial support, including supportive communication and problem solving [DCP-E]*	◉ Psychosocial support, including supportive communication and problem solving [DCP-E]*	◉ Psychosocial support, including supportive communication and problem solving [DCP-E]*	
★ Community based prevention programmes for gender-based violence [DCP-H]		★ Clinical assessment for survivors of violence, including documentation and evidence collection as appropriate	★ Clinical assessment for survivors of violence, including documentation and evidence collection as appropriate	★ Clinical assessment for survivors of violence, including documentation and evidence collection as appropriate	
			◉ Provide medical and psychological care for victims of sexual violence, including PEP	◉ Provide medical and psychological care for victims of sexual violence, including PEP	
			◉ Special programme for violence mitigation	◉ Special programme for violence mitigation	
				★ Management of complications following FGM [DCP-E]	

Source: Ministry of Health and Human Services, Federal Republic of Somalia 2020.

Note: DCP-E = DCP Essential UHC; DCP-H = DCP highest priority package; DCP-P = DCP package; FGM = female genital mutilation; IM = intramuscular; IV = intravenous; UHC = universal health coverage; WHO = World Health Organization. Arrows indicate services optimally delivered at a lower-level platform. Other symbols indicate priority or sequencing.

Figure 17.4 Afghanistan Package of Essential Health Services, 2019: Local Information on Platforms and Staffing Norms to Guide Decisions and Foreground Feasibility Considerations

Ministry of Public Health, Afghanistan

Integrated Package of Essential Health Services 2019: Health, Medical, and Surgical Interventions

Table 1. Health, medical, and surgical interventions

*Please note that both the number of each type of facility and the staffing levels shown listed in first two rows of this table were as of December 2018. The Ministry is now examining the implications of the IPEHS and so the numbers and types of staff may change over time. Updates can be obtained from the MoPH Monitoring & Evaluation and Health Information System General Directorate.

Community health post 16,510*	Mobile health teams 309*	Sub-health centre (SHC) 1,001*	Basic health centre (BHC) 874*	Comprehensive health centre (CHC) 433*	District hospital 85*	Provincial hospital 27*
2 Community health workers (CHWs), one female and one male	Doctor do Doctor (where possible),	*Staff: 1 male nurse; 1 community midwife; 1 cleaner/guard	*Staff: 1 male nurse; 1 community midwife; 1 laboratory technician; 1 cleaner/guard	*Staff: 1 male nurse; 1 female nurse; 2 community midwives; 1 community health supervisor; 2 vaccinators; 1 male physician; 1 female physician; 1 laboratory technician; 1 pharmacy technician; 1 psychosocial counsellor; 1 administrator; 4 cleaners/guards; 1 driver	*Staff: 2 male physicians general; 2 female physicians; 1 surgeon; 1 anaesthetist; 1 paediatrician; 1 dentist; 5 male nurses; 5 female nurses; 4 midwives; 1 community health supervisor; 1 pharmacist; 2 vaccinators; 2 laboratory technicians; 1 dental technician; 1 x-ray technician; 1 physiotherapist; 6 cleaners/guards; 1 driver	*Staff: 2 surgeons; 1 anaesthetist; 2 obstetrician /gynaecologists; 2 paediatricians; 2 medical specialists; 7 general practitioners; 1 dentist; 5 nurses; 8 midwives; 12 ward nurses; 2 anaesthetic nurses; 4 nurses for emergency room and outpatient department; 1 physiotherapist; 2 pharmacists; 2 x-ray technicians; 4 laboratory technicians; 1 dental technician; 2 vaccinators; 2 technical assistants; driver

Source: Ministry of Public Health Afghanistan: Integrated Package of Essential Health Services 2019. Provided by the Ministry.

Note: IPEHS = Integrated Package of Essential Health Services; MoPH = Ministry of Public Health. The asterisks link the number of health workers mentioned under the facility to the types of health workers.

CEA and Integration: The Whole and the Sum of Its Parts

Countries have increasing interest in including interventions that are proven to be effective and cost-effective, but there is some mismatch between the techniques and goals of CEA for a specific intervention in a defined context and the techniques and goals of defining a package of priority services for UHC (Bertram et al. 2021; Eregata et al. 2021; Jeet et al. 2021). Challenges with the development and use of CEA data have been described by Baltussen et al. (2023), but this chapter focuses on some of the challenges the use of those data raises for implementation.

CEA evidence can be used effectively to define choices that provide the most benefit within a limited resource envelope, but there are important limitations. Trial-based CEA studies are typically oriented to support decisions about incremental additions to an existing system and are necessarily highly contingent on context. Although CEA evidence transferred to another setting can provide directional indication of the likely relative cost-effectiveness of interventions, CEA cannot provide an absolute quantification of likely costs and benefits across contexts. In recent years, the focus has shifted to model-based CEA studies that typically estimate CEA across populations within the jurisdiction for which the decision is being made (usually national but sometimes cross-country), using data from trials and other sources.

In addition, the CEA literature does not cover the full possible list of services that countries should consider for a UHC package. Given that CEA is often commissioned for new interventions. with potentially high budget impacts, the evidence base on the cost-effectiveness of foundational services that make up the bulk of promotive and demand-driven primary cases is highly limited. A large proportion of facility visits is never linked to a specific diagnosis but is based on symptoms that are assessed, managed, and often resolved without a diagnosis ever being made (Finley et al. 2018; Fontil et al. 2022; Stephenson et al. 2021; Treasure and Jones 2016). Such foundational services are (or are often considered to be) so widely available in well-resourced settings that they do not require a decision on inclusion; in resource-scarce settings, however, they are an important foundational cost that the health sector needs to invest in to achieve UHC. Even for specific conditions, there is a mismatch between the burden of disease and the volume of CEA evidence available (figure 17.5). Among the 218 interventions included in the Disease Control Priorities 3 (DCP3) Essential UHC package, 89 lack adequate supporting CEA evidence.[2]

Bringing together a range of incremental services, particularly when skewed toward newer and emerging services, neither creates a coherent whole nor provides a solid foundation for package development in limited-resource settings. A UHC package will need to include many services even if they have not been—or cannot be— quantified through a cost-effectiveness lens.

Figure 17.5 Number of CEAs versus Disease Burden for Selected Diseases, Selected Regions

a. Latin America and the Caribbean

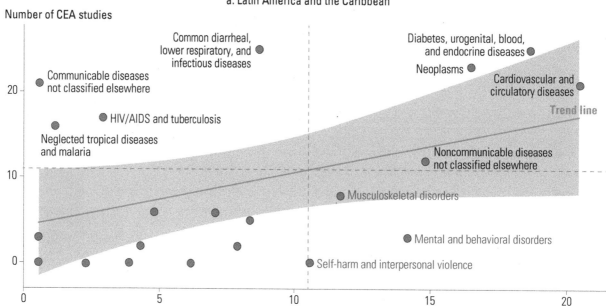

b. Middle East and North Africa

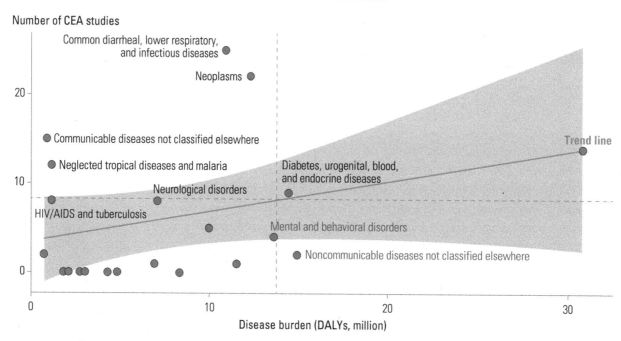

Source: Adapted from Do et al. 2021.

Note: CEA = cost-effectiveness analysis; DALYs = disability-adjusted life years.

Country-Led Priority Setting for Health | Ala Alwan, Mizan Kiros Mirutse, Pakwanja Desiree Twea, and Ole F. Norheim

Several of the countries in this volume have tried to address this gap, by either modeling additional CE estimates or using expert opinion together with information on cost and probable cost-effectiveness. There is also growing literature on adaptive methods for evidence synthesis in CEA to address these gaps, but there remains a need to validate these different approaches. Currently, however, there is a danger that if only existing peer-reviewed cost-effectiveness evidence is used as a prerequisite for package inclusions, a wide range of highly effective services may be excluded.

Consideration for integrated service delivery and its benefits through economies of scope and scale is also important. While there is a general body of evidence (notably around integration of HIV and tuberculosis services, and around integration of HIV services with sexual and reproductive health services), evidence is not widely available for most service combinations. Attention to the economic gains linked to integrated service delivery is essential, and we must build the evidence base on efficiency gains from integration.

Building coherent and implementable packages for UHC requires thinking early on about their ultimate use and complementing CEA considerations by incorporating service delivery considerations into prioritization, as well as into the structure and content of UHC packages themselves.

CONCLUSION

Packages of priority services are intrinsic to the idea of UHC and are powerful mechanisms for influencing service delivery. Despite increasing attention to service package development, however, countries continue to struggle with implementation. Delivering a package means bridging the gap from development to implementation, and that delivery process starts with the package itself. Critical translational work is needed to move from criteria-driven formulations to packages designed to support implementation.

Effective package design will not, of course, ensure effective implementation—designing an implementable package is a necessary but not sufficient step on the road to UHC. Countries can make key strategic choices in package design to facilitate successful delivery, and this chapter aggregates some key ideas from country experiences. Based on these experiences, WHO has developed the UHC Compendium of health interventions and the associated Service Planning, Delivery & Implementation tool,[3] which incorporates the content and structural elements described in this chapter to support countries to take a structured approach to building implementable packages. Approaches to service prioritization, and the package documents that result, should orient to impact and incorporate the terminology, content, and structure that will best support implementation, creating packages aligned with the way countries use them and that improve the care people receive.

ACKNOWLEDGMENTS

This work was supported by the Bill & Melinda Gates Foundation. This chapter is part of a series to be published as a supplement coordinated by the DCP3 Country Translation Project at the London School of Hygiene & Tropical Medicine, which is funded by the Bill & Melinda Gates Foundation. The sponsor had no involvement in the project design; collection, analysis, and interpretation of the data; or the writing of the chapter.

NOTES

1. World Health Organization, Universal Health Coverage, https://www.who.int/health-topics/universal-health-coverage#tab=tab_12022 (accessed August 19, 2022).
2. University of Washington, Department of Global Health, DCP3 Annexes, http://dcp-3.org/chapter/2708/annexes (accessed August 19, 2022).
3. World Health Organization, WHO UHC Service Planning, Delivery & Implementation (SPDI) Platform, https://uhcc.who.int/uhcpackages/.

REFERENCES

Alwan, A., R. Majdzadeh, G. Yamey, K. Blanchet, A. Hailu, M. Jama, K. A. Johansson, et al. 2023. "Country Readiness and Prerequisites for Successful Design and Transition to Implementation of Essential Packages of Health Services: Experience from Six Countries." *BMJ Global Health* 8 (Suppl 1): e010720.

Baltussen, R., O. Mwalim, K. Blanchet, M. Carballo, G. T. Eregata, A. Hailu, M. Huda, et al. 2023. "Decision-Making Processes for Essential Packages of Health Services: Experience from Six Countries." *BMJ Global Health* 8 (Suppl 1): e010704. https://doi.org/10.1136/bmjgh-2022-010704.

Bertram, M. Y., D. Chisholm, R. Watts, T. Waqanivalu, V. Prasad, and C. Varghesee. 2021. "Cost-Effectiveness of Population Level and Individual Level Interventions to Combat Non-communicable Disease in Eastern Sub-Saharan Africa and South East Asia: A WHO-CHOICE Analysis." *International Journal of Health Policy and Management* 10 (11): 724–33. https://doi.org/10.34172/IJHPM.2021.37.

Danforth, K., A. M. Ahmad, K. Blanchet, M. Khalid, A. R. Means, and S. T. Memirie. 2023. "Monitoring and Evaluating the Implementation of Essential Packages of Health Services." *BMJ Global Health* 8 (Suppl 1): e010726. https://doi.org/10.1136/bmjgh-2022-010726.

Do, L. A., P. G. Synnott, S. Ma, and D. A. Ollendorf. 2021. "Bridging the Gap: Aligning Economic Research with Disease Burden." *BMJ Global Health* 6 (6): e005673. https://doi.org/10.1136/bmjgh-2021-005673.

Eregata, G. T., A. Hailu, Z. A. Geletu, S. T. Memirie, K. A. Johansson, K. Stenberg, M. Y. Bertram, et al. 2020. "Revision of the Ethiopian Essential Health Service Package: An Explication of the Process and Methods Used." *Health Systems and Reform* 6 (1): e1829313. https://doi.org/10.1080/23288604.2020.1829313.

Eregata, G. T., A. Hailu, K. Stenberg, K. A. Johansson, O. F. Norheim, and M. Y. Bertram. 2021. "Generalised Cost-Effectiveness Analysis of 159 Health Interventions for the Ethiopian Essential Health Service Package." *Cost Effectiveness and Resource Allocation* 19 (1): 2.

Finley, C. R., D. S. Chan, S. Garrison, C. Korownyk, M. R. Kolber, S. Campbell, D. T. Eurich, et al. 2018. "What Are the Most Common Conditions in Primary Care? Systematic Review." *Canadian Family Physician* 64 (11): 832–40.

Fontil, V., E. C. Khoong, C. Lyles, N. A. Rivadeneira, K. Olazo, M. Hoskote, and U. Sarkar. 2022. "Diagnostic Trajectories in Primary Care at 12 Months: An Observational Cohort Study." *Joint Commission Journal on Quality and Patient Safety* 48 (8): 395–402. https://doi.org/10.1016/j.jcjq.2022.04.010.

Gaudin, S., W. Raza, J. Skordis, A. Soucat, K. Stenberg, and A. Alwan. 2023. "Using Costing to Facilitate Policy Making towards Universal Health Coverage: Findings and Recommendations from Country-Level Experiences." *BMJ Global Health* 8 (Supplement 1): e010735.

Jamison, D. T., H. Gelband, S. Horton, P. Jha, R. Laxminarayan, C. N. Mock, and Rachel Nugent, eds. 2018. *Disease Control Priorities* (third edition), Volume 9, *Disease Control Priorities: Improving Health and Reducing Poverty*. Washington, DC: World Bank. https://documents.worldbank.org/en/publication/documents-reports/documentdetail/527531512569346552/disease-control-priorities-improving-health-and-reducing-poverty.

Jeet, G., E. Masaki, A. Vassall, and S. Prinja. 2021. "Costing of Essential Health Service Packages: A Systematic Review of Methods from Developing Economies." *Value in Health* 24 (11): 1700–13. https://doi.org/10.1016/j.jval.2021.05.021.

Lange, I. L., F. Feroz, A. J. Naeem, S. A. Saeedzai, F. Arifi, N. Singh, and K. Blanchet. 2022. "The Development of Afghanistan's Integrated Package of Essential Health Services: Evidence, Epertise and Ethics in a Priority Setting Process." *Social Science & Medicine* 305: 115010. https://doi.org/10.1016/j.socscimed.2022.115010.

Mallender, J. A., M. Bassett, and J. Mallender. 2020. "Health System Benefit Package Design & Provider Payment Mechanisms: Essential Health Benefits Package Technical Report." Economics By Design. https://sudan-ehbp.com/wp-content/uploads/2021/01/WHO_EBD_EHBP-Technical-Report.pdf.

Ministry of Health and Human Services, Federal Republic of Somalia. 2020. "Appendix: EPHS 2020 interventions." In "Essential Package of Health Services (EPHS) Somalia" (p. 64). Mogadishu, Somalia.

Mohamed, I. S., J. S. Hepburn, B. Ekman, and J. Sundewall. 2022. "Inclusion of Essential Universal Health Coverage Services in Essential Packages of Health Services: A Review of 45 Low- and Lower-Middle Income Countries." *Health Systems & Reform* 8 (1): e2006587. https://doi.org/10.1080/23288604.2021.2006587.

MoHHS (Somalia, Ministry of Health and Human Services). 2021. "Essential Package of Health Services (EPHS) Somalia 2020." Federal Government of Somalia. https://reliefweb.int/report/somalia/essential-package-health-services-ephs-somalia-2020.

MoPH (Afghanistan, Ministry of Public Health). 2020. "Normative Costing of the Integrated Package of Essential Health Services (IPEHS)." Government of Afghanistan. https://moph.gov.af/sites/default/files/2020-12/IPEHS%20Costing%20Report_Sep%2002-2020.pdf.

Siddiqi, S., W. Aftab, A. V. Raman, A. Soucat, and A. Alwan. 2023. "The Role of the Private Sector in Delivering Essential Packages of Health Services: Lessons from Country Experiences." *BMJ Global Health* 8: e010742. https://doi.org/10.1136/bmjgh-2022-010742.

Sohail, S., G. Wajid, and S. Chaudhry. 2021. "Perceptions of Lady Health Workers and Their Trainers about Their Curriculum for Implementing the Interventions Identified for Essential Package of Health Services for Pakistan." *Pakistan Journal of Medical Science* 37 (5): 1295–1301. https://doi.org/10.12669/pjms.37.5.4175.

Soucat, A., A. Tandon, and E. Gonzales Pier. 2023. "From Universal Health Coverage Services Packages to Budget Appropriation: The Long Journey to Implementation." *BMJ Global Health* 8: e010755. https://doi.org/10.1136/bmjgh-2022-010755.

Stephenson, E., D. A. Butt, J. Gronsbell, C. Ji, B. O'Neill, N. Crampton, and K. Tu. 2021. "Changes in the Top 25 Reasons for Primary Care Visits during the COVID-19 Pandemic in a High-COVID Region of Canada." *PLoS One* 16 (8): e0255992. https://doi.org/10.1371/journal.pone.0255992.

Treasure, W., and R. Jones, eds. 2016. *Diagnosis and Risk Management in Primary Care: Words That Count, Numbers That Speak.* London: CRC Press.

Verguet, S., A. Hailu, G. T. Eregata, S. T. Memirie, K. A. Johansson, and O. F. Norheim. 2021. "Toward Universal Health Coverage in the Post-COVID-19 Era." *Nature Medicine* 27 (3): 380–87. https://doi.org/10.1038/s41591-021-01268-y.

WHO (World Health Organization). 2021. *Principles of Health Benefit Packages.* Geneva: WHO.

Wright, J., and J. Holtz. 2017. "Essential Packages of Health Services in 24 Countries: Findings from a Cross-Country Analysis." Health Finance and Governance Project, Bethesda, MD. https://www.hfgproject.org/ephs-cross-country-analysis/.

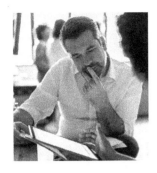

18

The Role of the Private Sector in Delivering Health Benefits Packages: Lessons from Country and Economy Experiences

Sameen Siddiqi, Wafa Aftab, A. Venkat Raman, Agnès Soucat, and Ala Alwan

ABSTRACT

To implement universal health coverage, many countries are adopting essential packages of health services (EPHSs), mostly financed and delivered by the public sector, leaving the potential role of the private sector untapped. Many low- and lower-middle-income countries have devised EPHSs but have limited guidance on translating the package into quality, accessible, and affordable services. This chapter explores the role of the private health sector in achieving universal health coverage, identifies key concerns, and presents experience of the Disease Control Priorities 3 Country Translation Project in Afghanistan, Ethiopia, Pakistan, Somalia, Sudan, and the semiautonomous region of Zanzibar.

Key challenges to engaging the private sector include the complexity and heterogeneity of private providers, their operation in isolation of the health system, limitations of population coverage and equity when leaving private providers to their own choices, and higher overall cost of care for privately delivered services. Irrespective of the strategies employed to involve the private sector in delivering EPHSs, it is necessary to identify private providers in terms of their characteristics and contribution and their response to regulatory tools and incentives.

Strategies for regulating private providers include better statutory control to prevent unlicensed practice, self-regulation by professional bodies to maintain standards of practice, and accreditation of large private hospitals and chains. Additionally, purchasing delivery of essential services by engaging private providers can be an effective regulatory approach to modify provider behavior. Despite existing experience, more research is needed to better explore and operationalize the role of the private sector in implementing EPHSs in low- and lower-middle-income countries.

INTRODUCTION

Private health sector providers are a major actor for provision of health services in low- and lower-middle-income countries. Although private providers operate primarily with commercial and market-oriented motives, enormous scope exists for them to play a key role in the progress toward achieving universal health coverage (UHC) in most countries.

Many countries use essential packages of health services (EPHSs) to progressively implement UHC. Although the public sector mostly delivers such packages, the private sector has a potentially useful, and still untapped, role. Increasingly normative and practical guidance on the development of benefits packages is available to countries (Glassman et al. 2016; WHO 2021). Processes of deliberation for development of benefits packages are maturing, and the need for institutionalization of the process at national and subnational levels is being increasingly asserted (Gopinathan and Ottersen 2017; WHO 2014). According to Glassman and Chalkidou (2012), at least 63 low- and middle-income countries had devised explicit EPHSs, and that number has progressively increased—particularly after the endorsement of UHC as a target in the Sustainable Development Goals.

Limited guidance exists, however, on how to translate a benefits package through effective implementation into quality, accessible, and affordable health care services. Current literature on country experiences provides little information about how to align the objectives and interests of various actors, especially the private health sector, to implement EPHSs and accelerate progress on UHC. The low- and lower-middle-income countries that need to implement such packages have diverse contexts that elude attempts at standardization of implementation approaches—in contrast with the relatively more standard approaches now available for setting UHC packages and increasingly on the deliberative processes of prioritization of health services (Gopinathan and Ottersen 2017; Jansen et al. 2018).

Many low- and lower-middle-income countries currently implementing EPHSs have complex, mixed health systems. Along with a public sector of varying capacity and breadth, those countries often have an extensive and heterogenous private health sector, with varying degrees of governance effectiveness. The mixed structure of their health systems may make it impossible for countries to provide universal access to essential health services without the effective involvement of the private sector, but engaging that sector in the provision of publicly funded packages raises key questions of accountability, quality, efficiency, and governance, which are yet to be appropriately answered (De Wolf and Toebes 2016; Horton and Clark 2016).

This chapter argues that the delivery of services by the private health sector must be broadly understood within the context of the overall health system rather than just by looking at the private providers in isolation (McPake and Hanson 2016). A comprehensive strategy for achieving universal access to health services should strategically review the role of the public and private sectors in service provision so that the two complement each other in achieving health sector goals. Drawing on existing literature and review of country experiences, this chapter explores the role the private health sector could play in achieving UHC, presents the experiences of countries in engaging that sector, and identifies key areas of concern and how they might be approached systematically while implementing an EPHS.

TYPOLOGY AND CHARACTERISTICS OF PRIVATE SECTOR PROVIDERS IN MIXED HEALTH SYSTEMS

In many low- and lower-middle-income countries, a key barrier to a policy approach to the private health sector is the inability of policy makers and planners to accurately characterize the sector. That barrier arises because the sector is often heterogenous and provides a broad array of services—from small shops selling medicines to independent practitioners, including unlicensed providers, to large private hospitals and private insurers (Mackintosh et al. 2016). Different types of providers serve different types of populations, provide different kinds of services, and crucially require different kinds of regulatory strategies to better align their activities with the overall goals of the health system (Stallworthy et al. 2014). Strategically leveraging the role of the private health sector should start with an assessment of the sector's diversity, composition, and contribution (Marten et al. 2014; Stallworthy et al. 2014; Tung and Bennett 2014). Although it is challenging to classify private providers in well-defined categories in low- and lower-middle-income countries, this chapter adapts the categories of private providers as defined by McPake and Hanson (2016) (table 18.1).

Table 18.1 Typology of Private Health Sector Providers in Low- and Lower-Middle-Income Countries

Category	Description
Unqualified and underqualified providers	Sometimes the main providers of health services to poor people, these providers include outlets such as traditional healers, faith healers, unqualified or unlicensed caregivers, and non-formulary-based drugs shops.
Not-for-profit providers	This heterogenous group of providers includes large NGOs, faith-based providers, and donor-funded organizations frequently contracted to provide services such as family planning or primary care in specific locations or to reach out to disadvantaged populations.
Formally registered small to medium private practices	In some low- and lower-middle-income countries, such practices make up a large proportion of the private health sector. They usually provide fee-for-service clinical interventions; however, they may have questionable quality and cost-effectiveness, and they normally exclude those who cannot pay. Governments may have the option to influence the range and quality of services through strategic purchasing or social franchising for special packages of services.[a]
Corporate commercial hospital sector	Although rapidly growing, this sector still plays a minor part in provision of health services in low- and lower-middle-income countries even where it is well developed. The cost of health services provided makes them inaccessible for most households in low- and lower-middle-income countries. Although these hospitals provide good-quality services to the affluent population, they play a limited role in achieving universal access to services because large-scale purchasing cannot be undertaken.[b]

Source: Original table compiled for this publication based on data from multiple sources, including McPake and Hanson 2016.

Note: NGOs = nongovernmental organizations.

a. McPake and Hanson 2016; Sundari Ravindran and Fonn 2011; Tangcharoensathien et al. 2015.

b. McPake and Hanson 2016.

PREVIOUS EVIDENCE ON THE ROLE OF THE PRIVATE SECTOR IN EPHS IMPLEMENTATION

Much of the existing literature on EPHSs focuses on package development, with less information available on country experiences regarding implementation and even less on the role of the private health sector, except in certain areas such as health insurance and commodity supply (PMNCH and SIDA 2019). More pertinent information is available regarding public-private partnerships (PPPs) through outsourcing of publicly financed health services to the private health sector, although that information does not often relate specifically to the delivery of EPHSs (Odendaal et al. 2018; Palmer et al. 2006; Siddiqi, Masud, and Sabri 2006). Previous experience with implementing packages comes mostly from countries in crisis and from postconflict states that receive significant donor funding for health, such as Afghanistan (Newbrander et al. 2014), Cambodia (Bloom et al. 2006), Mozambique, Timor-Leste, and Uganda (Vaux and Visman 2005). The following paragraphs provide two illustrative examples from Afghanistan and Cambodia.

Around the year 2000, Afghanistan had some of the world's worst health indicators and a devastated health system. The public health sector was largely dysfunctional, with services delivered by a multitude of national and international nongovernmental organizations (NGOs). In parallel with the development of the country's basic package of health services (BPHS) in 2003, the Ministry of Public Health (MoPH) decided to contract with NGOs to provide those services (MoPH 2009; Newbrander et al. 2014). Despite concerns that health service delivery was a function of the state, the donors encouraged contracting with well-established NGOs for provision of the BPHS in defined geographic areas (Loevinsohn and Sayed 2008). The NGOs received payment according to budgets they submitted, with full payment depending on achievement of agreed-on goals. The institutionalization of a Grants and Contracts Management Unit within MoPH allowed the ministry to lead the nationwide implementation of the BPHS, which was instrumental in increased access, better access for women, and increased use of services for deliveries (Newbrander et al. 2014).

In 1999, Cambodia contracted out management of public sector primary care facilities to NGOs in five randomly selected districts (Bloom et al. 2006; Odendaal et al. 2018). The contracts specified targets for maternal and child health service improvement. The program increased the availability of 24-hour service, reduced provider absence, and increased supervisory visits. It involved increased public health funding and led to offsetting reductions in private expenditure as residents in treated districts switched from unlicensed drug sellers and traditional healers to government clinics. Concurrently, the Asian Development Bank piloted two models of contracting for health services: (1) *contracting out*, whereby contractors had full responsibility for delivery of all district health services in accordance with the Health Coverage Plan; and (2) *contracting in*, whereby contractors managed only district health care services, with the remaining staff consisting of Ministry of Health civil servants. An evaluation found that contracting to NGOs was feasible, cost-effective, high performing, and equitable, and that it effectively targeted and benefited the poor (ADB 2004).

FEASIBILITY OF ENGAGING THE PRIVATE SECTOR IN EPHS IMPLEMENTATION: COUNTRY AND ECONOMY EXPERIENCES

More recently, the Disease Control Priorities 3 (DCP3) Country Translation Project reviewed the experiences of Afghanistan, Ethiopia, Pakistan, Somalia, Sudan, and Zanzibar in setting and implementing EPHSs using the DCP3 evidence and model packages (Jamison et al. 2018). All six countries and economies have a mix of public and private providers. Formally registered providers operating as individuals or small to medium facilities seem to provide the bulk of services in the private sector, especially in urban areas. Despite its importance, the private health sector does not play a major role in EPHS delivery. As mentioned, Afghanistan is an outlier, with most of its basic and essential benefits packages delivered mainly by NGOs through outsourcing of services. Notwithstanding its short-term benefits, outsourcing is unlikely to be sustainable because of the unpredictability and increasing scarcity of external aid for health (Sabri et al. 2007).

All six countries and economies have a wide range of private health care providers—from large tertiary hospitals and qualified practitioners to unqualified providers. In all countries and economies, policy and regulatory frameworks exist to varying degrees to govern the private health sector, but no country systematically uses that sector in the delivery of EPHSs. Even in countries with social health insurance programs, such as Pakistan and Sudan, benefits packages in those programs are not linked with the EPHS.

All have policy frameworks that support PPPs, with contracting used as the predominant mechanism for engaging the private health sector. PPPs are being used in Afghanistan, Pakistan, and Somalia to enhance delivery of services. The countries and economies show only limited use of social marketing and franchising in delivery of the benefits packages, except for services such as family planning in Pakistan and family planning and nutrition in Afghanistan; but Zanzibar is actively considering such elements. All have substantial out-of-pocket expenditure as a percent of total health expenditure—except Zanzibar, where it is less than 20 percent. Table 18.2 summarizes the feasibility of engaging the private sector in EPHS implementation and presents information on related health financing and service use indicators in the six cases.

Table 18.2 Status of Private Health Sector Arrangements and Feasibility of Engagement in EPHS Implementation, Selected Countries and Economies

	Afghanistan	Ethiopia	Pakistan	Somalia	Sudan	Zanzibar
Types of private providers and Private Health Sector policy framework						
Types of PHS providers and their contribution to delivery of services	• HBPs are provided by NGOs through contracting out to some not-for-profit hospitals. • Unqualified and underqualified providers practice mainly in rural areas. • Limited corporate commercial hospital sector exists.	• Formally registered providers, corporate commercial sector, and some practitioners of traditional medicine	• Private providers include qualified GPs, secondary and tertiary hospitals, and unqualified or underqualified providers. • Some private hospitals are empaneled and implement national health insurance packages.	• NGOs are the largest service providers. • Large numbers of unqualified providers, faith-based healers practice. • Small to medium secondary and tertiary hospitals exist mainly in urban areas.	• Many qualified small to medium private facilities exist. • Corporate sector is present in cities. • Faith healers, herbal medicine sellers, and traditional healers also provide services. • Many health facilities are run by charities and not-for-profits.	• Most providers are registered, licensed, and monitored. • Some unqualified practitioners work as traditional healers. • Private health facilities empaneled with national health insurance program implement benefits packages.
PHS policy framework	• National policy on PHS exists. • MoPH has PHS oversight authority.	• Policy and legal framework for PHS exists and is enforced by regulatory agency. • Licensing and registration system is present for providers.	• Various policies include the PHS. • Common regulatory framework for public and PHS facilities and providers is implemented by licensing and registration bodies.	• No specific policy exists for the PHS; a general law governs commercial sector. • National health sector strategy recognizes PHS, but no regulatory authority exists.	• No national policy framework or regulatory body exists for PHS. • Registration and licensing systems exist under different boards or bodies.	• Policy exists, but no legal framework exists for PHS. • Private Hospital Advisory Board and professional bodies register facilities and providers.
Current level of relationship/ partnership between the public and PHS	• Ministry of Finance manages PPP policy on health. • NGOs provide BPHS and EPHS countrywide via a contracting out model.	• Policy on engaging PHS for service delivery in cities exists. • PHS provides some services included in EPHS but is not obliged to do so. • Some pilot and small-scale PPPs are in place, and a PHS engagement unit exists in MoH.	• Some provinces and programs have PPP policies for service delivery and facility manaagement through contracting with NGOs. • Contracts are not always done through open competition or tied to results-based investments.	• Strategy exists for contracting service delivery to NGOs and private hospitals. • All NGOs are required to deliver EPHS regardless of who contracts them. • MoH has limited capacity to manage contracts.	• No policy exists for PHS engagement, but federal MoH is currently developing one.	• MoH has policy on PHS engagement for service delivery and some programs, and NGOs have PPP policies for health. • Private Hospital Advisory Board acts as the link between MoH and the private sector.

table continues next page

Table 18.2 Status of Private Health Sector Arrangements and Feasibility of Engagement in EPHS Implementation, Selected Countries (continued)

	Afghanistan	Ethiopia	Pakistan	Somalia	Sudan	Zanzibar
	Types of private providers and Private Health Sector policy framework					
Financial and service contribution of the PHS to the delivery of services						
Private expenditure as % of THE (year)	75 (2009) 77 (2019)	—	46.7[a]	—	70.3[b]	—
Out-of-pocket payment as % of THE	77[c]	—	56.48[a]	47	66.95[b]	16
Prepaid plans and social security as % of THE	..	—	0.9[a]	2	6.43 (SHI as % of THE) 24.62 (SHI as % of GGHE)[b]	—
PHS as % of annual total outpatient visits	n.a.	—	75–80 (mainly curative services)	60 (services provided by the PHS)	n.a.	47 (services by PHS mainly curative)
PHS as % of inpatient episodes or hospital visits (year)	n.a.	—	n.a. (bed density in PHS <3/10,000; in public sector 6/10,000)	—	n.a.	—
Policies and interventions used or piloted to engage the PHS in delivering health services and/or HBPs						
Outsourcing/ contracting out	• Delivery of BPHS and EPHS	• None	• Provinces contract out for delivery of primary and secondary services. • Provincial HBPs exist, but role of contracting not defined.	• Private for-profit sector provides more services not included in EPHS, particularly in curative and rehab care.	• NHIF contracts with private facilities to deliver listed services. • FMoH and NHIF codeveloped newly defined EPHS, which will be linked.	NHIF, Jubilee, and Strategies insurance company contract with private facilities to deliver services.
Social marketing or franchising	• Limited vertical projects on family planning, iodized salt, oral rehydration solution (ORS), iron, and folic acid	• Some	• Mainly in family planning through donor funding.	• Not included in the health benefits package.	• Benefits package includes role of social marketing and franchising.	n.a.

table continues next page

Table 18.2 Status of Private Health Sector Arrangements and Feasibility of Engagement in EPHS Implementation, Selected Countries (continued)

	Afghanistan	Ethiopia	Pakistan	Somalia	Sudan	Zanzibar
Types of private providers and Private Health Sector policy framework						
Social (health) insurance	n.a.	• No	• Sehat Sahulat program (health insurance program) covers selected inpatient tertiary and secondary services.	• Not included in the health benefits package.	• SHI covers > 82 %[d] population with own list of services and medicines.	n.a.
Demand-side interventions (vouchers or cash transfers)	• Pilot projects for RMNCH services in two provinces	• No	• Limited and mainly from NGOs, mostly through direct donor financing.	• Not included in the health benefits package.	• With support from World Bank and European Union, cash transfers have been provided intermittently in some areas.	n.a.

Source: Original table developed for this publication.

Note: BPHS = basic package of health services; EPHS = essential package of health services; FMoH = Federal Ministry of Health; GGHE = general government health expenditure; GPs = general practitioners; HBPs = health benefits packages; MoH = Ministry of Healthe; MoPH = Ministry of Public Health; NGOs = nongovernmental organizations; NHIF = National Health Insurance Fund; PHS = private health sector; PPP = public-private partnership; SHI = social health insurance; THE = total health expenditure; .. = negligible; n.a. = not applicable; — = not available.

a. National Health Accounts 2017–18.

b. Sudan System of Health Accounts 2018.

c. National Health Accounts 2019.

d. National Health Insurance Annual Report 2021.

The chapters on India and Nigeria in this volume provide examples of explicitly addressing the role of the private sector in providing defined services in a package, including simultaneous efforts to improve private sector regulation and strategically increase the sector's role in achieving universal access to essential health services.

India's regulatory framework governing the private sector, encompassing both quality control and pricing of services, is identified as weak. However, India's 2017 National Health Policy provides a clear vision for private sector engagement (chapter 10 in this volume). That policy advocates transitioning from input-based financing to output-based purchasing for secondary and tertiary services. India's Pradhan Mantri Jan Arogya Yojana program provides tax-financed noncontributary care to 40 percent of the population by purchasing services from empaneled public and private facilities for secondary and tertiary care. Furthermore, the refined and expanded health benefits package incorporates certain regulatory measures for specific hospital types (for example, public or tertiary hospitals) to mitigate fraud and ensure the delivery of services at the appropriate level.

For the Nigerian context, chapter 9 of this volume proposes enhanced resource management through strategic purchasing and highlights that the new National Health Insurance Authority Act 2022 provides a firm statutory basis for robust oversight and regulation of providers such as through health management organizations. The chapter also suggests a potential role for the private sector in pooling health funding through quasi-public or private entities as one potential way of aligning donor funding with national health priorities. Although recognizing the potential role of the private sector, the chapter advocates for stringent regulation considering the expected expansion of private sector involvement following the 2022 act.

KEY CHALLENGES TO ENGAGING THE PRIVATE HEALTH SECTOR: IMPLICATIONS FOR EPHS IMPLEMENTATION

Engaging the private sector in providing high-quality services as part of EPHS implementation comes with multiple challenges:

- First, understanding the complexity and heterogeneity of private providers is a prerequisite for devising a clear role for those providers in implementing the benefits package.
- Second, private health providers are part of complex mixed health systems and need to complement the public sector without operating in isolation. Box 18.1 elaborates various roles that the private sector plays in mixed health systems (Mackintosh et al. 2016).
- Third, equity and population coverage become challenges when the private health sector is left to its own choices. Without any public subsidy, the private health sector generally provides only a limited set of services and neglects crucial public health services. Private providers therefore are not geared to provide universal coverage of needed services even at the primary level without clear financing mechanisms, additional incentives, and performance monitoring (McPake and Hanson 2016).
- Fourth, challenges related to quality and performance exist. It is often asserted that people use health services from the private sector because of better perceived quality compared to the public sector (WHO 2012); however, perceived quality is often confused with technical quality and patient outcomes. In many cases, overall services are of low quality in both the public and the private sector (Morgan, Ensor, and Waters 2016).
- The final challenge relates to system inefficiency. Private health services may add to the overall costs of care through, for example, overuse of diagnostics and services and overuse of expensive medications leading to waste of resources and other system inefficiencies such as antibiotic resistance. For routine and simple ailments, the public sector is more efficient by limiting overuse of resources and treatments and by providing preventive and public health services (Morgan, Ensor, and Waters 2016).

Box 18.1

Categories of Mixed Health Systems in Low- and Lower-Middle-Income Countries and the Role of the Private Sector

Countries like India and Nigeria have health systems characterized by dominant private provision in primary and secondary care accompanied by high out-of-pocket expenditure. They also have low public expenditure on health. Fees and other charges in the public sector create an additional access barrier encouraging people to turn to private services, which include low-quality and unlicensed providers.

Countries and economies such as Ghana, Malawi, Nepal, and the semiautonomous region of Zanzibar show a stratified private health system with high out-of-pocket expenditure driven by private hospitals and clinics for the more well-off and extensive use by the poor of medicine-selling private shops. The public sector is characterized by varying levels of reliance on fees, which acts as a barrier to access, especially for the poor.

Countries such as Argentina and South Africa have a high-cost private health sector used predominantly by affluent patients, largely financed by private health insurance. The poor generally rely on the public sector, where there is little reliance on service charges.

In Sri Lanka and Thailand, the private sector complements a universalist public sector. Well-funded, high-quality public health systems limit the private sector to a complementary role. That role keeps out-of-pocket costs in check because they mainly relate to use of private services.

Transitioning systems, as in China, have a small private health sector. Such systems traditionally have high private expenditure because of a commercialized public sector, but ongoing reforms are causing that expenditure to fall.

Source: Mackintosh et al. 2016.

DISCUSSION

There is no denying the importance of engaging private health providers in the implementation of UHC packages in the context of low- and lower-middle-income countries. The rather limited evidence, however, makes it less clear how to do so. Using country experiences, the following paragraphs summarize the associated challenges and opportunities as well as possible options for governments to consider when implementing EPHSs in partnership with the private health sector.

Characterizing private providers is essential for understanding their composition, characteristics, and contribution to the overall provision of health care and in determining how the private sector will behave and respond to regulatory tools, incentives and disincentives, and market supply and demand dynamics. In systems with an inadequate or low-quality public sector, engaging the private sector in EPHS delivery seems a realistic option, at least in the short to medium term, for rapidly improving access to essential health services and enhanced financial protection (Ensor et al. 2002; Montagu and Goodman 2016). Private sector engagement has its challenges related to governance issues, such as dual practice of health providers

(WHO 2012); poor quality of care; regulatory compliance; and the limited number of private service providers, which creates a barrier to rapid increase of access to services.

A key takeaway is that, although private providers have an important role to play in such contexts, they are not a panacea to the problem of limited and poor-quality health care services or access to services (Mackintosh et al. 2016; Montagu and Goodman 2016). For instance, the current evidence is mixed about whether financial protection will be provided when services are offered by the private sector as part of a publicly funded benefits package (Ensor et al. 2002; WHO 2012). Although the private sector may play a significant role in the delivery of the publicly financed EPHS, concurrent improvement in the quality of public sector health care delivery in strategic and planned ways is imperative. Whatever strategies countries use to involve the private sector in the delivery of UHC packages, it is necessary to pay attention to the issues of performance and quality. In purchasing interventions from the private sector, countries will need various regulatory tools such as credentialing, accreditation, and use of key performance indicators, along with regular monitoring and enforcement (Montagu and Goodman 2016).

There can be several strategies used for regulating private providers, such as better statutory control to prevent unlicensed practice, self-regulation by professional bodies to maintain professional standards of practice, and accreditation, especially of large private hospitals and chains. Additionally, purchasing delivery of essential services by engaging private providers can serve as an effective regulatory approach to modify provider behavior.

Use of large-scale purchasing interventions has occurred mainly in postconflict situations. Although such purchasing may offer a useful strategy to quickly increase access to services, its long-term sustainability is questionable especially as donor interest fades over time (Ensor et al. 2002; Sabri et al. 2007). In Lebanon, the key challenges to contracting were found to be a weak enabling environment, weak clinical governance, and poor marketing and promotion of the package (Hemadeh, Hammoud, and Kdouh 2019). The Arab Republic of Egypt used PPPs to deliver services for its BPHS for child and maternal care, primary care, and laboratory services, directly managed by a Family Health Fund. Pakistan contracted with private providers to improve access to services in remote areas or to improve the functionality of existing public sector facilities (WHO 2012). However, the evidence for whether such efforts improve access and quality of services is mixed even for small portions of services (Odendaal et al. 2018).

Evidence for financial protection is also not clear. In Argentina and Nigeria, adequacy of funds has presented a problem: only a limited set of services could be provided, and financial sustainability of purchasing interventions has been questionable. In addition, most contracting initiatives in many low- and lower-middle-income countries have not had a pro-poor focus, which suggests inadequate focus on equity (WHO 2012). Therefore, given the evidence so far, it is not clear that large-scale purchasing represents an effective, efficient, or sustainable strategy to provide the larger number of services included in an EPHS.

One view is that a package can act as a tool or instrument for systematizing and aligning the interests of private providers with the overall goals of the health system. In turn, the package can be leveraged as a coordination tool for organizing the health care system and its components, such as financing, purchasing, provider payments, and the organization of service delivery, conceptualizing the role of the private sector within that framework. The explicit nature of the package also facilitates negotiation and conditions of contracts between providers and the government (Giedion, Bitrán, and Tristao 2014).

Although incentives to providers do not always explicitly align with EPHSs, in some countries evidence shows that purchasing strategies are used to ensure quality and efficiency in delivery of the packages. For instance, in Argentina, resources are linked to prioritized services and the outcomes obtained by the providers. By contrast, in Mexico, where resources to providers are not linked with the services in the EPHS, providers have limited incentives to provide services included in the package (Giedion, Bitrán, and Tristao 2014).

Given the urgency to meet the UHC goals, how can governments navigate the challenges of implementing EPHS and progressively achieving UHC while dealing with the uncertainty inherent in working with large, heterogenous, insufficiently documented, and poorly regulated private health sector providers? First, policy makers need to characterize and understand the public health sector in terms of service mix, health expenditure, distribution of services, and its interactions with the public sector as a prerequisite to involving it in EPHS implementation. Second, they must pay attention to supply-side factors—especially the availability of health providers of various categories because that availability can limit their role in rapid expansion of service delivery. Third, countries should conduct a systematic preassessment of private providers and facilities to identify any shortfalls in the infrastructure and personnel needed to provide services included in the EPHS (PMNCH and SIDA 2019). Delivery of EPHSs will not be realized unless countries address the gaps in their health systems (WHO 2021). Fourth, investment and capacity building will also be needed to develop high-quality monitoring and enforcement systems. Finally, increasing overall health expenditure is a must for effective engagement of the private sector in EPHS implementation.

Conflict, political instability, and underinvestment have devastated the health systems in three of the six countries assessed. They face unique challenges of coordinating and dealing with the fragmented aid system as well as with large numbers of NGOs supported by donors that have different approaches to planning, financing, implementing, monitoring, and evaluation. Their governance systems have either collapsed or become severely weakened, and financing health care largely depends on foreign aid. Nevertheless, opportunities exist to rebuild their health systems, including their choice of models for service delivery (for example, the adoption of public financing and private provision). Recent experience in the reviewed countries and economies shows a greater receptiveness of policy makers to positive change than one would encounter in transforming rigid and unyielding health systems, as seen in many low- and lower-middle-income countries.

CONCLUSION

In those systems with an inadequate or low-quality public sector, and in which the private health sector currently provides a substantial proportion of services, designing and implementing EPHSs without involving the private health sector is unrealistic at least in the short term. Such systems are the most likely to benefit from involving the private health sector in the institution and reliable delivery of EPHSs. With private sector involvement, countries may rapidly improve access to essential services and financial protection.

Despite the inevitability of private health sector involvement in UHC, countries need to consider the challenges that surround private health sector engagement before formulating a coherent strategy on such engagement. Better exploring the role of the private health sector in EPHS implementation will require more research, with some of the recommended options operationalized by developing a guide for engaging the private health sector, which can be adapted to the local context, and by piloting EPHS implementation at small subnational administrative levels (for example, by conducting a cluster-randomized trial in a district, assessing impact, and providing recommendations for scaling up implementation).

REFERENCES

ADB (Asian Development Bank). 2004. "Project Completion Report on the Basic Health Services Project in Cambodia." ADB, Mandaluyong. https://www.adb.org/sites/default /files/project-document/70061/pcr-cam-27410.pdf.

Bloom, E., I. Bhushan, D. Clingingsmith, R. Hong, E. King, M. Kremer, B. Loevinsohn, and J. B. Schwartz. 2006. "Contracting for Health: Evidence from Cambodia." Brookings Institution, Washington, DC. https://www.brookings.edu/wp-content/uploads /2016/06/20060720cambodia.pdf.

De Wolf, A. H., and B. Toebes. 2016. "Assessing Private Sector Involvement in Health Care and Universal Health Coverage in Light of the Right to Health." *Health and Human Rights* 18 (2): 79.

Ensor, T., P. Dave-Sen, L. Ali, A. Hossain, S. Begum, and H. Moral. 2002. "Do Essential Service Packages Benefit the Poor? Preliminary Evidence from Bangladesh." *Health Policy and Planning* 17 (3): 247–56.

Giedion, U., R. Bitrán, and I. Tristao. 2014. *Health Benefit Plans in Latin America: A Regional Comparison.* Inter-American Development Bank, Social Protection and Health Division. https://publications.iadb.org/en/health-benefit-plans-latin-america-regional-comparison.

Glassman, A., and K. Chalkidou. 2012. "Priority-Setting in Health: Building Institutions for Smarter Public Spending." Center for Global Development. https://www.cgdev.org /publication/priority-setting-health-building-institutions-smarter-public-spending.

Glassman, A., U. Giedion, Y. Sakuma, and P. C. Smith. 2016. "Defining a Health Benefits Package: What Are the Necessary Processes?" *Health Systems & Reform* 2 (1): 39–50. https://doi.org/10.1080/23288604.2016.1124171.

Gopinathan, U., and T. Ottersen. 2017. "Evidence-Informed Deliberative Processes for Universal Health Coverage: Broadening the Scope: Comment on 'Priority Setting for Universal Health Coverage: We Need Evidence-Informed Deliberative Processes, Not Just More Evidence on Cost-Effectiveness.'" *International Journal of Health Policy and Management* 6 (8): 473.

Hemadeh, R., R. Hammoud, and O. Kdouh. 2019. "Lebanon's Essential Health Care Benefit Package: A Gateway for Universal Health Coverage." *International Journal of Health Planning and Management* 34 (4): e1921–36. https://doi.org/10.1002/hpm.2850.

Horton, R., and S. Clark. 2016. "The Perils and Possibilities of the Private Health Sector." *The Lancet* 388 (10044): 540–41. https://doi.org/10.1016/S0140-6736(16)30774-7.

Jamison, D. T., A. Alwan, C. N. Mock, R. Nugent, D. Watkins, O. Adeyi, S. Anand, et al. 2018. "Universal Health Coverage and Intersectoral Action for Health: Key Messages from *Disease Control Priorities,* 3rd Edition." *The Lancet* 391 (10125): 1108–20. https://doi.org/10.1016/s0140-6736(17)32906-9.

Jansen, M. P., R. Baltussen, E. Mikkelsen, N. Tromp, J. Honotelez, L. Bijlmakers, and G. J. van der Wilt. 2018. "Evidence-Informed Deliberative Processes–Early Dialogue, Broad Focus and Relevance: A Response to Recent Commentaries." *International Journal of Health Policy and Management* 7 (1): 96. https://doi.org/10.15171/ijhpm.2017.88.

Loevinsohn, B., and G. D. Sayed. 2008. "Lessons from the Health Sector in Afghanistan: How Progress Can Be Made in Challenging Circumstances." *JAMA* 300 (6): 724–26. https://doi.org/10.1001/jama.300.6.724.

Mackintosh, M., A. Channon, A. Karan, S. Selvaraj, E. Cavagnero, and H. Zhao. 2016. "What Is the Private Sector? Understanding Private Provision in the Health Systems of Low-Income and Middle-Income Countries." *The Lancet* 388 (10044): 596–605. https://doi.org/10.1016/S0140-6736(16)00342-1.

Marten, R., D. McIntyre, C. Travassos, S. Shishkin, W. Longde, S. Reddy, and J. Vega. 2014. "An Assessment of Progress towards Universal Health Coverage in Brazil, Russia, India, China, and South Africa (BRICS)." *The Lancet* 384 (9960): 2164–71. https://doi.org/10.1016/S0140-6736(14)60075-1.

McPake, B., and K. Hanson. 2016. "Managing the Public–Private Mix to Achieve Universal Health Coverage." *The Lancet* 388 (10044): 622–30. https://doi.org/10.1016/S0140-6736(16)00344-5.

Montagu, D., and C. Goodman. 2016. "Prohibit, Constrain, Encourage, or Purchase: How Should We Engage with the Private Health-Care Sector?" *The Lancet* 388 (10044): 613–21. https://doi.org/10.1016/S0140-6736(16)30242-2.

MoPH (Afghanistan, Ministry of Public Health). 2009. *A Basic Package of Health Services for Afghanistan.* Government of Afghanistan. https://webgate.ec.europa.eu/europeaid/online-services/index.cfm?ADSSChck=1445120985854&do=publi.getDoc&documentId=94459&pubID=128652.

Morgan, R., T. Ensor, and H. Waters. 2016. "Performance of Private Sector Health Care: Implications for Universal Health Coverage." *The Lancet* 388 (10044): 606–12. https://doi.org/10.1016/S0140-6736(16)00343-3.

Newbrander, W., P. Ickx, F. Feroz, and H. Stanekzai. 2014. "Afghanistan's Basic Package of Health Services: Its Development and Effects on Rebuilding the Health System." *Global Public Health* 9 (Supplement 1): S6–S28. https://doi.org/10.1080/17441692.2014.916735.

Odendaal, W. A., K. Ward, J. Uneke, H. Uru-Chukwu, D. Chitama, Y. Balakrishna, and T. Kredo. 2018. "Contracting Out to Improve the Use of Clinical Health Services and Health Outcomes in Low- and Middle-Income Countries." *Cochrane Database of Systematic Reviews* 4 (4): Cd008133. https://doi.org/10.1002/14651858.CD008133.pub2.

Palmer, N., L. Strong, A. Wali, and E. Sondorp. 2006. "Contracting Out Health Services in Fragile States." *BMJ* 332 (7543): 718–21. https://doi.org/10.1136/bmj.332.7543.718.

PMNCH (Partnership for Maternal, Newborn & Child Health) and SIDA (Swedish International Development Cooperation Agency). 2019. "Prioritizing Essential Packages of Health Services in Six Countries in Sub-Saharan Africa: Implications and Lessons for SRHR." SIDA, Stockholm. https://evidentdesign.dk/wp-content/uploads/2020/06/53306-WHO-One-PMNCH-report-web.pdf.

Sabri, B., S. Siddiqi, A. M. Ahmed, F. K. Kakar, and J. Perrot. 2007. "Towards Sustainable Delivery of Health Services in Afghanistan: Options for the Future." *Bulletin of the World Health Organization* 85 (9): 712–18. https://pubmed.ncbi.nlm.nih.gov/18026628/.

Siddiqi, S., T. I. Masud, and B. Sabri. 2006. "Contracting but Not without Caution: Experience with Outsourcing of Health Services in Countries of the Eastern Mediterranean Region." *Bulletin of the World Health Organization* 84 (11): 867–75. https://www.ncbi.nlm.nih.gov /pmc/articles/PMC2627537/pdf/17143460.pdf/.

Stallworthy, G., K. Boahene, K. Ohiri, A. Pamba, and J. Knezovich. 2014. "Roundtable Discussion: What Is the Future Role of the Private Sector in Health?" *Globalization and Health* 10 (1): 1–5. https://globalizationandhealth.biomedcentral.com/articles /10.1186/1744-8603-10-55.

Sundari Ravindran, T. K., and S. Fonn. 2011. "Are Social Franchises Contributing to Universal Access to Reproductive Health Services in Low-Income Countries?" *Reproductive Health Matters* 19 (38): 85–101. https://doi.org/10.1016/S0968-8080(11)38581-3.

Tangcharoensathien, V., S. Limwattananon, W. Patcharanarumol, J. Thammatacharee, P. Jongudomsuk, and S. Sirilak. 2015. "Achieving Universal Health Coverage Goals in Thailand: The Vital Role of Strategic Purchasing." *Health Policy and Planning* 30 (9): 1152–61. https://doi.org/10.1093/heapol/czu120.

Tung, E., and S. Bennett. 2014. "Private Sector, For-Profit Health Providers in Low and Middle Income Countries: Can They Reach the Poor at Scale?" *Globalization and Health* 10 (1): 1–9.

Vaux, T., and E. Visman. 2005. "Service Delivery in Countries Emerging from Conflict." UK Department for International Development, London.

WHO (World Health Organization). 2012. *Role and Contribution of Private Sector in Moving towards Universal Health Coverage in the Eastern Mediterranean Region.* Geneva: WHO, Regional Office for the Eastern Mediterranean.

WHO (World Health Organization). 2014. *Making Fair Choices on the Path to Universal Health Coverage: Final Report of the WHO Consultative Group on Equity and Universal Health Coverage.* Geneva: WHO.

WHO (World Health Organization). 2021. *Principles of Health Benefit Packages.* Geneva: WHO.

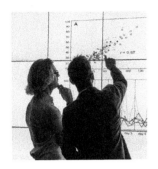

19

Monitoring and Evaluating the Implementation of Essential Packages of Health Services

Kristen Danforth, Ahsan Ahmad, Karl Blanchet, Muhammad Khalid,
Arianna Rubin Means, Solomon Tessema Memirie, Ala Alwan, and David A. Watkins

ABSTRACT

Essential packages of health services (EPHSs) are a critical tool for achieving universal health coverage, especially in low- and lower-middle-income countries; however, guidance and standards for monitoring and evaluation (M&E) of EPHS implementation are lacking. This chapter assesses current approaches to EPHS M&E, including case studies of M&E approaches in Ethiopia, Pakistan, and Somalia. It proposes a step-by-step process for developing a national EPHS M&E framework, starting with a theory of change that links to the specific health system reforms the EPHS aims to accomplish and includes explicit statements about the "what" and "for whom" of M&E efforts. Monitoring frameworks need to consider the additional demands such efforts could make on weak and already-overstretched data systems, and they must put in place processes that enable quick action on emergent implementation challenges. Evaluation frameworks could learn from the field of implementation science; for example, they could adapt the Reach, Effectiveness, Adoption, Implementation, and Maintenance framework to policy implementation. Although each country will need to develop its own locally relevant M&E indicators, all countries are encouraged to include a set of core indicators that align with the Sustainable Development Goal 3 targets and indicators. The chapter concludes with a call to reprioritize M&E more generally and to use the EPHS process as an opportunity for strengthening national health information systems. It also calls for an international learning network on EPHS M&E to generate new evidence and exchange best practices.

INTRODUCTION

Essential packages of health services (EPHSs) have risen to prominence in low- and middle-income countries (LMICs) as a means of delivering on Sustainable Development Goal (SDG) target 3.8 and national commitments to achieve universal health coverage (UHC) (Waddington 2013; Watkins et al. 2017). A major threat to the usefulness of EPHSs is that development and implementation processes have historically paid little attention to monitoring and evaluation (M&E) efforts (Glassman et al. 2016). Consequently, few empirical, country-derived precedents exist on how to conceptualize and execute M&E activities specific to EPHS-related reforms. Resource-limited countries face unique challenges in tracking the implementation and impact of their EPHSs. At the same time, the proliferation of stakeholders with different M&E requirements—for example, external donors, national ministries of health, district health administrative offices, and international normative bodies—limits the transferability of lessons from high-resource settings (Thomas et al. 2021).

This chapter emerged from a series of meetings on capturing lessons learned from country-level efforts to translate the model EPHS recommended in the third edition of *Disease Control Priorities* (*DCP3*). Drawing on the experience of *DCP3* projects in Ethiopia, Pakistan, and Somalia, the chapter summarizes the state of the evidence on M&E for EPHSs. Ethiopia and Pakistan were chosen from among the seven case study countries and economies (others being Afghanistan, Kenya, Somalia, Sudan, and the semiautonomous region of Zanzibar) because they were the farthest along in development of their EPHS M&E frameworks. Somalia was chosen as one of the case studies included in the *Disease Control Priorities,* fourth edition, country and economy experiences series. The chapter proposes a generic framework for EPHS M&E, including reflections on key indicator features. That framework is intended as a starting point for developing local frameworks, and it will need reviewing and updating as experience with EPHS M&E accumulates in the coming years. The chapter also identifies high-priority areas for future research and collective action in this area, with the intention of stimulating new dialogue and laying out a learning agenda for practitioners, project sponsors, researchers, and policy makers.

WHY A NEW APPROACH?

The individual interventions and services within an EPHS exist within the larger health ecosystem, and monitoring and evaluation of those health services come in many varieties. Interventions addressing high-burden communicable conditions are captured by disease-specific M&E efforts, frequently within the context of donor-funded initiatives. Other basic services, such as obstetric care, are tracked by routine health management information systems (HMISs). For a very low-resource country with a limited set of interventions in its EPHS, the combination of such activities may allow for monitoring of all the included services, though in a fragmented, uncoordinated way. At the policy level, national and condition-specific strategy revision processes often include retrospective analyses of health targets, implicitly or explicitly tied to services in an EPHS. Those analyses provide countries with opportunities to take stock and inform changes to the next iteration of strategic plans. Separately, one-off or periodic evaluations of major system areas such as through health sector performance assessments can provide additional insights.

Those myriad efforts are invaluable but are insufficient to capture the implementation and impact of EPHSs in the context of UHC in LMICs. An EPHS is a specific policy tool intended to motivate the rationalization of resource allocation and change the composition of services delivered. In the context of UHC, it is also a tool to advance progressive universalism by expanding the types of health conditions for which care is available. Growing numbers of EPHSs in LMICs include interventions for high-burden noncommunicable diseases, like cardiovascular disease and cancer, as well as acute but complex issues like emergency and surgical care.

To understand whether EPHSs as currently designed are an effective policy mechanism for service delivery reforms will require new approaches for M&E. Those approaches will need to draw on existing theory while integrating classical targets of evaluation, such as commodities and measures of health status, along with measures of policy implementation. The latter is especially important in determining whether the EPHS effectively influences activities throughout different departments of the Ministry of Health, rather than simply sitting on a shelf in the planning department. The new approach is not meant to duplicate the immense M&E efforts already under way, but rather to interrogate the data they collect in a way that allows for determining whether the resource-intensive processes involved in health benefits package revision are producing the desired impact on resource allocation, equity, and ultimately the scope of care available to patients at little to no cost. The following sections briefly review relevant literature on EPHS M&E, reflect on EPHS M&E experiences in Ethiopia, Pakistan, and Somalia (three countries that recently underwent EPHS revision processes), and outline how other countries could develop their own frameworks.

M&E OF HEALTH SERVICES PACKAGES IN THE UHC ERA

Information to supplement the experiences of the *DCP3* country projects and place them in context came from searches of Pubmed, PAIS, and a few gray literature sources known to contain information on EPHS M&E. The original search, conducted in January 2022 and updated in January 2023, focused on studies published after 2002. (Refer to online annex 19A for additional information regarding the methods used [https://dcp4.w.uib.no/volumes/volume-1-country-led -priority-setting-for-health].)

Monitoring

High-income country analogues of EPHSs are benefits packages and medicine formularies that act primarily as tools for determining provider payments and controlling drug costs (Ulmer et al. 2012). In LMICs, however, EPHSs have a mandate to rationalize the entire suite of health services currently (or potentially) provided in the country. Countries often link EPHSs to national strategic planning exercises and, as such, use them to outline a vision for health reforms that can help progressively realize UHC by expanding the range of publicly financed health services (for example, to address emerging challenges like cancer or cardiovascular disease) as available budgets for health increase (Soucat, Tandon, and Gonzales Pier 2023). High-quality, timely monitoring is essential for accountability and management of health facilities, and findings from the literature support the need to leverage existing data collection efforts to the greatest extent possible, even if they provide an incomplete picture of EPHS adoption, implementation, and impact (Global Health Cluster and WHO EPHS Task Team 2018).

Current monitoring efforts in LMICs emerged from specific programs or disease areas (such as HIV/AIDS, family planning, and vaccination campaigns) and efforts to strengthen national HMISs generally (Thomas et al. 2021). In settings where resource constraints effectively limit EPHSs to donor-financed interventions delivered in community and primary care settings, a robust HMIS could capture the alignment of service delivery outputs with EPHS priorities. HMISs alone, however, cannot monitor whether an EPHS as a policy mechanism is being implemented as intended (for example, EPHS dissemination, or changes in financial flows following EPHS revisions). Little monitoring guidance exists for complex, integrative policy efforts such as those related to UHC, though emerging work from the field of policy implementation science offers promise (Bullock et al. 2021). Compounding the challenge is the fragmentation of financing and service provision mechanisms. For example, the most recent resource-mapping exercise in Malawi identified 185 sources of funding, which flowed through 226 implementing agents (Yoon et al. 2021). Existing approaches to routine monitoring—tied to specific development projects and global health initiatives—may not be meaningful for EPHS M&E.

Evaluation

The search yielded seven publications evaluating EPHSs in LMICs. Six studies either compared the contents of an EPHS to a normative set of recommended services (Akazili et al. 2020; Hepburn et al. 2021; Shekh Mohamed et al. 2022) or assessed the extent to which the EPHS development process reflected an overarching set of aims (such as human rights) (Chapman, Forman, and Lamprea 2017; Kapiriri 2013; Mbau et al. 2023). One study assessed a set of service delivery indicators to understand the impact of EPHS on clinical or health outcomes (Bowie and Mwase 2011). Beyond systematic evaluations, information on EPHS effectiveness surfaced in case studies and program reports (Phoya et al. 2014; Wright and Holtz 2017). The publications on EPHS implementation discussed one-time evaluation activities that occur after policy adoption and use a range of methods. The search did not find any instances of the integration of formal impact evaluations into EPHS planning and design; however, to the extent that such integration occurred, it would likely have been captured within national policy processes and thus not picked up by the search method.

COUNTRY EXPERIENCES

The following subsections summarize the experiences with EPHS M&E in three *DCP3* country projects, illustrating different potential approaches.

EPHS M&E Approach in Ethiopia

Ethiopia took a parsimonious approach to M&E that relies heavily on population surveys (Eregata et al. 2020; FMoH 2021) and trends in health outcomes reported by the Global Burden of Disease study. Other countries with resource-limited information systems might choose such an approach, which is feasible in nearly all contexts and requires limited setup or additional EPHS-specific M&E investment. Still, imperfect survey coverage makes it difficult to reliably correlate changes in deaths and disability-adjusted life years to specific EPHS measures, making the approach suboptimal.

Ethiopia's Federal Ministry of Health completed an EPHS revision process in 2019. That process involved 35 consultative workshops with numerous stakeholders and resulted in a list of about 1,000 interventions to be included in the EPHS, with just over half deemed high priority and thus free of charge. (Unlike in Afghanistan and Pakistan, the process in Ethiopia drew on a range of sources for candidate interventions, beyond the model lists from *DCP3*.) Refer to Eregata et al. (2020) for a summary of the deliberative process and outcomes.

Development of M&E plans occurred later in the EPHS reform process, with M&E for the EPHS nested in a larger M&E framework for all of Ethiopia's Health Sector Strategic Plan goals (FMoH 2021). Ethiopia's framework relies heavily on population-based surveys supplemented by other data sources like health information systems and National Health Accounts data (refer to online annex 19B, https://dcp4.w.uib.no/volumes/volume-1-country-led-priority-setting -for-health).

To track the EPHS's objectives related to universal health coverage, the Ministry of Health chose 16 tracer service coverage indicators that aligned with the World Health Organization Service Coverage Index and with SDG indicator 3.8.1. It also included financial risk protection indicators (online annex 19B). The overarching M&E framework also includes a proposed list of tracer indicators to explicitly monitor equity of service provision across several dimensions (including sex, wealth, and geography) during the EPHS implementation time frame (FMoH 2021).

The Ministry intends to evaluate the impact of the EPHS by tracking annual estimates of age-standardized death and disability-adjusted life-year rates using estimates from the Global Burden of Disease study, with 2019 as the baseline year for evaluation (online annex 19B). The framework also includes mechanisms for assessing how the EPHS has been adopted within various strategy and planning activities, such as the national essential drugs list and development/revision of clinical guidelines.

EPHS M&E Approach in Pakistan

Pakistan is pursuing a more ambitious approach (Shekh Mohamed et al. 2022). Its M&E efforts will use a broader array of domestically generated, service delivery–focused indicator data collected via existing, strengthened national and subnational health information systems. The monitoring data will be aggregated up to evaluative metrics. Other countries considering this approach would need to ensure sufficient resources for developing and maintaining such a system. For Pakistan, the increased costs are balanced by the potential benefits of (1) leveraging the EPHS process to strengthen much-needed existing health information system infrastructure at the local and national levels, and (2) generating data that provide a compelling case for the benefits of the EPHS on equity, financial risk protection, societal trust, and health outcomes.

Over 2017–18, Pakistan's Ministry of National Health Services, Regulations & Coordination led a two-year process to develop a national-level EPHS. Because of the federal and decentralized design of its health system, Pakistan intended the EPHS as a model for contextualized, provincial-level EPHSs. That process was under way as of 2021, with early-stage implementation in selected districts. As in Ethiopia, the national M&E framework is intended to align with Pakistan's global commitments, principally to SDG indicators 3.8.1 (service coverage index) and 3.8.2 (financial protection).

The EPHS M&E framework development process involved detailed consultations with provincial governments, development partners (including United Nations agencies), and international academic institutes such as the London School of Hygiene and Tropical Medicine. Development of the M&E framework, organized around a results chain model that includes the six components of the World Health Organization health systems framework, used the following cardinal principles:

- The district as the primary unit of implementation and of M&E
- Enhanced use of district-level routine data (that is, existing HMISs) or monitoring, complemented by provincial- and national-level data
- A careful approach to selection and use of monitoring indicators, ensuring they can all be collected and reviewed regularly
- Monthly, quarterly, and yearly benchmarks for EPHS monitoring
- Use of rapid and targeted special data collection activities in the yearly monitoring activities; examples include short client exit surveys, community catchment surveys across the served populations of primary health care facilities, and other data to assess effective coverage
- Taking a systemwide approach to monitoring rather than focusing on the EPHS; the rationale for this approach was to integrate efforts related to universal health coverage into the existing health system, including its M&E function.

The principles apply particularly to monitoring. A detailed evaluation, planned after three years of implementation, will involve additional survey data collection (for example, facility surveys, client exit surveys, and qualitative assessments of process indicators). Refer to online annex 19C for more on Pakistan's approach (https://dcp4.w.uib.no/volumes/volume-1-country-led-priority-setting-for-health).

Somalia's Experience in Revising Its EPHS M&E Framework

The prolonged conflict in Somalia has hampered the country's progress on its health system objectives. Despite the challenges facing it, the country has sought to continue its efforts for improving population health by defining EPHSs. The initial EPHS, developed in 2009, allowed the country to expand service delivery through targeted demand creation and health system investments. The process of revising the package started in 2020 and aimed to address the shortfalls of the earlier work through an implementable package that incorporates a comprehensive approach to service delivery and enhances health system responsiveness. (Chapter 6 in this volume details Somalia's experience during the 2020 revision of its EPHS.)

The revision of the EPHS included the development of an M&E framework. Until that point, Somalia lacked a standardized health information system, necessitating the establishment of a system capable of generating routine and consistent data. As part of that process, it defined a standard list of key indicators. The data sources for those indicators included surveys, community-based surveillance systems, and a routine District Health Information System. The M&E framework aims to monitor multiple dimensions including service delivery, quality of health services, and overall impact of the EPHS. To ensure transparency and accountability, an independent agency is involved in conducting the M&E activities.

KEY ISSUES AND UNKNOWNS IN EPHS M&E PROCESSES

Logic models, used in both Ethiopia's and Pakistan's EPHS monitoring plans, and theories of change commonly used in program monitoring more broadly provide a starting point for EPHS monitoring but suffer from two limitations (Rogers 2014; Sharp 2021; W. K. Kellogg Foundation 2004). On the one hand, the simplified, linear approaches used to track single disease initiatives are inadequate for effectively monitoring the complex, systems-level objectives of health benefits packages. On the other hand, the existing EPHS-specific guidance from better-resourced countries requires extensive, highly detailed data that are often unavailable in lesser-resourced countries.

When it comes to evaluation, available empirical data are even more scarce. The cross-sectoral, decentralized nature of an EPHS makes an integrated evaluation unlikely because the EPHS is not any one department's domain, as underscored by the lack of existing literature and empirical examples. Unlike monitoring, however, existing evaluation and implementation models and tools could be readily adapted to an EPHS.

Applying current M&E frameworks to an EPHS runs the risk of going straight from policy formulation to measuring changes in service coverage and health outcomes, thereby skipping the intermediary processes essential for understanding and improving the implementation of EPHSs. Developing effective EPHS M&E frameworks requires a better understanding of the mechanisms of EPHS operation on health systems and the determinants of EPHS implementation, as distinct from broader health system and socioeconomic factors.

PROPOSED APPROACH TO EPHS M&E

Given the lack of a systematic approach to monitoring and evaluating the implementation of EPHSs, this chapter proposes the following stepwise approach.

Step 1. Develop Theories of Change

Figure 19.1 presents examples of simple theories of change that illustrate how EPHS-related reforms might influence health and systems processes and outcomes that M&E activities ought to capture. It shows the types of questions a detailed theory of change might ask relating to priority areas for UHC and the EPHS, such as essential medicines, equitable financing, and management of chronic diseases like hypertension. Local theories of change will need to include the roles and obligations of nongovernment actors as applicable. For example, external partners may provide financial support for EPHS interventions, or private sector physician groups might have a contractual arrangement with the government to provide certain essential services. Overall, the theory-of-change exercise aims to help the Ministry of Health determine what is being monitored or evaluated, and for whom (that is, the government or otherwise).

Step 2. Create an EPHS M&E Framework

The most common approach to M&E framework development is a results chain or logic model, which links program inputs, activities, outputs, outcomes, and impact(s) in a linear and causal manner (UNAIDS 2010; W. K. Kellogg Foundation 2004). Such an approach is ideal for standalone health programs of low to moderate complexity (Institute of Medicine 2013; Nutbeam et al. 2015); however, it is unclear how applicable this linear, unidirectional approach is for whole-system reforms such as those implied in EPHS exercises. A retrospective look at Pakistan's experience in coming years could provide insight into the usefulness of the approach.

Figure 19.1 Sample Questions or Tracer Indicators Based on Theories of Change for EPHS Reform

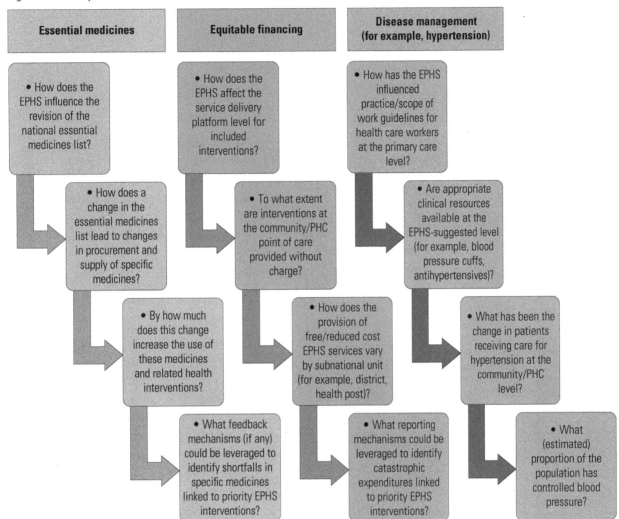

Source: Original figure for this publication.

Note: EPHS = essential package of health services; PHC = primary health care.

The framework for EPHS monitoring and the framework for EPHS evaluation should be distinct and separate documents, but they should align with each other as well as with the overall health sector M&E strategy. Monitoring is understood as an ongoing effort that uses routine data and existing staff to ensure that EPHS reforms are being implemented and corrected as needed to achieve the intended objectives. Thus, the EPHS monitoring framework should place relatively greater emphasis on policy processes and intermediate indicators to enable quick identification and remediation of emergent implementation shortfalls. By contrast, evaluation is understood as a periodic effort, usually covering a period of at least 12 months, that builds onto monitoring activities with specialized and one-off data collection to ensure that the planned reforms are achieving their intended outcomes. Thus, the EPHS evaluation framework should place relatively greater emphasis on measures of service coverage, health status, client satisfaction, and so on, to build a coherent understanding of the effectiveness of the EPHS reforms and their effect on populations and health system performance.

Monitoring

Monitoring frameworks should start from the recognition that much work has been done to strengthen health information systems in LMICs and that many countries regularly review and revise their national and subnational indicators (Aqil, Lippeveld, and Hozumi 2009; Belay, Azim, and Kassahun 2014; Mutale et al. 2013). EPHS monitoring needs to determine how those existing data collection efforts, along with expensive ongoing surveys and health indicator databases, can be combined to understand EPHS implementation, rather than create novel indicators, as discussed in step 3 (Global Health Cluster and WHO EPHS Task Team 2018). Developing recommendations on procedures for identifying tracer indicators, for example, would be beneficial.

Monitoring of the EPHS should occur in multiple dimensions (refer to the earlier discussion on theory of change). Ministries need to monitor the content of the package itself as well as the process used for its development. Relevant characteristics to consider include responsiveness to local needs, inclusiveness, the extent to which the delivery and organization of services match the implementation arrangements with the health system, and feasibility (Glassman, Giedion, and Smith 2017). Without capturing these metrics over time, countries will find it difficult to determine whether implementation failures are due to a lack of acceptability or adoption of the EPHS (for example, among subnational planning teams), to limited demand for mismatched services, to insufficient resources, or to other factors.

The EPHS is fundamentally an evidence-informed tool to advance the UHC agenda, primarily via client interactions with the health care system. Prior retrospective assessments of EPHSs focused on nationally defined packages (Hepburn et al. 2021; Kapiriri 2013) but did not consider adaptations made, formally or informally, at subnational levels of service planning, or did not consider the EPHSs' impact on use or out-of-pocket costs. Not only is EPHS development an ongoing, adaptive process, but national and subnational health contexts will likely change over the EPHS life course (5–10 years), altering the assessment of feasibility, costs, and so on. Ongoing monitoring of policy adaptation is critical.

Pakistan's experience shows the importance of tracking quality of care as an early bellwether for monitoring client experience and health system responsiveness. Traditional quantitative monitoring approaches may not be fit for this purpose. Consequently, understanding how to integrate qualitative methods into routine monitoring efforts will require more theoretical work.

Evaluation

Insights from the field of implementation science can help fill the gap in linking the EPHS to changes in resource allocation, service delivery, and ultimately health outcomes. For example, many country- and disease-specific applications have used the Reach, Effectiveness, Adoption, Implementation, and Maintenance (RE-AIM) framework. RE-AIM seeks to identify and, when possible, quantify the "active ingredients" of a program that translate directly into favorable outcomes of UHC for the populations served (Glasgow, Vogt, and Boles 1999). RE-AIM could be applied to the implementation of the EPHS in general (that is, understanding how district managers use it) or to a series of specific tracer interventions (such as safe delivery) linked to the selected indicators (table 19.1).

Table 19.1 General and Specific Application of RE-AIM for EPHS Evaluation, Using the Example of the Maternal Health Services Tracer "Safe Delivery"

Construct	Application to EPHS in general	Application to specific service, safe delivery
Reach	% of population covered[a] by facilities that use EPHS	% of population in need[a] receiving safe delivery services
Effectiveness	Change in service delivery (qualitative[b]) + OOP costs (quantitative)	Change in mortality and OOP costs for facility delivery (quantitative)
Adoption	% of units[c] adopting EPHS	% of units[c] adopting safe delivery service
Implementation	Level of fidelity to EPHS overall (for example, % of services provided)	Level of fidelity (quality) of core components of safe delivery
Maintenance	Sustainment of adoption/implementation over time	Sustainment of adoption/implementation over time

Source: Adapted from Glasgow, Vogt, and Boles 1999.

Note: EPHS = essential package of health services; OOP = out of pocket; RE-AIM = Reach, Effectiveness, Adoption, Implementation, and Maintenance.

a. Calculation of coverage would be a population-weighted average based on utilization data and measures of adoption.

b. Because an EPHS reform might continue some interventions from a previous EPHS and add or remove others, "effectiveness" would need to be a holistic, qualitative assessment of how effective the EPHS reform was in *actually* changing clinical practice.

c. Units can refer to districts, facilities, or individual providers depending on the needs of the particular application.

Although RE-AIM does not usually include a specific assessment of equity impact, such an assessment could flow naturally out of the application of RE-AIM across different subnational units. Specifically, population levels of each of the (quantitative) RE-AIM indicators could be disaggregated by province/state or a comparable measure of socioeconomic/demographic status, such as through a geospatial analysis of HMIS or Demographic and Health Survey data. In principle, results could also be stratified by gender, income, or other dimensions (depending on the service area), though such stratifications would probably require additional client-level data collection via population surveys (for example, benefit incidence analysis), which could prove costly and labor intensive in some circumstances (McIntyre and Ataguba 2010). Establishing or expanding health records systems that can cover the entire population could also provide additional insights into the equity impact of the EPHS, though at a considerable cost.

Step 3. Select Indicators

The modern concept of an EPHS is that of a policy instrument that helps achieve the SDGs, including target 3.8 relating to UHC. All countries are expected to report on two indicators related to that target: SDG 3.8.1 (service coverage index) and SDG 3.8.2 (financial protection)—refer to box 19.1 (UNSD 2023a, 2023b). Pakistan and Ethiopia have integrated the two measures into their M&E frameworks, but many countries do not currently track even these most basic indicators, so efforts to improve national-level EPHS monitoring and reporting must start here.

Box 19.1

Sustainable Development Goal 3 Universal Health Coverage Indicators

3.8.1. Coverage of essential health services (defined as the average coverage of essential services based on tracer interventions that include reproductive, maternal, newborn and child health, infectious diseases, non-communicable diseases and service capacity and access, among the general and the most disadvantaged population).

3.8.2. Proportion of population with large household expenditures on health as a share of total household expenditure or income.

Source: UN General Assembly 2017, 7.

This chapter proposes that M&E of EPHS implementation should use two sets of indicators. The first set, or "core" indicators, would be based on the indicators for SDG target 3.8, including the indicators used to compute the World Health Organization's Service Coverage Index, and used in nearly all countries unless compelling epidemiological reasons suggest otherwise. The second set, or "dynamic" indicators, would be based on the local context and reflect the specific reforms the EPHS aims to achieve. For example, although not included in the Service Coverage Index, breast cancer has increasingly become a priority for many countries. A country that introduces or significantly expands a breast cancer program as part of an EPHS process might then include a dynamic indicator related to breast cancer screening or treatment access. Several sources of available UHC indicators used in research and implementation in LMICs could serve as a starting point (Haas et al. 2012; Lozano et al. 2020).

Regardless of the sources of core and dynamic indicators, they should leverage ongoing data collection activities whenever possible, and the M&E needs of the EPHS should be seen as an opportunity to improve routine data collection systems. The challenges countries have experienced in reporting on the SDG indicators highlight the depth of the need for greater investment in human, technological, and financial resources (WHO and World Bank 2021). Further, to minimize the risk of adding to already high data collection burdens, countries could focus on a limited number of tracer conditions and components not related to service delivery (for example, supply chain strengthening and financing system) along with their associated signal indicators. The choice of dynamic indicators should also be linked to the theory of change created during the EPHS development process (refer to step 1).

In the context of UHC and the EPHS, M&E of financial protection outcomes is particularly important. Measures of financial protection need to align with the reality of fragmented, nonfungible health resource flows in many countries. For example, most catastrophic health expenditure worldwide is for noncommunicable diseases (Essue et al. 2017), but EPHSs may not include many of the most expensive (and highest-financial-risk) interventions, especially in low-income countries. Efforts need to be made to estimate out-of-pocket spending on interventions included in the EPHS rather than out-of-pocket spending in general, because the latter may not capture the intended effect of the EPHS—that is, to reduce out-of-pocket spending on interventions in the package.

Finally, the set of measures necessary for routine tracking of the provision of comprehensive, high-quality health care to all citizens—the M&E function of the health system in general—must be distinguished from the much smaller subset of indicators required to monitor the implementation and effectiveness of an EPHS as a policy tool. As a complement to aggregate, quantitative indicators, countries should also institutionalize data collection activities that capture policy processes and the rollout of new services (that is, early policy implementation). Examples of those activities include key informant interviews conducted among EPHS implementers to better understand how the EPHS is being used (or not) and what determinants of nonuse are amenable to intervention.

The framework described in this chapter is intended to be a first, not a final, offering on how to extend M&E theory to understand EPHS impact. Integrating equity considerations more fully at each step will require additional theoretical work. The theory and its components will also need validation through empirical work in countries revising their EPHSs.

A CALL TO ACTION

Most guidance on M&E in LMICs either aims at strengthening national health data collection systems or follows from standalone health programs that address specific topics like HIV/AIDS (UNAIDS 2010) or child health (Bryce et al. 2004). Little published to date on M&E offers specific guidance for understanding the impact of EPHSs. Current M&E tools are inadequate for providing practical, actionable direction on how to evaluate the design and implementation of EPHSs as policy instruments and monitor their ongoing rollout in an affordable, timely way. Consequently, departments tasked with EPHS M&E risk defaulting to broad health data collection efforts with limited adaptation or integration into an EPHS-specific theory of change and M&E framework.

This chapter lays out an approach to developing EPHS M&E frameworks intended to keep these needs front and center. Ideally, political buy-in for EPHS-related reforms could provide an opportunity to mobilize additional government resources to build out routine information systems, both supporting EPHS implementation and benefiting the M&E function more broadly. Countries can leverage strong HMISs for evaluations, so efforts to build HMIS capacity should be coordinated with EPHS-specific process and implementation data needs (Wagenaar et al. 2016). Additionally, considering the paucity of evidence on the relationship between EPHSs and improved health outcomes in LMICs, global health research funders should consider supporting a limited number of high-quality external evaluations of EPHSs.

The approach in this chapter has several practical and theoretical limitations. A full systematic search of the literature on EPHS M&E was beyond the team's remit, which creates a weakness of the findings presented here. Considering the scarcity of publications in the peer-reviewed literature, a comprehensive review that focuses particularly on gray literature and policy documentation would be immensely valuable and fill an important gap in understanding the different tools being applied to EPHS policy implementation M&E in practice. The chapter is further limited by the focus on seven *DCP3* country and economy projects. Future efforts integrating lessons from non-*DCP3* countries, particularly those with longer EPHS histories like Malawi and Thailand, would provide valuable insight into effective strategies for EPHS implementation M&E. The proposed way forward underscores the need for a learning agenda built around the experiences of countries undertaking EPHS reforms. International organizations and philanthropies committed to supporting national EPHS development should strongly consider investing in an international learning network that could help harmonize methods, tools, and reporting on country projects and help identify and disseminate best practices.

ACKNOWLEDGMENTS

This work was supported by Bill & Melinda Gates Foundation grant number OPP1201812. This chapter builds on a paper (Danforth et al. 2023) for a series of papers coordinated by the DCP3 Country Translation Project at the London School of Hygiene & Tropical Medicine. The sponsor had no involvement in chapter design; collection, analysis, and interpretation of the data; and the writing of the chapter.

REFERENCES

Akazili, J., E. W. Kanmiki, D. Anaseba, V. Govender, G. Danhoudo, and A. Koduah. 2020. "Challenges and Facilitators to the Provision of Sexual, Reproductive Health and Rights Services in Ghana." *Sexual and Reproductive Health Matters* 28 (2): 1846247.

Aqil, A., T. Lippeveld, and D. Hozumi. 2009. "PRISM Framework: A Paradigm Shift for Designing, Strengthening and Evaluating Routine Health Information Systems." *Health Policy and Planning* 24 (3): 217–28.

Belay, H., T. Azim, and H. Kassahun. 2014. "Assessment of Health Management Information System (HMIS) Performance in SNNPR, Ethiopia." USAID/MEASURE Evaluation, Carolina Population Center, University of North Carolina at Chapel Hill.

Bowie, C., and T. Mwase. 2011. "Assessing the Use of an Essential Health Package in a Sector Wide Approach in Malawi." *Health Research Policy and Systems* 9: 4.

Bryce, J., C. G. Victora, J.-P. Habicht, J. P. Vaughan, and R. E. Black. 2004. "The Multi-country Evaluation of the Integrated Management of Childhood Illness Strategy: Lessons for the Evaluation of Public Health Interventions." *American Journal of Public Health* 94 (3): 406–15.

Bullock, H. L., J. N. Lavis, M. G. Wilson, G. Mulvale, and A. Miatello. 2021. "Understanding the Implementation of Evidence-Informed Policies and Practices from a Policy Perspective: A Critical Interpretive Synthesis." *Implementation Science* 16 (1): 18.

Chapman, A. R., L. Forman, and E. Lamprea. 2017. "Evaluating Essential Health Packages from a Human Rights Perspective." *Journal of Human Rights* 16 (2): 142–59.

Danforth, K., A. M. Ahmad, K. Blanchet, M. Khalid, A. R. Means, and S. T. Memirie. 2023. "Monitoring and Evaluating the Implementation of Essential Packages of Health Services." *BMJ Global Health* 8 (Suppl 1): e010726. https://doi.org/10.1136/bmjgh-2022-010726.

Eregata, G. T., A. Hailu, Z. A. Geletu, S. T. Memirie, K. A. Johansson, K. Stenberg, M. Y. Bertram, et al. 2020. "Revision of the Ethiopian Essential Health Service Package: An Explication of the Process and Methods Used." *Health Systems and Reform* 6 (1): e1829313. https://doi.org/10.1080/23288604.2020.1829313.

Essue, B. M., T. Laba, F. Knaul, A. Chu, H. Minh, T. Nguyen, and S. Jan. 2017. "Economic Burden of Chronic Ill Health and Injuries for Households in Low- and Middle-Income Countries." In *Disease Control Priorities* (third edition), Volume 9, *Disease Control Priorities: Improving Health and Reducing Poverty*, edited by D. T. Jamison, H. Gelband, S. Horton, P. Jha, R. Laxminarayan, C. N. Mock, and Rachel Nugent. Washington, DC: World Bank.

FMoH (Federal Ministry of Health of Ethiopia). 2021. *Health Sector Tranformation Plan— HSTP II: 2020/21–2024/25*. Addis Ababa: Government of Ethiopia.

Glasgow, R. E., T. M. Vogt, and S. M. Boles. 1999. "Evaluating the Public Health Impact of Health Promotion Interventions: The RE-AIM Framework." *American Journal of Public Health* 89 (9): 1322–27.

Glassman, A., U. Giedion, Y. Sakuma, and P. C. Smith. 2016. "Defining a Health Benefits Package: What Are the Necessary Processes?" *Health Systems & Reform* 2 (1): 39–50.

Glassman, A., U. Giedion, and P. C. Smith. 2017. *What's In, What's Out? Designing Benefits for Universal Health Coverage*. Washington, DC: Center for Global Development. https://www.cgdev.org/publication/whats-in-whats-out-designing-benefits-universal-health-coverage.

Global Health Cluster and WHO EPHS Task Team. 2018. "Working Paper on the Use of Essential Packages of Health Services in Protracted Emergencies." WHO, Geneva. https://healthcluster.who.int/publications/m/item/working-paper-on-the-use-of-essential-packages-of-health-services-in-protracted-emergencies.

Haas, S., L. Hatt, A. Leegwater, M. El-Khoury, and W. Wong. 2012. "Indicators for Measuring Universal Health Coverage: A Five-Country Analysis (DRAFT)." Draft report prepared for the Health Systems 20/20 Project, Abt Associates Inc., Bethesda, MD.

Hepburn, J. S., I. Shekh Mohamed, B. Ekman, and J. Sundewall. 2021. "Review of the Inclusion of SRHR Interventions in Essential Packages of Health Services in Low- and Lower-Middle Income Countries." *Sexual and Reproductive Health Matters* 29 (1): 1985826.

Institute of Medicine (Institute of Medicine of the National Academies). 2013. *Evaluation of PEPFAR*. Washington, DC: National Academies Press. 848.

Kapiriri L. 2013. "How Effective Has the Essential Health Package Been in Improving Priority Setting in Low Income Countries?" *Soc Sci Med* 85: 38–42. https://doi.org/10.1016/j.socscimed.2013.02.024.

Lozano, R., N. Fullman, J. E. Mumford, M. Knight, C. M. Barthelemy, C. Abbafati, H. Abbastabar, F. Abd-Allah, M. Abdollahi, A. Abedi, and H. Abolhassani. 2020. "Measuring Universal Health Coverage Based on an Index of Effective Coverage of Health Services in 204 Countries and Territories, 1990–2019: A Systematic Analysis for the Global Burden of Disease Study 2019." *The Lancet* 396 (10258): 1250–84.

Mbau, R., K. Oliver, A. Vassall, L. Gilson, and E. Barasa. 2023. "A Qualitative Evaluation of Priority-Setting by the Health Benefits Package Advisory Panel in Kenya." *Health Policy and Planning* 38 (1): 49–60.

McIntyre, D., and J. E. Ataguba. 2010. "How to Do (or Not to Do) ... a Benefit Incidence Analysis." *Health Policy and Planning* 26 (2): 174–82.

Mutale, W., N. Chintu, C. Amoroso, K. Awoonor-Williams, J. Phillips, C. Baynes, et al. 2013. "Improving Health Information Systems for Decision Making across Five Sub-Saharan African Countries: Implementation Strategies from the African Health Initiative." *BMC Health Services Research* 13 (Supplement 2): S9.

Nutbeam, D., S. S. Padmadas, O. Maslovskaya, and Z. Wu. 2015. "A Health Promotion Logic Model to Review Progress in HIV Prevention in China." *Health Promotion International* 30 (2): 270–80.

Phoya, A., T. Araru, R. Kachale, J. Chizonga, and C. Bowie. 2014. "Setting Strategic Health Sector Priorities in Malawi." Working Paper #9 for *Disease Control Priorities in Developing Countries*, third edition, World Bank, Washington, DC. https://www.dcp-3.org/resources/setting-strategic-health-sector-priorities-malawi#:~:text=The%20Planning%20Department%20in%20the,the%20increasing%20health%20needs%20of.

Rogers, P. 2014. "Theory of Change." Methodological Briefs: Impact Evaluation 2, UNICEF Office of Research, Florence.

Sharp, S. 2021. "Logic Models vs. Theories of Change." *CERE Blog*, March 15, 2021. https://cere.olemiss.edu/logic-models-vs-theories-of-change/.

Shekh Mohamed, I., J. S. Hepburn, B. Ekman, and J. Sundewall. 2022. "Inclusion of Essential Universal Health Coverage Services in Essential Packages of Health Services: A Review of 45 Low- and Lower- Middle Income Countries." *Health Systems and Reform* 8 (1). https://doi.org/10.1080/23288604.2021.2006587.

Soucat, A., A. Tandon, and E. Gonzales Pier. 2023. "From Universal Health Coverage Services Packages to Budget Appropriation: The Long Journey to Implementation." *BMJ Global Health* 8: e010755. https://doi.org/10.1136/bmjgh-2022-010755.

Thomas, J. C., K. Doherty, S. Watson-Grant, and M. Kumar. 2021. "Advances in Monitoring and Evaluation in Low- and Middle-Income Countries." *Evaluation and Program Planning* 89 (December): 101994.

Ulmer, C., J. Ball, E. McGlynn, and S. Bel Hamdounia, eds. 2012. *Essential Health Benefits: Balancing Coverage and Cost.* Washington, DC: National Academies Press.

UNAIDS (Joint United Nations Programme on HIV/AIDS). 2010. "Basic Terminology and Frameworks for Monitoring and Evaluation." UNAIDS Monitoring and Evaluation Fundamentals Series, UNAIDS, Geneva.

UN (United Nations) General Assembly. 2017. Resolution adopted by the General Assembly on Work of the Statistical Commission pertaining to the 2030 Agenda for Sustainable Development (A/RES/71/313). United Nations, New York. https://documents.un.org/doc/undoc/gen/n17/207/63/pdf/n1720763.pdf.

UNSD (United Nations Statistics Division). 2023a. SDG Indicator Metadata: Metadata 03-08-01. United Nations, New York. https://unstats.un.org/sdgs/metadata/files/Metadata-03-08-01.pdf.

UNSD (United Nations Statistics Division). 2023b. SDG Indicator Metadata: Metadata 03-08-02. United Nations, New York. https://unstats.un.org/sdgs/metadata/files/Metadata-03-08-02.pdf.

Waddington C. 2013. "Essential Health Packages: What Are They For? What Do They Change?" HLSP Institute, London. https://www.mottmac.com/download/file /6125?cultureId=127.

Wagenaar, B. H., K. Sherr, Q. Fernandes, and A. C. Wagenaar. 2016. "Using Routine Health Information Systems for Well-Designed Health Evaluations in Low- and Middle-Income Countries." *Health Policy and Planning* 31 (1): 129–35.

Watkins, D. A., D. T. Jamison, A. Mills, R. Atun, K. Danforth, A. Glassman, S. Horton, et al. 2017. "Universal Health Coverage and Essential Packages of Care." In *Disease Control Priorities* (third edition), Volume 9, *Disease Control Priorities: Improving Health and Reducing Poverty,* edited by D. T. Jamison, H. Gelband, S. Horton, P. Jha, R. Laxminarayan, C. N. Mock, and R. Nugent. Washington, DC: World Bank.

WHO (World Health Organization) and World Bank. 2021. *Global Monitoring Report on Financial Protection in Health 2021.* Geneva: World Health Organization and Washington, DC: World Bank. https://www.who.int/publications/i/item/9789240040953.

W. K. Kellogg Foundation. 2004. "Logic Model Development Guide." W. K. Kellogg Foundation, Battle Creek, MI.

Wright, J., and J. Holtz. 2017. "Essential Packages of Health Services in 24 Countries: Findings from a Cross-Country Analysis." Health Finance and Governance Project, Bethesda, MD. https://www.hfgproject.org/ephs-cross-country-analysis/.

Yoon, I., P. Twea, S. Heung, S. Mohan, N. Mandalia, S. Razzaq, L. Berman, et al. 2021. "Health Sector Resource Mapping in Malawi: Sharing the Collection and Use of Budget Data for Evidence-Based Decision Making." *Global Health: Science and Practice* 9 (4): 793–803.

Part **3**

Other Experiences in Setting and Implementing Selected Packages

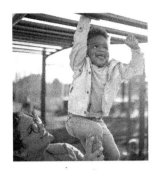

20

Cross-National Experiences on Child Health and Development during School Age and Adolescence: The Next 7,000 Days

Linda Schultz, Peter Hangoma, Dean T. Jamison, and Donald A. P. Bundy on behalf of the Authors' Writing Group

ABSTRACT

The *Disease Control Priorities* series has increasingly addressed the health and development of school-age children and adolescents across its four editions, recognizing the growing momentum of support for national programs and a growing understanding of the underlying science and economics in this area. This chapter continues that focus by exploring how countries have adopted national school-based health and nutrition programs and providing the latest update on the value-for-money choices that policy makers can make in the context of the health and development of school-age children and adolescents.

The authors dedicate this chapter to Professor George C. Patton, MB, BS, MD, FAAHMS, whose research as an adolescent psychiatrist and psychiatric epidemiologist improved the health of adolescents around the globe. His contribution to global health was defined by the 2016 Lancet Commission on Adolescent Health and Wellbeing, a seminal body of work he led that has galvanized investments and a surge of research interest in adolescent health and well-being. He served as an editor of the *Disease Control Priorities*, third edition's *Child and Adolescent Health and Development* volume, and it is thanks to his leadership that the volume emphasized adolescence as a unique developmental stage within the life course. If his life had not been cut short, he would certainly have been part of the team contributing to this chapter in the fourth edition of *Disease Control Priorities*. He was a friend and colleague to many authors of this chapter, and we remember him not only for his academic contributions but also for his collaborative approach and the sincere interest he showed in mentoring early career researchers.

INTRODUCTION

The Disease Control Priorities (DCP) series was created to help guide policy makers in making value-for-money choices to improve the human condition in low-resource settings. The DCP series was introduced as a more in-depth companion to the influential World Bank *World Development Report 1993: Investing in Health*, which pointed to the possibility for focused investments in health to advance human welfare more rapidly than could income growth alone. Since then, the DCP analyses have been revisited approximately every 10 years to update that guidance. The first and all subsequent editions have addressed health and development of school-age children and adolescents. This chapter continues that theme and provides the latest update on the value-for-money choices that policy makers can make in the context of the health and development of school-age children and adolescents.

The first edition of DCP (*DCP1*), also published in 1993, raised the importance of good health for development during school age and adolescence in the context of the ubiquitous yet underrecognized importance of helminth infection in school-age children, and how simple, safe, and low-cost interventions could affect cognition, education, and development in ways now recognized as important for human capital (Warren et al. 1993). One important conclusion then was that major health and development returns could be achieved by addressing health insults that occurred at key stages in human development, especially if those health issues were prevalent across a population.

A look back across the 30 years of publishing DCP provides insights into the evolution of school health and nutrition programming as a health and development intervention. Implementation science suggests that it takes an average of 13–17 years for an area of research investigation to influence programming (Grant et al. 2000; Grant et al. 2003; Morris, Wooding, and Grant 2011), so the DCP editions, published at approximately 10-year intervals, should help illustrate how earlier ideas were translated into policy.

As the DCP series has evolved over the past 30 years, so has the interest in cost-efficient approaches to improve the well-being and development of school-age children and adolescents (figure 20.1). The second edition (*DCP2*), published in 2006, expanded the scope to include dedicated chapters on school-based health and nutrition as well as on adolescent health programs. The expanded footprint reflected the growing strength of evidence that schools can safely deliver routine health interventions as well as a recognition that the Millennium Development Goals had increased enrollment in primary schools to nearly universal, enhancing the cost-efficiency of using schools as a platform to reach a substantial majority of school-age children (Bundy et al. 2006; Hotez et al. 2006; Lule et al. 2006). That period saw increasing development partner interest in the topic: for example, in 2006 the World Health Organization created its first department for neglected tropical diseases, which prioritized school-based deworming for the reasons expanded upon in *DCP1* and *DCP2*; and in 2009 the World Bank published a report on the developmental value of investing in the health and nutrition of school-age children. That report,

Rethinking School Feeding, was associated with a renaissance in interest in national school health and nutrition programs, best documented for China and the Russian Federation (Bundy et al. 2009).

DCP3, published between 2015 and 2018, for the first time dedicated an entire volume to the health and development of children and adolescents (Bundy, de Silva, Horton, Jamison, and Patton 2017), supported by other relevant chapters across the broader nine-volume series focused on the well-being of schoolchildren. A key conclusion from *DCP3* was the endorsement of the prevailing view that investment in the "first 1,000 days"—the period spanning conception to two years of age—is crucial for survival and to lay the foundation for subsequent healthy development. Moreover, that continuing investment through the "next 7,000 days"—or through to the early 20s—is essential to sustain and build upon the gains achieved from earlier intervention and to secure well-being into adult life and for the next generation (Bundy, de Silva, Horton, Patton et al. 2017; Gray et al. 2022). That conclusion has increasingly been adopted as a mainstream view, for example in the Non-Communicable Disease Risk Factor Collaboration published in 2020, which recommends that "global and national nutrition and health programmes should extend to children and adolescents in school years to consolidate gains in children younger than 5 years and enable healthy growth through the entire developmental period" (Rodriguez-Martinez et al. 2020, 1512).

The historical treatment of school health and nutrition in the *DCP* series suggests a growing momentum of support for national programs and a growing understanding of the underlying science and economics in this area. This chapter moves beyond the narrative of school health and nutrition as a specific intervention area to explore how countries have adopted such interventions to develop broader system-level approaches to improve the well-being of the learner.

This chapter is organized in three sections. The first section explores changes in research focused on the next 7,000 days and spotlights how new evidence on biological changes during school age and adolescence[1] informs investments to strengthen human capital formation. The second section summarizes the decade of growth of school health and nutrition programs globally and looks at the way interest has expanded in development and normative agencies, as evidenced by new publications offering guidance in this area. The second section also explores the extraordinary momentum from governments, largely in response to school closures during the COVID-19 pandemic, and best illustrated by the more than 100 countries that have created the School Meals Coalition. That coalition has the twin aims of reopening schools and rebuilding more resilient school-based health systems; within 24 months it restored global school health and nutrition programs to levels seen before the COVID-19 pandemic and dramatically increased coverage even in low-resource countries, notably Benin, Honduras, and Rwanda. The final section of the chapter explores the subsequent programmatic performance of the school-age package proposed in *DCP3* and updates the policy guidance for each intervention in light of programmatic experience.

Figure 20.1 Evolving and Increasing Focus on the Condition of School-Age Children and Adolescents across the DCP Series

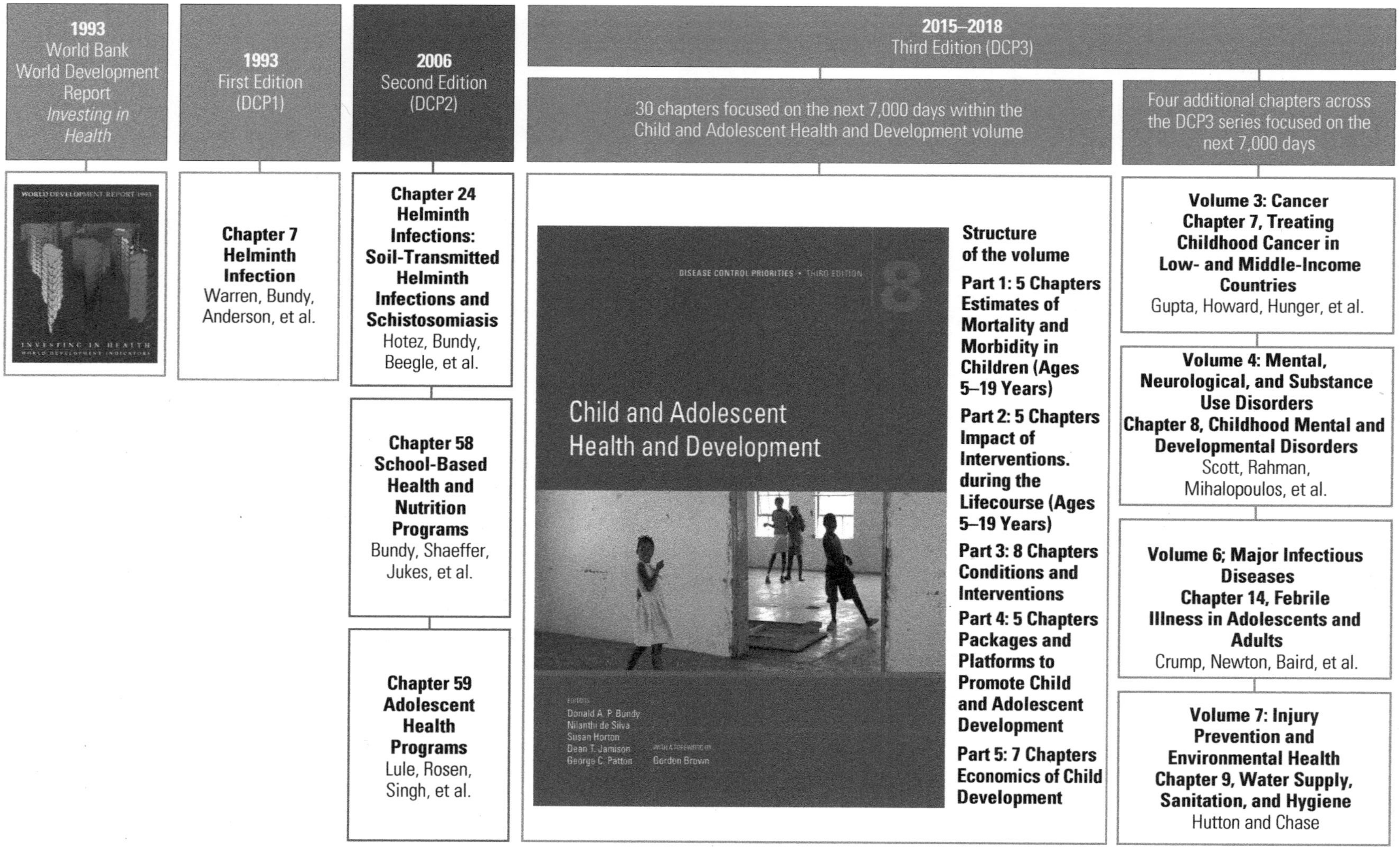

1993 World Bank World Development Report *Investing in Health*	1993 First Edition (DCP1)	2006 Second Edition (DCP2)	2015–2018 Third Edition (DCP3)

1993
World Bank World Development Report *Investing in Health*

1993
First Edition (DCP1)

Chapter 7
Helminth Infection
Warren, Bundy, Anderson, et al.

2006
Second Edition (DCP2)

Chapter 24
Helminth Infections: Soil-Transmitted Helminth Infections and Schistosomiasis
Hotez, Bundy, Beegle, et al.

Chapter 58
School-Based Health and Nutrition Programs
Bundy, Shaeffer, Jukes, et al.

Chapter 59
Adolescent Health Programs
Lule, Rosen, Singh, et al.

2015–2018
Third Edition (DCP3)

30 chapters focused on the next 7,000 days within the Child and Adolescent Health and Development volume

Four additional chapters across the DCP3 series focused on the next 7,000 days

Structure of the volume

Part 1: 5 Chapters
Estimates of Mortality and Morbidity in Children (Ages 5–19 Years)

Part 2: 5 Chapters
Impact of Interventions. during the Lifecourse (Ages 5–19 Years)

Part 3: 8 Chapters
Conditions and Interventions

Part 4: 5 Chapters
Packages and Platforms to Promote Child and Adolescent Development

Part 5: 7 Chapters
Economics of Child Development

Child and Adolescent Health and Development

Volume 3: Cancer
Chapter 7, Treating Childhood Cancer in Low- and Middle-Income Countries
Gupta, Howard, Hunger, et al.

Volume 4: Mental, Neurological, and Substance Use Disorders
Chapter 8, Childhood Mental and Developmental Disorders
Scott, Rahman, Mihalopoulos, et al.

Volume 6: Major Infectious Diseases
Chapter 14, Febrile Illness in Adolescents and Adults
Crump, Newton, Baird, et al.

Volume 7: Injury Prevention and Environmental Health
Chapter 9, Water Supply, Sanitation, and Hygiene
Hutton and Chase

Source: Original figure created for this publication.

In line with the DCP series generally, this chapter does not intend to replicate textbooks and technical guidelines on these issues. The chapter focuses specifically on a package of school-based interventions and how that package has, or has not, been delivered as part of government programs.

ADVANCES IN THE CONCEPTUAL UNDERSTANDING OF SCHOOL HEALTH AND NUTRITION SINCE DCP3

Research and investment over the first 8,000 days have historically focused on children under five years, leaving older children and adolescents largely neglected. This section explores how that bias in research has changed since 2000 and the emerging efforts within nutrition and elsewhere to better account for school-age children and adolescents in research. This section also distills nuanced and advanced understandings of human development and nutrition over the first 8,000 days, and it makes the case for delivering well-timed school health and nutrition interventions during this developmental period.

A Historically Neglected Area of Research

A significant conclusion from DCP3 is that both research and investment for children concentrate on children younger than five years, with a concomitant relative absence of research on the needs of older children and adolescents. A DCP3 review of publications by subject age on mortality, cause of death, and health for children and young people over the age range 0–19 years shows a severe bias in publications between 2005 and 2016 toward children under 5 years, with 99 percent of publications in Google Scholar and 95 percent in PubMed databases focusing on that age range (Bundy, de Silva, Horton, Patton et al. 2017).

Revisiting the same issues using more detailed search questions and databases confirms that the youngest children are the priority subjects for research and that school-age children are neglected but also reveals a more nuanced story. Overall between 2001 and 2020, the number of publications per year on subjects in the age range of 0–19 years showed a sustained increase for all four age quintiles and topic areas (figure 20.2). As found by the review published in DCP3, most publications focus on children under age 5 but with a declining, and possibly accelerating, trend in the proportion of publications on that youngest quintile and a rising trend for publications on older adolescents (15–19 years). Overall, some 50–80 percent of all publications focus on children under 5 years, and some 20–40 percent on older adolescents, confirming yet again that school-age children and young adolescents are the most neglected in all research on young people. One might conclude that efforts to stimulate research on adolescence, such as the 2011 State of the World's Children focused on adolescence (UNICEF 2011) and the Lancet Commission of 2016 (Patton et al. 2016), have contributed to more research on older adolescents but that school-age children remain extraordinarily underrepresented.

Figure 20.2 Number of Publications on Subjects in Age Range 0–19 Years, by Age Cohort and Year Range, 2001–20

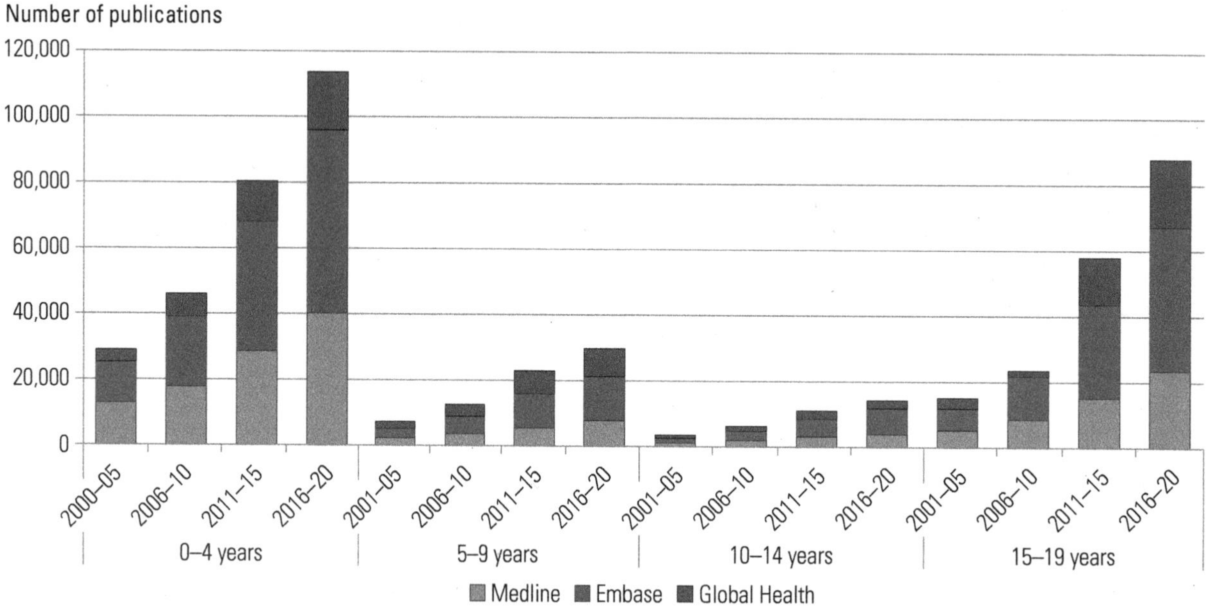

Number of publications

Source: Original figure created for this publication.

Note: The figure shows data for health, based on a search of three Ovid databases: Embase, Global Health, and Medline.

The neglect of research on school-age children and young adolescents is hard to reconcile with their numerical and developmental importance to the overall population, particularly in low-income settings. As shown in figure 20.3, school-age children and adolescents constitute nearly 40 percent of the population in Sub-Saharan Africa, where the median age of the population is often less than 20 years. In Europe and North America, where the median age exceeds 40 years, the cohort represents 16–18 percent of the population but nevertheless is the source of future human capital in those populations.[2] Demographic projections suggest that Sub-Saharan Africa will retain its youthful age structure through 2030, whereas declining or stagnant fertility rates in countries like Brazil, China, and India will result in school-age children and adolescents accounting for a shrinking proportion of the overall population (UN DESA 2015). The latter settings will require continued high levels of public sector investment in the next generation of school-age children, adolescents, and youth to sustain the social safety net for an aging population.

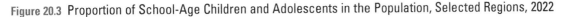

Figure 20.3 Proportion of School-Age Children and Adolescents in the Population, Selected Regions, 2022

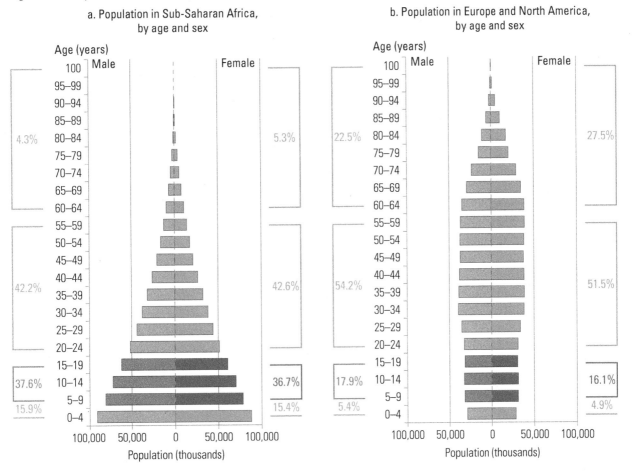

a. Population in Sub-Saharan Africa, by age and sex

b. Population in Europe and North America, by age and sex

Source: United Nations Population Division, UN Population Division Data Portal, https://population.un.org/dataportal/home (accessed January 16, 2023).

Nutrition studies provide an example of how the age-specific pattern of research neglect has affected practice and how the scientific community has begun reacting to address that neglect. The closure of schools during the COVID-19 pandemic and the subsequent global focus on rebuilding systems to support the well-being of schoolchildren spotlighted the near absence of nutrition and dietary indicators for school-age children and adolescents, among other areas, such as for well-being and mental health (Khan et al. 2022; Tzioumis and Adair 2014; Tzioumis et al. 2016; Wrottesley et al. 2023). Consequently, the US National Institutes of Health convened global nutritionists around the Biomarkers of Nutrition for Development-Knowledge Indicating Dietary Sufficiency (BOND-KIDS) project[3] in 2022, and concluded:

> [The nutrition community has focused] considerable attention on the most vulnerable groups and critical periods of human development, starting with the "first 1,000 days" covering pregnancy and the first two years of life. However, another critical period of development, the "next 7,000 days" extending from age 2 through age 21, has received less attention in terms of efforts to inform our understanding of the role of nutrition in

the health and development of children. While significant effort has gone into providing nutrition support to school-aged children (particularly via school-based programs), this lack of evidence has constrained our ability to assess the functional impact of these programs on health and development (Raiten et al., 2024).

Similarly, the Nutrition Society, based in the United Kingdom, identified the same gap in available guidance and technical support to ensure quality nutrition interventions for school-age children and created two special interest groups in 2022 to help strengthen research on neglected age groups. The work of those efforts aligns with the recommendations of the Non-Communicable Disease Risk Factor Collaboration, which identified heterogeneous age trajectories and time trends of height and body mass index in late childhood and adolescence across 200 countries between 1985 and 2019, suggesting the need to rethink nutrition guidelines targeted to school-age children and adolescents (Rodriguez-Martinez et al. 2020). At the same time, *The Lancet* published a series on adolescent nutrition, which brought attention to the previous failure of the nutrition and health communities to come together (Patton et al. 2022).

The important new developments in nutrition are being mirrored in other research areas focused on school-age children, including eye health, physical exercise, mental health, and menstrual health. Any detectable effect of such research on the publication of evidence, however, will inevitably take some years.[4]

Recognition of the Developmental Importance of the "Next 7,000 Days"

Three main phases crucial to health and development occur during ages 5–19 years, and each requires condition-specific and age-specific responses (Bundy, de Silva, Horton, Patton et al. 2017). Children in middle childhood, ages 5–9, undergo steady physical growth and development of sensorimotor brain functions. Younger adolescents, ages 10–14, experience their second most rapid period of linear and brain growth, allowing for interventions to support optimal physical growth and development of lifelong health and nutrition habits. During puberty (usually between ages 8 and 16), young people usually gain 15–25 percent of adult height and 50 percent of adult weight, with the potential of overcoming growth deficits from early childhood. In older adolescents, ages 15–19, and young adults, ages 20–24, areas of the brain that are important for social development mature and adolescents establish lifelong behaviors, offering opportunities to mitigate risk-taking and socio-emotional behaviors (Bundy and Horton 2017; Orben, Tomova, and Blakemore 2020).

Recent studies of human development and nutrition further emphasize the opportunity to intervene during this developmental period (Raiten et al. 2024). For example, middle childhood is marked by the activation of the adrenal glands, which have an effect on brain development along sexually differentiated trajectories and on many of the psychological changes of this phase (Del Giudice 2018). Periods of rapid growth, especially the adolescent growth spurt, are sensitive to increased nutrient requirements to support cell replication, differentiation, and expansion (figure 20.4). Children with particular vulnerabilities—including the estimated 240 million children globally with physical, developmental, behavioral, or sensory impairments—may experience challenges to their development and so can benefit from additional attention and intervention (UNICEF 2021).

Figure 20.4 Developmental Stages Sensitive to Intervention across the First 8,000 Days of Life

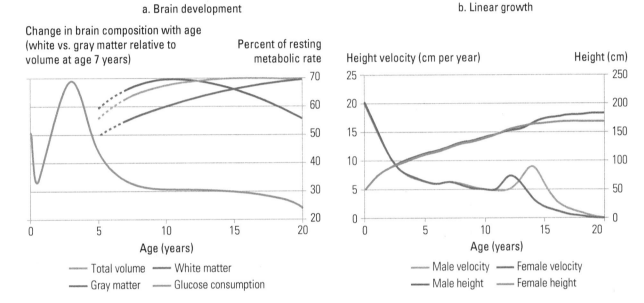

a. Brain development

Change in brain composition with age (white vs. gray matter relative to volume at age 7 years)

Percent of resting metabolic rate

Age (years)

— Total volume — White matter
— Gray matter — Glucose consumption

b. Linear growth

Height velocity (cm per year)

Height (cm)

Age (years)

— Male velocity — Female velocity
— Male height — Female height

c. Physical activity

Adjusted difference in counts per minute (95% CI)

Age (years)

— Male — Female

Sources: Bogin 1999, figure 5 (linear growth); Cooper et al. 2015, figure 1 (physical activity); Giedd and Rapoport 2010, figure 1 (brain development); Kuzawa et al. 2014, figure 1 (brain development).

Note: The composite graphs in this figure illustrate the multiple changes with age in organ function and size and in physical activity. All scales are relative and illustrative. The individual parameters were measured using different units: brain region volumes were measured in cubic centimenters (cm); glucose consumption as a percentage of resting metabolic rate; and total physical activity as accelerator counts per minute (cpm). CI = confidence interval; cm = centimeters.

Throughout the first 8,000 days of life, and not only during the first 1,000-day period, children and adolescents have high and sustained energy expenditure well above adult levels, and a concomitant demand for a nutrient-dense diet (Pontzer et al. 1979). That pattern changes continuously after age 5 years and well into the 20s, with physical activity declining and sedentary time increasing at rates that are gender-dependent but nevertheless with energy demands that remain above later levels (Cooper et al. 2015). A more nuanced understanding of human biology and behavior should inform the design of age-specific school-based health and nutrition interventions, including those intended to prevent and control overweight and obesity of school-age children and adolescents and into adulthood.

New Understanding of the Central Contribution of Well-Being at School Age to Human Capital Accumulation

Schools offer the opportunity to reach a majority of children with school-based or school-linked health services, thereby reducing implementation costs and maximizing cost efficiency by building on existing infrastructure and systems (Baltag and Saewyc 2017). Incorporating health and nutrition education into school lessons can also amplify health services within national education sector plans (Bundy, Schultz, et al. 2017). Although countries have yet to meet the goal of universal primary education, first set in 1980, global access to education has never been higher. The out-of-school rate among children of primary school age has halved globally from 19 percent in 2000 to 9 percent in 2020 (Dharamshi et al. 2022). Attendance among children and adolescents of primary and secondary school age (about 6–17 years) has reached an estimated 84 percent worldwide and continues to rise.[5]

The sustained increase in primary and secondary school enrollment, together with the young demographic in low- and lower-middle-income countries (map 20.1), suggests that schools remain the most efficient platform for reaching a majority of school-age children and adolescents. Despite that potential, addressing the needs of children who are frequently excluded from schools, such as children with disabilities, and those who prematurely end schooling will require additional efforts.

Map 20.1 School-Age Children and Adolescents as a Proportion of Country Population, 2022

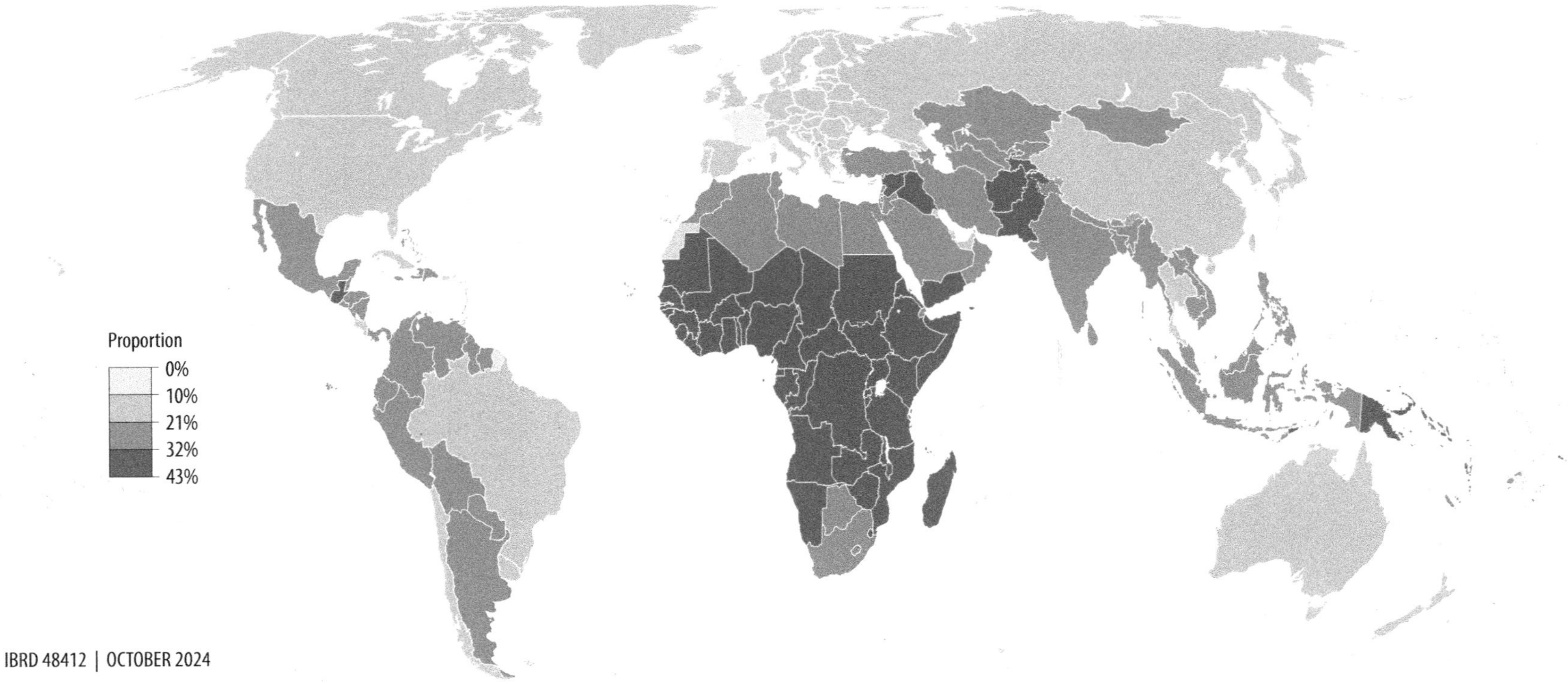

Proportion

0%
10%
21%
32%
43%

IBRD 48412 | OCTOBER 2024

Source: United Nations Population Division, UN Population Division Data Portal, https://population.un.org/dataportal/home (accessed January 16, 2023).

Targeting investments to children and adolescents presents an opportunity to grow human capital and contribute to economic prosperity and global stability in high- and low-income countries alike (Gatti et al. 2018). The Human Capital Index (HCI), introduced by the World Bank, shows that 70–80 percent of the wealth of high-income countries is attributable to human capital but that shares can be as low as 30–40 percent in low-income countries. Of the 30 countries with the lowest global rankings in terms of human capital, 25 are on the continent of Africa (Lange, Wodon, and Carey 2018; World Bank 2019). Countries with low rankings on the HCI suffer a double deficit: their young people are less able to achieve their full potential as adults, and the countries are less likely to realize the potential contribution of their human resource to national development and growth.

A key conclusion from DCP3 and several subsequent analyses was that the condition of learners is essential to their learning, and that the well-being of students is essential to the creation of human capital, through direct effects on cognitive engagement and indirect effects such as incentivizing attendance at school (Global Financing Facility 2021a; Schultz, Appleby, and Drake 2018; UNESCO 2023). That issue remains important today because, although school enrollment has increased worldwide over the past decades, low and stagnant learning levels persist in many low- and middle-income countries (Angrist et al. 2021; Gatti et al. 2018; Pritchett 2013). A recent and growing evidence base identifies reforms that can improve both schooling and learning (Angrist et al. 2025). Learning-adjusted years of schooling—a new unified metric that captures the health, education, and nutrition status of school-age children—helps quantify that benefit, and recent research suggests that some health interventions can improve cognitive skills and education outcomes by a similar order of magnitude as more direct education interventions (Angrist et al. 2023; Angrist et al. 2025) (figure 20.5). Those findings, together with findings from recent studies on the effect of school meals on learning outcomes, suggest that investments in school health and nutrition can significantly leverage the current interventions in education (Aurino et al. 2023; Chakraborty and Jayaraman 2019). The mental health and well-being of the learner, and how school health gains can help boost learning outcomes, have become an important new area of research into transforming education interventions.

Figure 20.5 Cost-Effectiveness Comparison of Selected Education Interventions and School-Based Malaria Chemoprevention in Enhancing Cognitive Skills and Education Outcomes

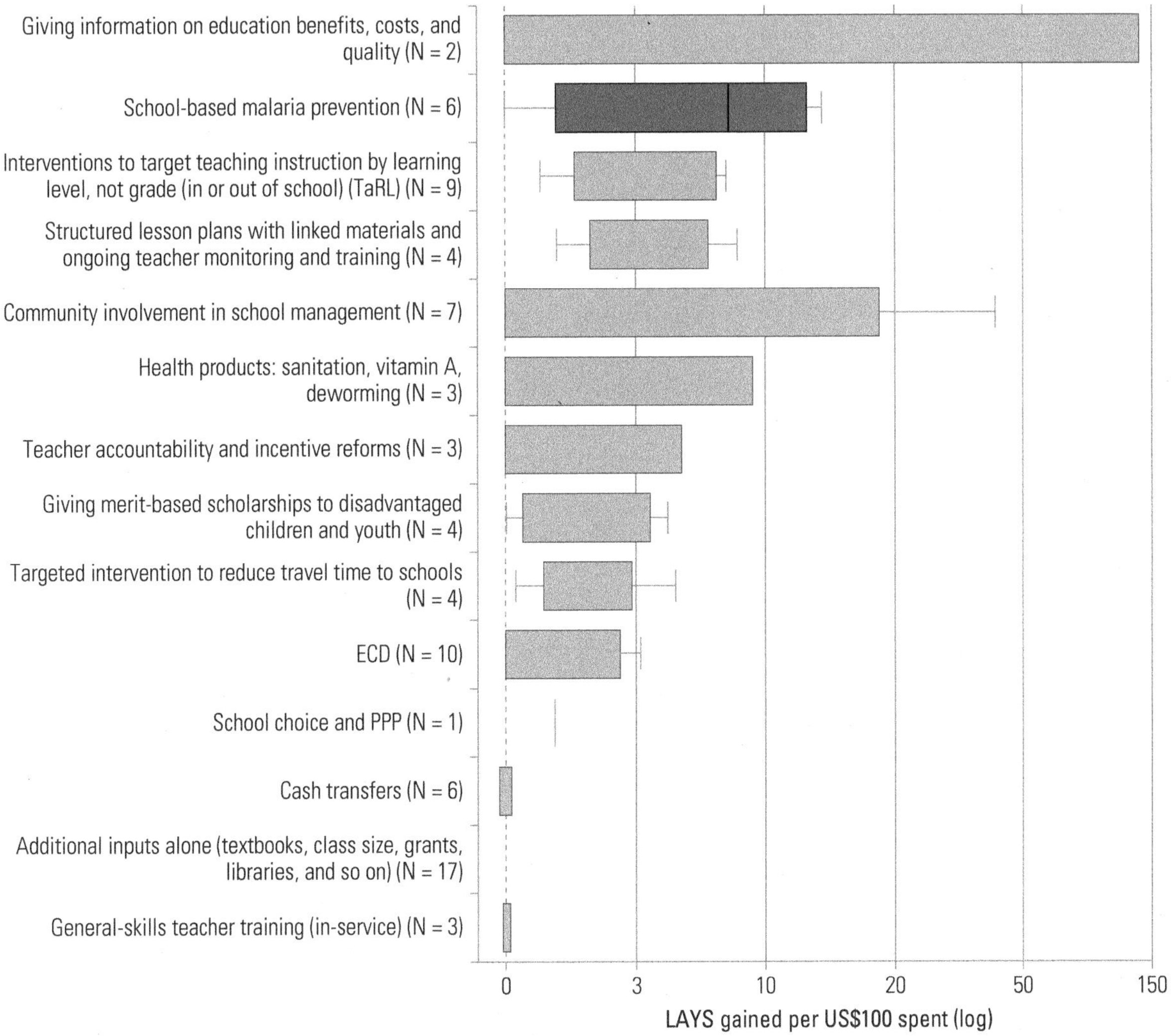

Source: Adapted from Angrist et al. 2025.

Note: Angrist et al. (2025) include over 150 impact evaluations grouped into various categories, ranging from "additional inputs (such as grants to schools, and computers)" to "early childhood development." The blue box and whisker plot emphasize the cost-effectiveness of a school-based health intervention, in this case to prevent malaria, compared to more traditional education interventions. ECD = early childhood development; LAYS = learning-adjusted years of schooling; PPP = public-private partnership; TaRL = Teaching at the Right Level.

Wider Adoption of a Multisectoral Approach to Strengthen Human Capital

Recent research suggests that school health and nutrition programs can offer substantial spillover effects that extend beyond the education and health sectors. This subsection explores the benefits to three sectors: gender empowerment, social protection, and the local agricultural economy. On gender, school meals both improve girls' attendance and can be an enabling factor for adolescent girls to remain in school. Each additional year of schooling has protective benefits for future generations: the longer girls remain in school, the later women begin childbearing, which lowers the risk of child mortality. Effects are robust even in the absence of learning outcomes, and the effects are stronger with improved levels of education quality (Oye, Pritchett, and Sandefur 2016).

School health and nutrition also have strong implications for social protection. Because the poorest and most marginalized children often have the most to gain from targeted education and health interventions (Marmot et al. 2008), 73 percent of national school health and nutrition programs have a social safety net role as one of their explicit objectives (Singh, Park, and Dercon 2014). School meals as a form of social assistance have historically been introduced or scaled during periods of social or economic shocks. In India, for instance, the midday meals scheme compensated for the negative impacts of drought on nutritional outcomes of children (Singh, Park, and Dercon 2014). In conflict-affected settings, school meals can increase participation in school and reduce the need for school-age girls to join the labor market by 10 percentage points more than general food assistance (Aurino et al. 2018).

Local agriculture, particularly for women and smallholder farmers, can enjoy major returns from school meals programs through local purchase and stable demand, which explains why the agriculture sector leads school meals programs in some countries. For example, the US federal school meals program emerged in the 1930s recession as a market stimulus, and the US Department of Agriculture continues to lead the program today (Radday 2020). Home-grown school feeding programs, which rely on domestically sourced food, can support food sovereignty, offer nutritious diets to students, trigger improved access to nutritious food for other community members, and create local jobs (Gelli et al. 2020). A recent survey finds that school meals programs create 1,000–2,000 jobs for every 100,000 children fed, with most jobs held by women (WFP 2023).

STRENGTHENING OF NATIONAL SCHOOL HEALTH AND NUTRITION PROGRAMS AND POLICY GUIDANCE SINCE DCP3

This section explores the significant expansion of national school health and nutrition programs over the past decade, and the breadth of policy tools and multisectoral programmatic guidance to support priority setting in this area. This section also follows the emergence of a global coalition that emerged from the COVID-19 pandemic with the goal of restoring school health and nutrition programs to prepandemic levels and to increasing their scale and quality.

A Decade of Expansion of National School Health and Nutrition Programs

National school health and nutrition programs have undergone a sustained decade of growth, with many delivering practical and affordable interventions at scale. By 2020, nearly every country in the world offered some form of school-based or school-linked health service to improve the physical health and nutritional status of school-going young people. More than 100 countries offered school-based vaccination programs, nearly all countries integrated health education into their curriculum, and more than 450 million school-age children have been dewormed every year in schools in low- and middle-income countries, with some 3.3 billion school-based deworming treatments delivered since 2010 (Baltag, Pachyna, and Hall 2015; Montresor et al. 2020; UNESCO 2023).

Those changes have been tracked longitudinally with the Systems Approach for Better Education Results (SABER) policy tool developed by the World Bank in 2010 to help countries respond to the 2008 food, fuel, and financial crisis (World Bank 2013). That tracking role intensified in 2013 when the United Nations (UN) World Food Programme (WFP) adopted SABER to provide targeted technical assistance to strengthen the relevant systems, policies, and implementation capacity as countries progress toward national programmatic ownership (WFP 2013). At least 81 SABER School Health and School Feeding surveys have now been conducted across 59 countries, with 32 percent of those exercises conducted in low-income countries and 49 percent in lower-middle-income countries (Schultz et al. 2024)—figure 20.6.

Figure 20.6 Cumulative Number of SABER School Health and Feeding Surveys, Sub-Saharan Africa and the Rest of the World, 2012–23

Number of reports

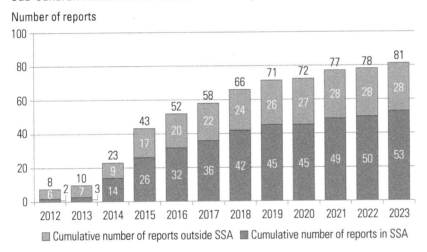

Source: Schultz et al. 2024.

Note: Figure shows the cumulative number of Systems Approach for Better Education Results (SABER) School Health and School Feeding exercises completed since 2012 globally and in Sub-Saharan Africa (SSA), by year. The 81 reports include 67 SABER School Feeding exercises conducted in 52 countries and 14 SABER School Health exercises in 14 countries. Twenty-two of those countries either repeated an exercise or conducted both the School Health and the School Feeding exercises.

The WFP report *State of School Feeding Worldwide 2020* estimates that, in the 85 survey countries with national school meals programs, 93 percent of governments also implement complementary health and nutrition interventions, and nearly 30 percent of those governments deliver an integrated school health package of at least seven interventions, most corresponding to the DCP3 essential package. The largest programs in the world, delivered in Brazil, China, India, Russia, and South Africa, all provide integrated school health and nutrition packages (figure 20.7). In January 2020, school meals programs delivered meals to more children in more countries than at any time in human history, reaching an estimated 388 million children daily—equivalent to about 69,840 billion meals in total (WFP 2020). Similarly, an estimated 186 million children received free school meals daily through universal school meals programs in the 2022–23 academic year (Cohen et al. 2023). By 2022, the most common programs delivered alongside school meals included handwashing (77 percent), deworming (38 percent), weight and height measurement (34 percent and 32 percent, respectively), eye testing (22 percent), dental/oral hygiene (22 percent), hearing testing (16 percent), and anemia testing (11 percent), among others (WFP 2023).

Figure 20.7 Complementary School Health and Nutrition Activities Implemented in Conjunction with School Meals, by Number of Interventions and Country Income Level

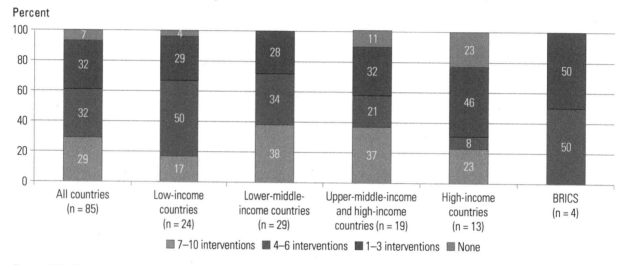

Source: WFP 2020.

Note: BRICS = Brazil, Russian Federation, India, China, and South Africa.

School meals programs have become the world's most extensive social safety net (Bundy et al. 2024), and more than 80 percent of such national programs enjoy the support of formally adopted national policies. An estimated 98 percent of those meals are supported by governments using domestic funds, totaling about US$43 billion globally, further illustrating national commitment. By contrast, official development assistance investment amounts to about US$300 million annually (Sustainable Financing Initiative 2022), reflecting the contradiction between the value that governments have placed on the current well-being of their children and the continuing relative neglect in this area by development agencies.

Increasing Availability of Cross-Sectoral Policy Guidance

This subsection explores the development of policy guidance, with a focus on three major issues: the link between education and health, the role of diets and food systems, and the contribution to development and human capital. Figure 20.8, which uses the publication of the DCP3 Child and Adolescent Health and Development volume as an arbitrary starting point, illustrates sustained and growing emphasis on the role of school health and nutrition in child and adolescent development.

Figure 20.8 Examples of Position Papers Published by Bilateral, Multilateral, and United Nations Agencies Focused on School-Age Children and Adolescents, 2017–23

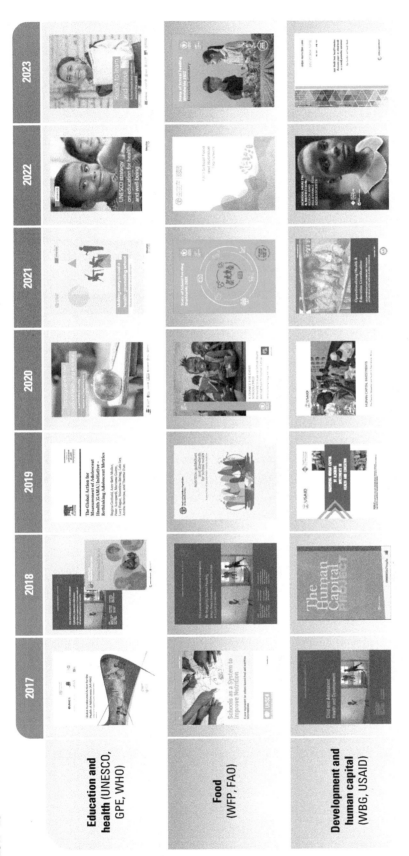

Source: Original figure created for this publication.

Note: FAO = Food and Agriculture Organization of the United Nations; GPE = Global Partnership for Education; UNESCO = United Nations Educational, Scientific and Cultural Organization; USAID = United States Agency for International Development; WBG = World Bank Group; WFP = World Food Programme; WHO = World Health Organization.

Education and health. In 2017, the United Nations Standing Committee on Nutrition emphasized the role of schools in supporting the health and well-being of children (Hunter et al. 2017). In 2021, the World Health Organization and United Nations Educational, Scientific and Cultural Organization developed the first standards for health-promoting schools, with accompanying guidance and new guidelines for school health services (WHO and UNESCO 2021a, 2021b, 2021c). The latter organization, taking the lead in coordinating a partnership across the UN agencies, published an overview of the status of school health and nutrition programming worldwide (UNESCO 2023). The first report of the Lancet Commission for Adolescent Health and Wellbeing suggested that secondary education was among the best investments for advancing adolescent health and well-being (Patton et al. 2016). At the same time, UN agencies published guidance to promote adolescent health and well-being and proposed a minimum set of populatable indicators to measure and track those changes (Guthold et al. 2019; Marsh et al. 2022; WHO 2019; WHO UNAIDS, UNFPA, UNICEF, the World Food Programme, and PMNCH 2023). UN agencies and partners have since agreed upon a definition and conceptual framework for adolescent well-being (Ross et al. 2020), followed up with a collection of articles on adolescent well-being[6] and endorsed by academics and leaders of key UN agencies, professional associations, and youth organizations (Clark et al. 2021).

Diet and food systems. Both WFP, the world's largest humanitarian agency, and the Global Partnership for Education, a partnership fund that supports education policy and implementation in more than 100 countries, repackaged the DCP3 Child and Adolescent Health and Development volume for social protection and education audiences, respectively (Bundy, de Silva, et al. 2018a; Bundy, de Silva, et al. 2018b). The Global Partnership for Education subsequently released further guidance on the delivery of integrated school health programs (GPE 2018). WFP publishes biennial reports on the status of school meals programs globally; in the absence of a reliable year-on-year database of school health and nutrition programmatic indicators, those reports serve as the primary source of country-level data (WFP 2020, 2023). WFP has also launched a "Data and Monitoring Initiative" with the goal of creating and sustaining a global database on national school health and nutrition programming.

Development and human capital. The World Bank, which publishes the *Disease Control Priorities* series, launched its HCI in 2018 to quantify the degree to which individuals can meet their health, education, and nutrition potential, as well as their ability to apply their soft skills and training to income-generating activities. The HCI assesses country indicators at critical periods throughout the life course, including during the school years, recognizing that investment decisions made today will determine how effectively countries reach their economic growth potential (Gatti et al. 2018). Similarly, the Global Financing Facility for Every Woman and Every Child, a catalytic fund hosted by the World Bank for maternal, newborn, child, and adolescent health, published operational briefs and decision tools to guide the inclusion of school health and nutrition investments within World Bank investments (Global Financing Facility 2021a, 2021b, 2021c, 2021d), recognizing the downstream and intergenerational outcomes, like lifetime fertility preferences and childhood stunting (Semba et al. 2008). Likewise, the United States Agency for International Development, the largest bilateral contributor to official development assistance globally, commissioned guidance on coordinating its education and health investments to maximize human capital in countries the agency supports (Schultz, Appleby, and Drake 2018; Schultz, Bundy, and Drake 2019; Schultz and Shors 2021).

Growing Global Momentum to Rebuild National School Health and Nutrition Programs after Prolonged Pandemic-Related School Closures

The outbreak of the COVID-19 pandemic and the subsequent closure of schools worldwide precipitated the largest education crisis in history, with more than 1.6 billion children deprived of schooling.[7] It was the first time that so many schools worldwide had synchronized closure; closures had not happened on such a scale even during the World Wars. In high-income countries, generations of children have lost out on educational opportunities, with lifelong consequences, and the World Bank estimates that the already very poor level of educational achievement in low-income countries has deteriorated further: the proportion of 10-year-old children unable to read a simple age-appropriate sentence increased to 70 percent in low- and middle-income countries, up from 54 percent before the pandemic (World Bank, UNESCO, and UNICEF 2021).

From the perspective of children's well-being, school closures dealt a blow that brought an end to nearly a decade of global growth in school meals programs and other health services. At the height of the crisis in April 2020, about 370 million children were suddenly deprived of their daily school meal.[8] Moreover, 100 million people were driven into poverty in 2020, falling under the US$1.90 threshold, especially in Africa. Those losses highlight the importance of schools as protective spaces where children receive not only an education but also other types of intervention, such as school meals that support their health, nutrition, well-being, and future.

In reaction, national political leaders formed a coalition at the 2021 UN Food System Summit with the specific aims of rebuilding the school-based services severely damaged by the pandemic closures and of ensuring the well-being of current and future generations of schoolchildren. Today, more than 105 countries, representing more than 67 percent of the world's population (map 20.2), have joined a School Meals Coalition with three specific goals: (1) to restore national school meals and complementary school health programs to prepandemic coverage by 2023; (2) to develop new approaches to reach, by 2030, an additional 73 million of the most in-need children who had not previously been reached; and (3) to raise the quality of school health and nutrition programs globally by 2030.[9] The more than 105 member states are delivering on those goals; remarkably, the number of children fed in 2022 rebounded to 418 million, exceeding the 388 million reported in January 2020 before COVID-19 (WFP 2023).

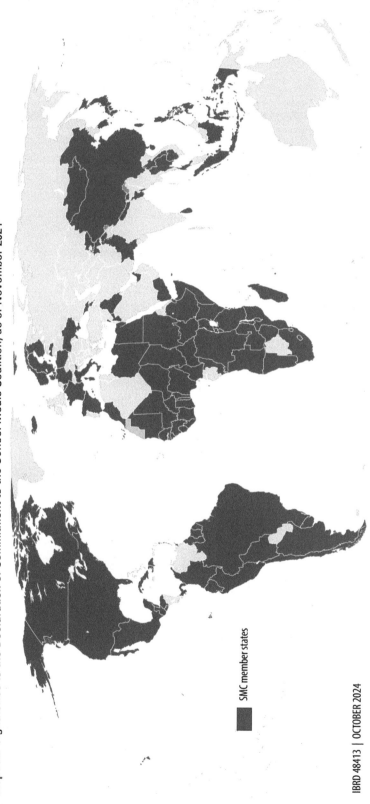

Map 20.2 Signatories to the Declaration of Commitment to the School Meals Coalition, as of November 2024

SMC member states

IBRD 48413 | OCTOBER 2024

Source: Original map created for this publication.

Note: The map shows the 108 countries that have signed the Declaration. SMC = School Meals Coalition.

Despite constraints on public finances due to the health and economic costs of the COVID-19 pandemic, low-income countries have increased the proportion of their domestic budgets dedicated to school meals: up to 45 percent from 30 percent before the pandemic. Benin, for example, has announced a national budget commitment of US$270 million over the next five years to scale up the national program, which in 2022 had already reached 75 percent coverage. Rwanda reached universal coverage of school meals, increasing its support for 640,000 children in 2020 to 3.8 million in 2022. High-income countries are similarly committing to more resilient school meals programs. France introduced a scheme to subsidize lunchtime meals for the most vulnerable students, with meals costing a maximum of €1; and the United States unveiled a new National Strategy on Hunger, Nutrition and Health, which includes the objective of expanding free school meals to all children.

REVISITING THE DCP3 ESSENTIAL PACKAGE OF CARE FOR SCHOOL-AGE CHILDREN AND ADOLESCENTS

The DCP3 Child and Adolescent Health and Development volume proposed a package of care for school-age children, which included interventions like school meals, deworming, vision screening, malaria prevention, vaccinations, and others to enhance the well-being of school-age children. Recent evidence supports the effectiveness of those initiatives, and this section builds on that enhanced understanding to explore the policy implications and practical consequence of delivering health and nutrition services through schools. Additionally, this section introduces interventions that require further analysis for inclusion in an expanded school health and nutrition package of care.

Advances in Understanding of the DCP3 School-Age Package of Care

In 2018, the DCP3 Child and Adolescent Health and Development volume proposed an essential school-based package of health services appropriate for school-age children (Fernandes and Aurino 2017) as well as an adolescent package delivered through schools, health clinics, and policy action (Horton et al. 2017). Both packages were identified as among the 21 essential universal health care packages from across the DCP3 nine-volume series, having met the criteria of (1) providing good value for money in multiple settings; (2) addressing a significant disease burden; and (3) being feasible to implement in a range of low- and lower-middle-income countries (Watkins et al. 2018). This section revisits the school-age package proposed in DCP3 to identify learnings from country implementation.

The evidence summarized in the DCP3 Child and Adolescent Health and Development volume shows that, for the conditions that are more prevalent among school-age children, schools provide a natural and cost-effective platform for harvesting these complementarities. The essential package for school-age children in DCP3 includes interventions to improve cognition and learning, provision of deworming tablets in endemic settings, vision screening and provision of spectacles, promotion of oral health, promotion of the use of insecticide-treated bed nets in malaria-endemic areas, and delivery of nutrition education and healthy school meals. In addition, the package protects against vaccine-preventable conditions in adulthood and among future offspring by including tetanus toxoid and human papillomavirus vaccinations. Table 20.1 summarizes the benefits from the interventions included within the school-age package.

Table 20.1 Essential Health Services Appropriate for Children and Adolescents as Proposed by DCP3

	Primary health center	School	Benefits of intervention delivery in schools
Physical health			
Deworming	Deworming	Deworming	In endemic areas, regular deworming (following WHO guidelines) can be done inexpensively in schools since most deworming drugs are donated; benefits in school attendance have been reported as a result
Insecticide-treated net promotion	Insecticide-treated net promotion	Insecticide-treated net promotion	Education about the use of insecticide-treated nets in endemic areas is important because schoolchildren tend to use nets less often than mothers and small children
Tetanus toxoid and HPV vaccination	Tetanus toxoid and HPV vaccination	Tetanus toxoid and HPV vaccination	Schools can be a good venue for administration of tetanus boosters, which benefit young people and babies born to those young women
Oral health promotion	Oral health promotion and treatment	Oral health promotion	Education on oral health is important; poor households generally cannot afford dental treatment
Correcting refractive error	Vision screening and provision of glasses	Vision screening and provision of glasses	Vision screening and provision of inexpensive ready-made glasses boost school performance
Diet			
Micronutrient supplementation	n.a.	Micronutrient supplementation	Supports learning
Multifortified foods	n.a.	Multifortified foods	Supports learning
Food provision	n.a.	School feeding	School meals promote attendance and education outcomes

Source: Bundy et al. 2018c.

Note: DCP3 = *Disease Control Priorities*, third edition; HPV = human papillomavirus; WHO = World Health Organization; n.a. = not applicable.

Since the publication of DCP3, new guidance has emerged for all health conditions proposed in the essential package for school-age children. None of the new evidence contradicts the earlier findings but rather reinforces them. Table 20.2 summarizes the changes in guidance and their policy relevance.

Some new evidence and policy guidance have significant implications for practice. One of the most important is the new malaria guidance that, for the first time, provides specific guidance on treatment for malaria in schools. The absence of such guidance was specifically highlighted as an important missing element of the normative guidance for malaria (WHO 2022a). There is now a robust understanding of the potential for school health and nutrition policies to improve the well-being of the learner along with recognition of the potential impact of those policies on the environment, biodiversity, food sovereignty, and climate. As described in the next subsection, school meals policies have the potential to improve reach and scope of national programs as well as to drive positive changes in energy usage, food wastage, and related agricultural practices.

Table 20.2 Updates to Guidance on Health Conditions Addressed by the DCP3 School-Age Package

	New evidence and normative guidance	Potential policy implications	Potential practical consequences
Physical health			
Deworming	• WHO road map for NTDs sets out global NTD policy from 2021 to 2030, calling for increasing transition to country leadership of national NTD programs, largely as part of a community focused universal health care approach (WHO 2021a).	• There is an increasing focus on deworming programs that are domestically led and financed. The donation of pharmaceutical drugs has enabled most endemic countries to scale up deworming programs.	• Although WHO coordinates deworming drugs free of charge to countries, extensive within-country distribution is required, necessitating domestic budget and personnel commitments. Implementation experience shows that school staff are effective in distributing deworming tablets and well received by the community in this role.
Insecticide-treated net promotion, now supported by intermittent preventive treatment for malaria	• New WHO guidance on malaria chemoprevention includes a recommendation for intermittent preventive treatment in school-age children (WHO 2022a). • LAYS analysis shows effectiveness of malaria control on cognitive skills and education outcomes (Angrist et al. 2023).	• The new guidance emphasizes the importance of malaria treatment for school-age children and, for the first time, provides specific guidance on the use of malaria treatment in schools, as specifically called for in DCP3. It is the first time that WHO normative advice has indicated that schools can and should intervene against malaria. • In addition to the recognized known health benefits, there is now credible evidence for substantial benefits to education.	• The guidance permitting the use of treatment for malaria is an important new development. DCP3 had indicated that it would be a much more cost-effective approach as part of a school health and nutrition program in an area endemic for malaria. The new guidance makes that approach possible.

table continues next page

	New evidence and normative guidance	Potential policy implications	Potential practical consequences
Tetanus toxoid and HPV vaccination	**Tetanus toxoid vaccination** • In 2017, WHO updated its recommendations for vaccination against diphtheria and tetanus. The tetanus and diphtheria components of the TD vaccine serve as booster doses to both vaccines, thus prolonging the duration of protection from both diseases. In addition to 3 doses of DTP given to infants during their first 6 months, 3 additional booster doses of the TD-containing vaccine should be given at ages 12–23 months, 4–7 years, and 9–15 years (WHO and UNICEF 2018a). **HPV vaccination** • WHO updated its recommendations for the vaccine, stating that a single-dose schedule, referred to as an alternative, off-label single-dose schedule, can provide a comparable efficacy and durability of protection to a two-dose regimen (WHO 2022b).	**Tetanus toxoid vaccination** • There is nominal price difference between the tetanus toxoid and TD vaccine and no programmatic impact on schedule, target group, or cold chain capacity. **HPV vaccination** • Delivering a single dose to a specific age or grade rather than two separate visits targeting different age groups offers significant potential cost savings.	• Older children and adolescents have limited contact with health facilities, making schools an attractive setting to deliver the second and third DTP vaccine boosters and the HPV vaccine. Cost savings from the updated HPV vaccination guidance may enable a ministry of health to finance the delivery of HPV vaccinations to both males and females. Parents, teachers, and school nurses can be a useful resource in monitoring the uptake of school-based vaccinations (Feldstein et al. 2020).
Oral health	• New evidence suggests that school-based oral health prevention programs positively affect school attendance and performance, as well as cavity prevention (Guarnizo-Herreño, Lyu, and Wehby 2019; Starr et al. 2021). • In 2021, new dental medicines were added to the WHO Model List of Essential Medicines for Adults and Children, including fluoride toothpaste, silver diamine fluoride, and glass ionomer cement (WHO 2021b).	• Oral health in schools is included within new standards that guide countries in their efforts to improve the well-being of children and adolescents (WHO and UNESCO 2021d).	• This evidence strengthens the argument for considering oral health promotion as part of a whole-school approach to improving the well-being of school-age children and adolescents.
Correcting refractive error	• Although this health intervention is one of the most effective for children, new estimates from the 2021 Lancet Global Health Commission on Global Eye Health suggest that over 450 million children have poor vision globally (Burton et al. 2021). • Research in this area suggests that properly fitting spectacles improve educational performance by a similar order of magnitude as other health interventions (Glewwe, Park, and Zhao 2016; Ma et al. 2018).	• The estimated burden of poor vision is more precise and significantly higher than when the DCP3 school-age package was published, indicating the need to increase the annual cost of service delivery to meet the greater unmet need for spectacles.	• The potential to include school-based vision screening, including the provision of glasses for refractive error, strengthens the argument for considering this intervention as part of a comprehensive school health program to address most childhood vision impairment.

table continues next page

Table 20.2 Updates to Guidance on Health Conditions Addressed by the DCP3 School-Age Package (continued)

	New evidence and normative guidance	Potential policy implications	Potential practical consequences
Diet			
Micronutrient supplementation	• Evidence on micronutrient supplementation continues to suggest that supplementation reduces risks of low birth weight, childhood infections, and nutritional anemia, and promotes the growth and cognitive function of children and adolescents (Caut, Leach, and Steel 2020; Keats et al. 2021; Tam et al. 2020).	• The evidence signals the importance of scaling up micronutrient supplementation and multifortified foods interventions as short-term effective strategy to tackling the double burden of malnutrition within the first 1,000 days and promote the growth and development of children and adolescents.	• This evidence illustrates the importance of careful planning, monitoring, and education to ensure that the benefits of micronutrient supplementation and fortified foods outweigh the potential risks and negative consequences. Different contexts and populations require tailored approaches to ensure the best outcomes.
Multifortified foods	• Evidence on multifortified foods continues to demonstrate effectiveness in reducing risks of nutritional anemia and undernutrition, as well as improvement in child socio-emotional and cognitive development and learning (Tam et al. 2020).		
Food provision	• About one in two children worldwide receives a meal in school, with national programs largely funded through domestic resources. Most national school meals programs also deliver complementary school-based deworming along with other nutrition-sensitive interventions (WFP 2023).	• Political importance of school meals has increased, as evidenced by the commitments of more than 105 governments to improve the quality and scale of national school meals programs by 2030 and to strengthen the focus on the impact of these programs on the environment, biodiversity, food sovereignty, and climate.[a]	• The global coalition of more than 105 countries is working toward a shared objective of rebuilding more resilient school-based health systems, with a focus on strengthening the reach and quality of national school meals programs and complementary interventions by 2030.

Sources: As indicated in table.

Note: DCP3 = *Disease Control Priorities*, third edition; DTP = diphtheria, tetanus, pertussis; HPV = human papillomavirus; LAYS = learning-adjusted years of schooling; NTD = neglected tropical disease; TD = tetanus-diphtheria; WHO = World Health Organization.

a. School Meals Coalition, n. d. "A Healthy Meal Every Day for Every Child," https://schoolmealscoalition.org, accessed December 10, 2021.

Emerging Challenges: Potential Future Additions to the Essential School Health and Nutrition Package

Some of the new generation of school health and nutrition programs have considered expansion to include interventions beyond those proposed in the essential package for low-resource countries. In some cases, those interventions are already established in high- and middle-income countries but have yet to be adopted in more fiscally constrained circumstances. This subsection reviews some of the different areas, all candidates for further analysis.

Menstrual Health

Menstrual health[10] is increasingly recognized as an important issue at school age. The onset of menarche is a milestone marker of puberty and is associated with physiological and social changes that collectively signal sexual maturation, adulthood, and fertility. The mean age at menarche has lowered globally over the past century to about 13 years of age (Leone and Brown 2020), making considerations for menstrual health management increasingly relevant in both primary and secondary school settings.

Evidence suggests that the ability to manage menstruation in a school setting affects school participation, absenteeism, and dropout (Barrington et al. 2021; Hennegan et al. 2019; Kumbeni et al. 2021; Oster and Thornton 2011; van Eijk et al. 2016), and that interventions can potentially positively improve educational attainment, self-confidence, and quality of life (Kansiime et al. 2020; Sumpter and Torondel 2013). School-based menstrual health interventions include (1) psychosocial components, such as puberty education within comprehensive sexuality education (that starts in primary school before the onset of puberty) and efforts to address stigma; and (2) physical components, such as adequate water, sanitation, and hygiene infrastructure as well as provision of a choice of menstrual products and knowledge and provision of pain management strategies. Increasing numbers of countries— including Botswana, England, Kenya, Scotland, South Africa, and Uganda—now aim to provide free menstrual supplies (Ali 2018; South Africa, Department of Women 2019).[11] Their experiences will shape best practices for implementing and sustaining menstrual health policies in schools. School sanitation remains a major challenge: an estimated 620 million children have limited or no sanitation service at school, and over 850 million children have basic or no handwashing service at school (WHO and UNICEF 2018b).[12]

Mental Health

The DCP3 Mental, Neurological, and Substance Use Disorders volume suggested that childhood mental and developmental disorders would increase in significance because of the higher proportion of young people in low- and lower-middle-income countries (Scott et al. 2015), and that suggestion is borne out by new evidence. Several mental health conditions emerge in adolescence, with potential for lifelong health implications regardless of whether conditions and symptoms are temporary or persistent (Kessler et al. 2007). Gender is an important factor. Although anxiety and depression increase with puberty, adolescent girls are almost twice as likely to experience symptoms of anxiety and depression and have higher rates of intentional self-harm and eating disorders; by contrast, adolescent boys have significantly higher rates of autism, attention deficit hyperactivity disorder, and schizophrenia (UNICEF 2021). Adverse childhood experiences, including abuse and bullying, are associated with the onset of mental health conditions (Blakemore 2019).

Universal and targeted school-based socio-emotional learning interventions can promote social and emotional competencies, coping, and resilience (UNICEF 2021). Some evidence, especially from high-income countries, suggests that students who directly benefit from programs to support emotional well-being, such as antibullying initiatives, may achieve better exam results (Kristjansson et al. 2022);

but school-based services rarely include interventions to address mental health conditions (Baltag, Pachyna, and Hall 2015). Teachers play an important role in containing bullying between students, in reducing the stigma experienced by vulnerable students, and by being role models for inclusive education. Validated school-based assessments—such as the Global School Health Survey, Health Behaviours in School-Age Children Survey, Warwick Edinburgh Mental Wellbeing Scales, and the Measurement of Mental Health Among Adolescents at the Population Level initiative—may provide further evidence as to how mental health among adolescents is changing over time and in response to high-quality school-based programming (Carvajal et al. 2023; WHO Regional Office for Europe 2020).[13]

Disability

Since the publication of DCP3, awareness of the importance of childhood disability has grown, not least through the inclusion of disability measures in the recent United Nations Children's Fund Multiple Indicator Cluster Surveys. Recent estimates suggest that 240 million children around the world have disabilities—encompassing physical, developmental, behavioral, or sensory impairments—and that over 80 percent of those children live in low- and lower-middle-income countries (UNICEF 2021). Children with disabilities often have greater needs for developmental support and early intervention because they have higher risk of delayed development and are more likely to live in poverty. However, they are also frequently excluded from school, which limits their access to supportive interventions such as vaccinations and school meals. Children with disabilities also face great health inequities—they have a 10-fold higher chance of dying before the age of five years compared to their peers without disabilities—and so have an even more urgent need for attention (Olusanya et al. 2022). Nevertheless, only 2 percent of the US$79.1 billion spent on early childhood development between 2007 and 2016 was targeted at disability (Olusanya et al. 2022).

More precise data suggest the importance of expanding the package of care to include early detection and intervention to benefit children with disabilities. In addition to screening for sight and hearing at birth, school entry provides another time to screen for impairments. A "twin-track" approach may be most relevant to promote disability inclusion in such initiatives to ensure that children with disabilities can access mainstream programs (for example, providing vaccination or school meals at accessible locations). Children with disabilities may also benefit from targeted approaches, for instance, to reach those who are out of school with nutrition programs, provide disability-relevant services (for example, assistive products), or offer additional opportunities for early development stimulation (for example, through parent support groups).

Diets and Food Systems in the Context of School Meals

Since the publication of DCP3, several analyses have spotlighted the need to make school diets more nutritionally appropriate (for example, BOND-KIDS), and the recognition of the importance of climate change has signaled the need to source those diets through food systems that consider their potential impact on the environment, biodiversity, food sovereignty, and climate. In that context, it is surprising to note that food was first included on the agenda of the UN Climate Change Conference in 2022, 27 years after the first conference on climate.

School food systems offer an important opportunity to drive positive changes in nutrition and food systems transformation through both consumption and production because they operate at scale, guide agricultural procurement practices, and influence individual and community-wide dietary preferences. Importantly, the policy levers for such programs are mostly government led and nationally funded, meaning that positive changes can be made at will with nearly instantaneous effect. A recent white paper on rethinking food systems and school meals identifies three priority areas for policy action: energy, menu changes, and food waste prevention (Pastorino et al. 2023). For example, because approximately 80 percent of school meals in low- and lower-middle-income countries are prepared over open fires, the use of fuel-efficient stoves offers considerable potential to reduce greenhouse gas emissions (WFP 2021).

Many countries have already established the link between culturally appropriate school meals provision and local agricultural change, and approximately 40 percent of national school meals programs currently have agriculture policy objectives such as agrobiodiversity, food sovereignty, and climate-smart foods (GCNF 2022). Home-grown school meals programs, for example, can help regenerate local agriculture by creating stable markets for often neglected and underused local crops, cost-neutral biofortified foods, and climate-smart nutrient-dense foods from local small farmers. In Nepal, the switch to home-grown school feeding changed the crop supply patterns from three mainly imported crops to 18 largely indigenous sources (Singh and Conway 2021). A transition to home-grown school feeding could have significant benefit, because approximately 30 percent of food produced globally is wasted and accounts for 8 percent of carbon emissions (FAO 2012).

Early Intervention for Surgical Conditions

DCP3's Essential Surgery volume spotlighted the importance and potential of surgical intervention in low-income settings (Mock et al. 2015). The DCP3 Child and Adolescent Health and Development volume found substantially higher mortality of young people ages 5–19 years than previously thought, in part because of the lack of access to clinical services, including surgery, to address prevalent conditions that contribute to morbidity and mortality in that age group (Bundy, de Silva, Horton, Patton, et al. 2017; Hill, Zimmerman, and Jamison 2017). Recent research confirms those observations, and highlights the importance and substantive neglect of the role of children's surgery in schoolchildren and adolescents, especially to address correctable congenital anomalies (Seyi-Olajude et al. 2024; Sykes et al. 2022).

The lifelong consequences from untreated, partially treated, or unsuccessful surgical treatment of congenital disorders can lead to stigma and marginalization, disengagement from school, and undue burden on caregivers. Girls experience particularly severe complications from early pregnancy and sexual violence, with lifelong consequences of fistula being one example (Johnson and Moore 2016; Sully et al. 2020; WHO 2014). A basic package of children's surgery procedures in low- and lower-middle-income countries is cost-effective and has significant societal and economic benefits, with an incremental cost-effectiveness ratio ranging from US$4 to US$14 per incremental disability-adjusted life year (Saxton et al. 2016). Similarly, operating room installations for children's surgery have yielded an incremental cost-effectiveness ratio of US$6 per disability-adjusted life year averted (Yap et al. 2018). Despite those findings, close to 2 billion children and adolescents lack access to basic, safe, and lifesaving surgical care, primarily in low- and lower-middle-income countries (Mullapudi et al. 2019); and the COVID-19 pandemic exacerbated the previously expansive wait lists for children's surgery (Klazura et al. 2022). School-based interventions for the prevention of injuries have been piloted in several low-resource settings and require further exploration as part of a school-based intervention package (Price et al. 2021; Sinha et al. 2011).

CONCLUSIONS

Global interest in school-based health and nutrition interventions to promote cognitive skills and education outcomes has grown since the World Bank's *World Development Report 1993: Investing in Health* and throughout the DCP series. Countries have increasingly supported this area as an investment in human capital, with momentum accelerated by two major social shocks: the 2008 food, fuel, and financial crisis that initiated a global recession and the 2020 COVID-19 pandemic. Today, school health and nutrition programs reach about one in two of the world's primary schoolchildren and have become the world's most extensive safety net. This chapter identifies six key messages on the current status of research, programming, and financing in the area of school health and nutrition, recognizing that investments in school infrastructure and teacher quality underpin the effectiveness of those interventions.

Despite slowly increasing research attention on older adolescents, a remarkable neglect of research on school-age children ages 5–14 years persists. A review of the published literature on children's health research shows that 40–80 percent of publications focus on the needs of children under five years. Time series analysis shows a slow but steady decline in the proportion of research on children younger than five years over the past 20 years, matched by a slowly increasing body of literature on older adolescents (20–40 percent). School-age children (5 percent of research) and young adolescents (5 percent of research) remain the most neglected age groups in health research. That neglect is difficult to understand, given that those age groups are the main targets for education investment and are also most affected by the dramatic changes related to puberty. There is a clear need to stimulate a greater proportion of research focus in this age cohort.

Substantial evidence now shows that investment in the whole 8,000-day period of development is a necessary contribution to the creation of human capital. Investment in the first 1,000 days of life is crucial to addressing the youngest children's vulnerability and high risk of mortality, as well as to establishing a strong developmental trajectory. Increasingly detailed research, especially the analysis by the BOND-KIDS project, shows that investment in health and nutrition over the next 7,000 days of life is also essential to sustain the gains of the earlier investments, support the child or young person during vulnerable phases (especially puberty and brain development), and provide important opportunities for catch-up for those who missed out on earlier interventions. There is a particular need for specific research to better understand the needs of a young person during those next 7,000 days, especially during puberty given its implications for brain development and mental health across adolescence. Adolescent girls have particular importance in this context, not only because of the specific challenges they face in relationship to sexuality and early pregnancy but also with respect to their key role in the health of the next generation.

An increasing body of evidence shows that investment during the next 7,000 days of life offers returns not only to health and education but also to many other important sectors. The benefits of investment in school-age children and adolescents have been well documented for health and education outcomes, and consequently contribute to the creation of human capital. Value-for-money and benefit-cost analyses also now show substantial returns to a broad range of other sectors, including agriculture, social protection, and gender. The benefits of these multisectoral returns are typically additive and make investments in school health and nutrition particularly cost-effective.

Development partners increasingly recognize the importance of school health and nutrition investments, as reflected in a substantial increase in the quality and quantity of guidance and policy notes. Policy papers published by international technical bodies and bilateral and multilateral agencies since the publication of the DCP3 Child and Adolescent Health and Development volume show high-level support for cross-sectoral investments in recent years. The newly introduced World Bank Human Capital Index and the SABER School Health and School Feeding policy tools offer opportunities to assess how policies that facilitate cross-sectoral investments in school-age children and adolescents contribute to strengthened economies.

Coverage of programs worldwide has seen sustained increases, with even greater momentum spurred by the COVID-19 pandemic. Widespread school closures to limit the spread of COVID-19 infection served as a counterfactual to the important role that schools play in reaching populations with safe, effective, and routine health and nutrition interventions. Countries responded by forming a global School Meals Coalition to reestablish and scale their national school meals programs. Those efforts have already shown promise, with more children provided with daily school meals than before the pandemic. The substantial growth in national programs represents a major commitment by countries themselves, because domestic funds support more than 90 percent of programs, and that commitment goes beyond food to include complementary health interventions in more than 90 percent of current programs. The commitment to complementary interventions further highlights the importance of ensuring that policy makers have access to appropriate evidence to guide the establishment or strengthening of comprehensive and quality national programs during the next 7,000 days.

Evidence increasingly supports the relevance and effectiveness of the school health package proposed in DCP3 and encourages the inclusion of additional components. The essential package of care for the 5–19 years age group remains cost-effective, even more so in light of updated policy guidance. Further cost-effective components are also emerging and can be taken forward through policy levers; those components include social and emotional well-being, menstrual health, disability-inclusive schooling, planet-friendly school meals, and prevention, detection, and referral of some surgical conditions, along with referral to pediatric clinics. Social media and other digital platforms offer a new frontier for providing health messaging to adolescents beyond formal channels afforded through school settings. Despite the lack of sufficient evidence to suggest promising practices and interventions, it is anticipated that digital platforms will increasingly be leveraged to deliver health behavior and health education messaging that complements in-school instruction and reaches out-of-school adolescents.

Health and education, and well-being and learning, all benefit if they work together. The well-being and education of schoolchildren both depend on a strong school platform that delivers a quality education and promotes health and well-being. There is now a sound case for schools as a platform for health and nutrition interventions, but the benefits will accrue only if the education program keeps children in school. That need implies a learning agenda that engages, motivates, and inspires students; teachers who are knowledgeable, informed, and respectful of students; and school classes that are interesting and engaging. Education is a strong predictor of health outcomes, and health promotes well-being and learning. New-generation programs increasingly recognize that interdependency, and the challenge going forward is to discard the sectoral boundaries and focus instead on what the sectors can achieve together to support human capital development.

AUTHORS' WRITING GROUP MEMBERS

The Authors' Writing Group members are as follows: Robert Akparibo, University of Sheffield, Sheffield, UK; Emmanuel Ameh, National Hospital, Abuja, Nigeria; Noam Angrist, Oxford University, Oxford, UK; Youth Impact, Gaborone, Bostswana; Louise Banham, Foreign, Commonwealth & Development Office, UK; Biniam Bedasso, Center for Global Development, London, UK; Mary Brenan, University of Edinburgh, Edinburgh, UK; Donald A. P. Bundy, Research Consortium for School Health and Nutrition, London School of Hygiene and Tropical Medicine, London, UK; Carmen Burbano, World Food Programme, Rome, Italy; Margaret Anne Defeyter, Northumbria University, Newcastle, UK; Lesley Drake, Partnership for Child Development, Imperial College London, London, UK; Christina Economos, Tufts University, Boston, Massachusetts, US; Pratibha Gautam, Harvard T. H. Chan School of Public Health, Boston, Massachusetts, US; Ugo Gentilini, World Bank Group, Washington, DC, US; Boitshepo Giyose, AUDA-NEPAD, Johannesburg, South Africa; Peter Hangoma, Bergen Center for Ethics and Priority Setting, University of Bergen, Bergen, Norway; Dean T. Jamison, University of California San Francisco, San Francisco, California, US; Hannah Kuper, London School of Hygiene and Tropical Medicine, London, UK; Peiman Milani, Rockefeller Foundation, Nairobi, Kenya; Doruk Ozgediz, University of California San Francisco, San Francisco, California, US; David A. Ross, Institute for Life Course Health Research, Stellenbosch University, South Africa and Consultant to the Child Health Initiative of the FIA Foundation; Shwetlena Sabarwal, World Bank Group, Washington, DC, US; Susan Sawyer, Murdoch Children's Research Institute, Melbourne, Australia; Linda Schultz, Research Consortium for School Health and Nutrition, London School of Hygiene and Tropical Medicine, London, UK; Justina Seyi-Olajide, Lagos University Teaching Hospital, Lagos, Nigeria; Samrat Singh, Imperial College London, London, UK; Stéphane Verguet, Harvard T. H. Chan School of Public Health, Boston, Massachusetts, US; Kevin Watkins, London School of Economics, London, UK; and Helen Weiss, London School of Hygiene and Tropical Medicine, London, UK.

NOTES

1. This chapter carries forward the nomenclature for age groupings from the DCP3 Child and Adolescent Health and Development volume, aligning it with the definitions and age-specific terminology outlined in the 2016 Lancet Commission on Adolescent Health and Wellbeing. The chapter refers to children and adolescents between ages 5 years and 14 years as "school age" in recognition that students in low- and lower-middle-income countries are largely in primary school because of factors such as late school entry, grade repetition, and dropout. The nomenclature also aligns with the World Health Organization's definition of "young people," which extends between ages 10 and 24 years.
2. United Nations Population Division, UN Population Division Data Portal, https://population.un.org/dataportal/home (accessed January 16, 2023).
3. BOND-KIDS—led by the Eunice Kennedy Shriver National Institute of Child Health and Human Development, together with the United States Department of Agriculture, the Research Consortium for School Health and Nutrition, and the Academy for Nutrition and Dietetics—builds on the BOND platform to establish a common framework of

nutritional indicators to monitor the nutritional status of school-age children and adolescents.

4. London School of Hygiene & Tropical Medicine, Research Consortium for School Health and Nutrition, www.lshtm.ac.uk/shn

5. Global Education Monitoring Report, UNESCO Institute of Statistics. Visualizing Indicators of Education for the World (VIEW), https://education-estimates.org/out-of-school/data/ (accessed May 3, 2024).

6. BMJ, "Adolescent Wellbeing," https://www.bmj.com/adolescent-wellbeing.

7. UNESCO Institute of Statistics, Dashboards on the Global Monitoring of School Closures Causes by the COVID-19 Pandemic, https://covid19.uis.unesco.org/global-monitoring-school-closures-covid19/.

8. World Food Programme, Global Monitoring of School Meals during COVID-19 School Closures, https://cdn.wfp.org/2020/school-feeding-map/index.html.

9. School Meals Coalition, "A healthy meal every day for every child," https://schoolmealscoalition.org/ (accessed December 10, 2021).

10. Menstrual health is defined as a state of complete physical, mental, and social well-being and not merely the absence of disease or infirmity, in relation to the menstrual cycle.

11. Refer to Kenya's Ministry of Gender, Culture, the Arts and Heritage web page, https://gender.go.ke/sanitary-towels-program/; and UK Department for Education, "Guidance: Period product scheme for schools and colleges," https://www.gov.uk/government/publications/period-products-in-schools-and-colleges/period-product-scheme-for-schools-and-colleges-in-england.

12. Note that the Sustainable Development Goal indicators for water, sanitation, and hygiene in schools define *limited sanitation service* as "improved sanitation facilities at the school that are either not single-sex or not usable at the time of the survey" and *no sanitation service* as "unimproved sanitation facilities or no sanitation facilities at the school." *Limited hygiene services* is defined as "handwashing facilities with water but no soap available at the school at the time of the survey" and *no hygiene services* as "no handwashing facilities available or no water available at the school."

13. UNICEF, Measurement of Mental Health Among Adolescents at the Population Level (MMAP), https://data.unicef.org/resources/mmap-august-2019/ (accessed January 16, 2023).

REFERENCES

Ali, C. S. 2018. "Study on Implementation of the Ministry of Education and Sports Circular on Provision of Menstrual Hygiene Management Facilities for Girls and Female Teachers in Primary and Secondary Schools." IRC, Kampala. https://www.ircwash.org/sites/default/files/mhm_final_study_report_2018_0.pdf.

Angrist, N., S. Djankov, P. K. Goldberg, and H. A. Patrinos. 2021. "Measuring Human Capital Using Global Learning Data." *Nature* 592: 403–08. https://doi.org/10.1038/s41586-021-03323-7.

Angrist, N., D. K. Evans, D. Filmer, R. Glennerster, F. H. Rodgers, and S. Sabarwal. 2025. "How to Improve Education Outcomes Most Efficiently? A Comparison of 150 Interventions Using the New Learning-Adjusted Years of Schooling Metric." *Journal of Development Economics* 172: 103382. https://www.sciencedirect.com/science/article/pii/S0304387824001317.

Angrist, N., M. C. H. Jukes, S. Clarke, R. M. Chico, C. Opondo, D. A. P. Bundy, and L. M. Cohee. 2023. "School-Based Malaria Chemoprevention as a Cost-Effective Approach to Improve Cognitive and Educational Outcomes: A Meta-analysis." Working paper, https://arxiv.org/pdf/2303.10684.

Aurino, E., A. Gelli, C. Adamba, I. Osei-Akoto, and H. Alderman. 2023. "Food for Thought? Experimental Evidence on the Learning Impacts of a Large-Scale School Feeding Program." *Journal of Human Resources* 58 (1): 74–111.

Aurino, E., J. P. Tranchant, A. S. Diallo, and A. Gelli. 2018. "School Feeding or General Food Distribution? Quasi-Experimental Evidence on the Educational Impacts of Emergency Food Assistance during Conflict in Mali." *Journal of Development Studies* 55 (Supplement 1).

Baltag, V., A. Pachyna, and J. Hall. 2015. "Global Overview of School Health Services: Data from 102 Countries." *Health Behavior and Policy Review* 2 (4): 268–83.

Baltag, V., and E. Saewyc. 2017. "Pairing Children with Health Services: The Changing Role of School Health Services in the Twenty-First Century." In *International Handbook on Adolescent Health and Development: The Public Health Response*, edited by A. Cherry, V. Baltag, and M. Dillon, 463–77. Cham: Springer.

Barrington, D. J., H. J. Robinson, E. Wilson, and J. Hennegan. 2021. "Experiences of Menstruation in High Income Countries: A Systematic Review, Qualitative Evidence Synthesis and Comparison to Low- and Middle-Income Countries." *PLoS One* 16 (7): e0255001.

Blakemore, S. J. 2019. "Adolescence and Mental Health." *The Lancet* 393 (10185): 2030–31.

Bogin, B. 1999. "Evolutionary Perspective on Human Growth." *Annual Review of Anthropology* 28 (1): 109–53.

Bundy, D. A. P, C. Burbano, M. Grosh, A. Gelli, M. Jukes, and L. Drake. 2009. *Rethinking School Feeding: Social Safety Nets, Child Development, and the Education Sector*. Directions in Development Series. Washington, DC: World Bank.

Bundy, D. A. P., N. de Silva, S. Horton, D. T. Jamison, and G. C. Patton, eds. 2017. *Disease Control Priorities* (third edition), Volume 8, *Child and Adolescent Health and Development*. Washington, DC: World Bank.

Bundy, D. A. P., N. de Silva, S. Horton, G. C. Patton, L. Schultz, and D. T. Jamison. 2017. "Child and Adolescent Health and Development: Realizing Neglected Potential." In *Disease Control Priorities* (third edition), Volume 8, *Child and Adolescent Health and Development*, edited by D. A. P. Bundy, N. de Silva, S. Horton, D. T. Jamison, and G. C. Patton, 1–24. Washington, DC: World Bank.

Bundy, D. A. P., N. de Silva, S. Horton, D. T. Jamison, and G. Patton G. 2018a. "Re-Imagining School Feeding: A High-Return Investment in Human Capital and Local Economies." In *Child and Adolescent Health and Development: Disease Control Priorities*, edited by D. A. P. Bundy, N. de Silva, S. Horton, D. T. Jamison, and G. Patton G, xxiii. Washington, DC: World Bank.

Bundy, D. A. P., N. de Silva, S. Horton, D. T. Jamison, and G. Patton, eds. 2018b. *Optimizing Education Outcomes: High-Return Investments in School Health for Increased Participation and Learning*. Washington, DC: World Bank.

Bundy, D. A. P., N. de Silva, S. Horton, G. Patton, L. Schultz, and D. T. Jamison. 2018c. "Investment in Child and Adolescent Health and Development: Key Messages from Disease Control Priorities, 3rd Edition." *The Lancet* 391 (10121): 687–99.

Bundy, D. A. P., U. Gentilini, L. Schultz, B. Bedasso, S. Singh, Y. Okamura, H. T. M. M. Iyengar, and M. M. Blakstad. 2024. "School Meals, Social Protection and Human Development: Revisiting Global Trends, Evidence, and Practices with a Focus on South Asia." Social Protection & Jobs Paper No. 2401, World Bank, Washington, DC.

Bundy, D. A. P., and S. Horton. 2017. "Impact of Interventions on Health and Development during Childhood and Adolescence: A Conceptual Framework." In *Disease Control Priorities, Third Edition: Child and Adolescent Health and Development*, Volume 8, edited by D. A. P. Bundy, N. de Silva, S. Horton, D. T. Jamison, and G. C. Patton, 73–78. Washington, DC: World Bank.

Bundy, D. A. P., L Schultz, B. Sarr, L. Banham, P. Colenso, and L. Drake. 2017. "The School as a Platform for Addressing Health in Middle Childhood and Adolescence." In *Disease Control Priorities, Third Edition: Child and Adolescent Health and Development*, Volume 8, edited by D. A. P. Bundy, N. de Silva, S. Horton, D. T. Jamison, and G. C. Patton, 269–85. Washington, DC: World Bank.

Bundy, D. A. P., S. Shaeffer, M. Jukes, K. Beegle, A. Gillespie, L. Drake, et al. 2006. "School-Based Health and Nutrition Programs." In *Disease Control Priorities in Developing Countries* (second edition), edited by D. Jamison, J. G. Breman, A. R. Measham, G. Alleyne, M. Claeson, D. Evans, P. Jha, et al. Washington, DC: World Bank/Oxford University Press.

Burton, M. J., J. Ramke, A. P. Marques, R. R. A. Bourne, N. Congdon, I. Jones, S. Arunga, et al. 2021. "The Lancet Global Health Commission on Global Eye Health: Vision beyond 2020." *The Lancet Global Health* 9 (4): e489–551.

Carvajal, L., J. W. Ahs, J. H. Requejo, C. Kieling, A. Lundin, M. Kumar, N. P. Luteil, et al. 2023. "Measurement of Mental Health among Adolescents at the Population Level: A Multicountry Protocol for Adaptation and Validation of Mental Health Measures." *Journal of Adolescent Health* 72 (1S): S27–S33. https://pubmed.ncbi.nlm.nih.gov/36528384/.

Caut, C., M. Leach, and A. Steel. 2020. "Dietary Guideline Adherence during Preconception and Pregnancy: A Systematic Review." *Maternal & Child Nutrition* 16 (2): e12916.

Chakraborty, T., and R. Jayaraman. 2019. "School Feeding and Learning Achievement: Evidence from India's Midday Meal Program." *Journal of Development Economics* 139 (June): 249–65.

Clark, H., T. A. Ghebreyesus, A. B. Albrectsen, J. Alcocer, E. Alden, A. Azoulay, S. Billingsley, et al. 2021. "Uniting for Adolescents in COVID-19 and Beyond." *BMJ* 31: n719.

Cohen, J. F. W., S. Verguet, B. B. Giyose, and D. A. P. Bundy. 2023. "Universal Free School Meals: The Future of School Meal Programmes?" *The Lancet* 402 (10405): P831–33.

Cooper, A. R., A. Goodman, A. S. Page, L. B. Sherar, D. W. Esliger, E. M. van Sluijs, L. B. Andersen, et al. 2015. "Objectively Measured Physical Activity and Sedentary Time in Youth: The International Children's Accelerometry Database (ICAD)." *International Journal of Behavioral Nutrition and Physical Activity* 12 (1): 113.

Crump, J., P. Newton, S. Baird, and Y. Lubell. 2017. "Febrile Illness in Adolescents and Adults." In *Disease Control Priorities* (third edition), Volume 6, *Major Infectious Diseases,* edited by K. Holmes, S. Bertozzi, B. Bloom, and P. Jha. Washington, DC: World Bank.

Del Giudice, M. 2018. "Middle Childhood: An Evolutionary-Developmental Synthesis." In *Handbook of Life Course Health Development*, 95–107. Cham: Springer International Publishing.

Dharamshi, A., B. Barakat, L. Alkema, and M. Antoninis. 2022. "A Bayesian Model for Estimating Sustainable Development Goal Indicator 4.1.2: School Completion Rates." *Journal of the Royal Statistical Society Series C* 71 (5): 1822–64.

FAO (Food and Agriculture Organization of the United Nations). 2012. "Food Wastage Footprint & Climate Change." United Nations. https://www.fao.org/fileadmin/templates/nr/sustainability_pathways/docs/FWF_and_climate_change.pdf.

Feldstein, L. R., G. Fox, A. Shefer, L. M. Conklin, and K. Ward. 2020. "School-Based Delivery of Routinely Recommended Vaccines and Opportunities to Check Vaccination Status at School, a Global Summary, 2008-2017 HHS Public Access." Vaccine 38 (3): 680–89. https://doi.org/10.1016/j.vaccine.2019.10.054.

Fernandes, M., and E. Aurino. 2017. "Identifying an Essential Package for School-Age Child Health: Economic Analysis." In *Disease Control Priorities* (third edition), Volume 8, *Child and Adolescent Health and Development*, edited by D. A. P. Bundy, N. de Silva, S. Horton, D. T. Jamison, and G. C. Patton, 355–68. Washington, DC: World Bank.

Gatti, R. V., A. C. Kraay, C. Avitabile, M. E. Collin, R. Dsouza, and N. A. P. Dehnen. 2018. *The Human Capital Project*. Washington, DC: World Bank.

GCNF (Global Child Nutrition Foundation). 2022. "School Meals Programs around the World: Results from the 2021 Global Survey of School Meal Programs." GCNF, Seattle. https://survey.gcnf.org/2021-global-survey/.

Gelli, A., J. Donovan, A. Margolies, N. Aberman, M. Santacroce, E. Chirwa, et al. 2020. "Value Chains to Improve Diets: Diagnostics to Support Intervention Design in Malawi." *Global Food Security* 25: 100321.

Giedd, J. N., and J. L. Rapoport. 2010. "Structural MRI of Pediatric Brain Development: What Have We Learned and Where Are We Going?" *Neuron* 67 (5): 728–34.

Glewwe, P., A. Park, and M. Zhao. 2016. "A Better Vision for Development: Eyeglasses and Academic Performance in Rural Primary Schools in China." *Journal of Development Economics* 122: 170–82.

Global Financing Facility. 2021a. "School Health & Nutrition: Reach and Relevance for Adolescents." World Bank, Washington, DC.

Global Financing Facility. 2021b. "Sustaining Adolescent Health Service Delivery during Prolonged School Closures: Considerations in Light of COVID-19." World Bank, Washington, DC.

Global Financing Facility. 2021c. "Monitoring Adolescent School Health and Nutrition Programs and Interventions: Answering the Why, What, Who, and How." World Bank, Washington, DC.

Global Financing Facility. 2021d. "Adolescent School Health & Nutrition: Interactive Decision Trees." World Bank, Washington, DC.

GPE (Global Partnership for Education). 2018. "School Health for All: An Operational Manual for Integrating Inclusive School Health and Nutrition." World Bank, Washington, DC. https://www.globalpartnership.org/content/school-health-all.

Grant, J., R. Cottrell, F. Cluzeau, and G. Fawcett. 2000. "Evaluating 'Payback' on Biomedical Research from Papers Cited in Clinical Guidelines: Applied Bibliometric Study." *BMJ* 320: 1107–11.

Grant, J., L. Green, B. Mason, J. Grant, L. Green, and B. Mason. 2003. "Basic Research and Health: A Reassessment of the Scientific Basis for the Support of Biomedical Science." *Research Evaluation* 12 (3): 217–24.

Gray, N. J., N. A. Desmond, D. S. Ganapathee, S. Beadle, and D. A. P. Bundy. 2022. "Breaking Down Silos between Health and Education to Improve Adolescent Wellbeing." *BMJ* 27: e067683.

Guarnizo-Herreño, C. C., W. Lyu, and G. L. Wehby. 2019. "Children's Oral Health and Academic Performance: Evidence of a Persisting Relationship over the Last Decade in the United States." *Journal of Pediatrics* 209: 183–89.e2.

Gupta, S., S. Howard, S. Hunger, F. Antillon, M. Metzger, T. Israels, M. Harif, et al. 2015. "Treating Childhood Cancers in Low- and Middle-Income Countries." In *Disease Control Priorities* (third edition), Volume 3, *Cancer*, edited by H. Gelband, P. Jha, R. Sankaranarayanan, and S. Horton. Washington, DC: World Bank.

Guthold, R., A. B. Moller, P. Azzopardi, M. G. Ba, L. Fagan, V. Baltag, L. Say, et al. 2019. "The Global Action for Measurement of Adolescent Health (GAMA) Initiative— Rethinking Adolescent Metrics." *Journal of Adolescent Health* 64: 697–9.

Hennegan, J., A. K. Shannon, J. Rubli, K. J. Schwab, and G. J. Melendez-Torres. 2019. "Women's and Girls' Experiences of Menstruation in Low- and Middle-Income Countries: A Systematic Review and Qualitative Metasynthesis." *PLoS Medicine* 16 (5): e1002803.

Hill, K., L. Zimmerman, and D. T. Jamison. 2017. "Mortality at Ages 5 to 19: Levels and Trends, 1990–2010." In *Disease Control Priorities* (third edition), Volume 8, *Child and Adolescent Health and Development*, edited by D. A. P. Bundy, N. de Silva, S. Horton, D. T. Jamison, and G. C. Patton, 25–26. Washington, DC: World Bank.

Horton, S., E. De la Cruz Toledo, J. Mahon, J. Santelli, and J. Waldfogel. 2017. "Identifying an Essential Package for Adolescent Health: Economic Analysis." In *Disease Control* (third edition), Volume 8, *Child and Adolescent Health and Development*, edited by D. A. P. Bundy, N. de Silva, S. Horton, D. T. Jamison, and G. C. Patton, 369–84. Washington, DC: World Bank.

Hotez, P. J., D. A. P. Bundy, K. Beegle, S. Brooker, L. Drake, N. de Silva, et al. 2006. "Helminth Infections: Soil-Transmitted Helminth Infections and Schistosomiasis." In *Disease Control Priorities in Developing Countries* (second edition), edited by D. Jamison, J. G. Breman, A. R. Measham, G. Alleyne, M. Claeson, D. Evans, P. Jha, et al., 467–82. Washington, DC: World Bank/Oxford University Press.

Hunter, D., B. Giyose, A. PoloGalante, F. Tartanac, D. A. P. Bundy, A. Mitchell, et al. 2017. "Schools as a System to Improve Nutrition: A New Statement for School-Based Food and Nutrition Interventions." UNSCN Discussion Paper, United Nations System Standing Committee on Nutrition.

Hutton, G., and C. Chase. 2017. "Water Supply, Sanitation, and Hygiene." In *Disease Control Priorities* (third edition), Volume 7, *Injury Prevention and Environmental Health*, edited by C. N. Mock , R. Nugent, O. Kobusingye, and K. Smith. Washington, DC: World Bank.

Johnson, W., and S. E. Moore. 2016. "Adolescent Pregnancy, Nutrition, and Health Outcomes in Low- and Middle-Income Countries: What We Know and What We Don't Know." *BJOG* 123 (10): 1589–92.

Kansiime, C., L. Hytti, R. Nalugya, K. Nakuya, P. Namirembe, S. Nakalema, S. Neema, et al. 2020. "Menstrual Health Intervention and School Attendance in Uganda (MENISCUS-2): A Pilot Intervention Study." *BMJ Open* 10 (2): e031182.

Keats, E. C., J. K. Das, R. A. Salam, Z. S. Lassi, A. Imdad, R. E. Black, and Z. A. Bhutta. 2021. "Effective Interventions to Address Maternal and Child Malnutrition: An Update of the Evidence." *The Lancet Child & Adolescent Health* 5 (5): 367–84.

Kessler, R. C., G. P. Amminger, S. Aguilar-Gaxiola, J. Alonso, and S. Lee. 2007. "Age of Onset of Mental Disorders: A Review of Recent Literature." *Current Opinion in Psychiatry* 20 (4): 359–64.

Khan, D. S. A., J. K. Das, S. Zareen, Z. S. Lassi, A. Salman, M. Raashid, A. A. Dero, et al. 2022. "Nutritional Status and Dietary Intake of School-Age Children and Early Adolescents: Systematic Review in a Developing Country and Lessons for the Global Perspective." *Frontiers in Nutrition* 8. https://doi.org/10.3389/fnut.2021.739447.

Klazura, G., P. Kisa, A. Wesonga, M. Nabukenya, N. Kakembo, S. Nimanya, R. Naluyimbazi, et al. 2022. "Pediatric Surgery Backlog at a Ugandan Tertiary Care Facility: COVID-19 Makes a Chronic Problem Acutely Worse." *Pediatric Surgery International* 38 (10): 1391–97.

Kristjansson, E., M. Osman, M. Dignam, P. R. Labelle, O. Magwood, A. H. Galicia, et al. 2022. "School Feeding Programs for Improving the Physical and Psychological Health of School Children Experiencing Socioeconomic Disadvantage." *Cochrane Database of Systematic Reviews* 2022(8): CD014794.

Kumbeni, M. T., F. A. Ziba, J. Apenkwa, and E. Otupiri. 2021. "Prevalence and Factors Associated with Menstruation-Related School Absenteeism among Adolescent Girls in Rural Northern Ghana." *BMC Women's Health* 21 (1): 279.

Kuzawa, C. W., H. T. Chugani, L. I. Grossman, L. Lipovich, O. Muzik, P. R. Hof, et al. 2014. "Metabolic Costs and Evolutionary Implications of Human Brain Development." *Proceedings of the National Academy of Sciences* 111 (36): 13010–15.

Lange, G. M., Q. Wodon, and K. Carey. 2018. *The Changing Wealth of Nations 2018*. Washington, DC: World Bank.

Leone, T., and L. J. Brown. 2020. "Timing and Determinants of Age at Menarche in Low-Income and Middle-Income Countries." *BMJ Global Health* 5 (12): e003689.

Lule, E., J. E. Rosen, S. Singh, J. C. Knowles, and J. R. Behrman. 2006. "Adolescent Health Programs." In *Disease Control Priorities in Developing Countries* (second edition), edited by D. Jamison, J. G. Breman, A. R. Measham, G. Alleyne, M. Claeson, D. Evans, P. Jha, et al. Washington, DC: World Bank.

Ma, Y., N. Congdon, Y. Shi, R. Hogg, A. Medina, M. Boswell, S. Rozelle, and M. Iyer. 2018. "Effect of a Local Vision Care Center on Eyeglasses Use and School Performance in Rural China." *JAMA Ophthalmology* 136 (7): 731.

Marmot, M., S. Friel, R. Bell, T. A. Houweling, and S. Taylor. 2008. "Closing the Gap in a Generation: Health Equity through Action on the Social Determinants of Health." *The Lancet* 372 (9650): 1661–69.

Marsh, A. D., A. B. Moller, E. Saewyc, E. Adebayo, E. Akwara, P. Azzopardi, M. G. Ba, et al. 2022. "Priority Indicators for Adolescent Health Measurement – Recommendations from the Global Action for Measurement of Adolescent Health (GAMA) Advisory Group." *Journal of Adolescent Health* 71 (4): 455–65.

Mock, C., P. Donkor, A. Gawande, D. Jamison, M. Kruk, and H. Debas. 2015. "Essential Surgery: Key Messages of This Volume." In *Disease Control Priorities* (third edition), Volume 1, *Essential Surgery*, edited by H. Debas, P. Donkor, A. Gawande, D. T. Kruk, and C. N. Mock, 1–18. Washington, DC: World Bank.

Montresor, A., D. Mupfasoni, A. Mikhailov, P. Mwinzi, A. Lucianez, M. Jamsheed, E. Gasimov, et al. 2020. "The Global Progress of Soil-Transmitted Helminthiases Control in 2020 and World Health Organization Targets for 2030." *PLoS Neglected Tropical Diseases* 14 (8): 1–17.

Morris, Z. S., S. Wooding, and J. Grant. 2011. "The Answer Is 17 Years, What Is the Question: Understanding Time Lags in Translational Research." *Journal of the Royal Society of Medicine* 104 (12): 510–20.

Mullapudi, B., D. Grabski, E. Ameh, D. Ozgediz, H. Thangarajah, K. Kling, et al. 2019. "Estimates of Number of Children and Adolescents without Access to Surgical Care." *Bulletin of the World Health Organization* 97 (4): 254–58.

Olusanya, B. O., N. Y. Boo, M. K. C. Nair, M. E. Samms-Vaughan, M. Hadders-Algra, S. M. Wright, et al. 2022. "Accelerating Progress on Early Childhood Development for Children under 5 Years with Disabilities by 2030." *The Lancet Global Health* 10 (3): e438–44.

Orben, A., L. Tomova, and S. J. Blakemore. 2020. "The Effects of Social Deprivation on Adolescent Development and Mental Health." *The Lancet Child & Adolescent Health* 4 (8): 634–40.

Oster, E., and R. Thornton. 2011. "Menstruation, Sanitary Products, and School Attendance: Evidence from a Randomized Evaluation." *American Economic Journal: Applied Economics* 3 (1): 91–100.

Oye, M., L. Pritchett, and J. Sandefur. 2016. "Girls' Schooling Is Good, Girls' Schooling with Learning Is Better." Education Commission, Washington, DC.

Pastorino, S., M. Springmann, U. Backlund, M. Kaljonen, P. Milani, R. Bellanca, et al. 2023. "School Meals and Food Systems: Rethinking the Consequences for Climate, Environment, Biodiversity and Food Sovereignty." White paper prepared by the Research Consortium for School Health and Nutrition, an initiative of the School Meals Coalition, London.

Patton, G. C., L. M. Neufeld, S. Dogra, E. A. Frongillo, D. Hargreaves, S. He, et al. 2022. "Nourishing Our Future: The Lancet Series on Adolescent Nutrition." *The Lancet* 399 (10320): 123–25.

Patton, G., S. M. Sawyer, J. S. Santelli, D. A. Ross, R. Afifi, B. Nicholas, et al. 2016. "Our Future: A Lancet Commission on Adolescent Health and Wellbeing." *The Lancet* 387 (10036): 2423–78.

Pontzer, H., Y. Yamada, H. Sagayama, P. N. Ainslie, L. F. Andersen, L. J. Anderson, et al. 1979. "Daily Energy Expenditure through the Human Life Course." *Science* 373 (6556): 808–12.

Price, K., K. C. Lee, K. E. Woolley, H. Falk, M. Peck, R. Lilford, and N. Moiemen. 2021. "Burn Injury Prevention in Low- and Middle-Income Countries: Scoping Systematic Review." *Burns & Trauma* 9: tkab037.

Pritchett, L. 2013. *The Rebirth of Education: Schooling Ain't Learning.* Washington, DC: CGD Books.

Radday, K. 2020. *Federal Development of the National School Lunch Program from an Agricultural Support to a Child Welfare Program.* Baltimore: Notre Dame of Maryland University.

Raiten, D. J., D. A. Bundy, D. DeBernardo, A. Steiber, C. Papoutsakis, B. Jimenez, et al. 2024. "Biomarkers of Nutrition for Development—Knowledge Indicating Dietary Sufficiency (BOND-KIDS)." Executive Summary: A Working Paper of the BOND-KIDS Working Group.

Rodriguez-Martinez, A., B. Zhou, M. K. Sophiea, J. Bentham, C. J. Paciorek, M. L. Iurilli, et al. 2020. "Height and Body-Mass Index Trajectories of School-Aged Children and Adolescents from 1985 to 2019 in 200 Countries and Territories: A Pooled Analysis of 2181 Population-Based Studies with 65 Million Participants." *The Lancet* 396 (10261): 1511–24.

Ross, D. A., R. Hinton, M. Melles-Brewer, D. Engel, W. Zeck, L. Fagan, et al. 2020. "Adolescent Well-Being: A Definition and Conceptual Framework." *Journal of Adolescent Health* 67 (4): 472–76.

Saxton, A. T., D. Poenaru, D. Ozgediz, E. A. Ameh, D. Farmer, E. R. Smith, et al. 2016. "Economic Analysis of Children's Surgical Care in Low- and Middle-Income Countries: A Systematic Review and Analysis." *PLoS One* 11(10): e0165480.

Schultz, L., L. Appleby, and L. Drake. 2018. "Maximizing Human Capital by Aligning Investments in Health and Education." Health Finance & Governance, United States Agency for International Development.

Schultz, L., D. A. P. Bundy, and L. Drake. 2019. "Human Capital Investments: The Case for Education and Health in Sub-Saharan Africa." United States Agency for International Development, Washington, DC.

Schultz, L., A. Renaud, D. A. P. Bundy, F. B. M. Barry, L. Benveniste, C. Burbano de Lara, et al. 2024. "The SABER School Feeding Policy Tool: A Ten-Year Analysis of Its Use by Countries in Developing Policies for Their National School Meals Programs." *Frontiers in Public Health* 12. https://doi.org/10.3389/fpubh.2024.1337600.

Schultz, L., and L. Shors. 2021. "Operationalizing Health & Education Coordination: Recommendations Surfaced through Interviews with Africa Bureau Missions." United States Agency for International Development, Washington, DC.

Scott, J., A. Rahman, C. Mihalopoulos, H. Erskine, and J. Roberts. 2015. "Mental and Developmental Disorders." In *Disease Control Priorities* (third edition), Volume 4, *Mental, Neurological, and Substance Use Disorders,* edited by V. Patel, D. Chisholm, T. Dua, R. Laxminarayan, and M. E. Medina-Mora, 145–61. Washington, DC: World Bank.

Semba, R. D., S. de Pee, K. Sun, M. Sari, N. Akhter, and M. W. Bloem. 2008. "Effect of Parental Formal Education on Risk of Child Stunting in Indonesia and Bangladesh: A Cross-Sectional Study." *The Lancet* 371 (9609): 322–28.

Seyi-Olajide, J., A. Ali, W. F. Powell Jr., L. Samad, T. Banu, H. Abdelhafeez, et al. 2024. "Surgery and the First 8000 Days of Life: A Review." *International Health* [Internet]. November 18; https://academic.oup.com/inthealth/advance-article/doi/10.1093/inthealth/ihae078/7903051.

Singh, A., A. Park, and S. Dercon. 2014. "School Meals as a Safety Net: An Evaluation of the Midday Meal Scheme in India." *Economic Development and Cultural Change* 62 (2): 275–306.

Singh, S., and G. R. Conway. 2021. "Nutrient Output, Production Diversity, and Dietary Needs." Briefing Paper No. 6, Centre for Environmental Policy, Imperial College London.

Sinha, I., A. Patel, F. S. Kim, M. L. MacCorkle, and J. F. Watkins. 2011. "Comic Books Can Educate Children about Burn Safety in Developing Countries." *Journal of Burn Care & Research* 32 (4): e112–17.

South Africa, Department of Women. 2019. "Menstrual Hygiene Day Seeks to End More Than Just Period Poverty." News Release, May 28, 2019. https://www.gov.za/speeches/department-women-menstrual-hygiene-day-28-may-2019-0000.

Starr, J. R., R. R. Ruff, J. Palmisano, J. M. Goodson, O. M. Bukhari, and R. Niederman. 2021. "Longitudinal Caries Prevalence in a Comprehensive, Multicomponent, School-Based Prevention Program." *Journal of the American Dental Association* 152 (3): 224–33e.1.1.

Sully, E. A., A. Biddlecom, J. E. Darroch, T. Riley, L. S. Ashford, N. Lince-Deroche, et al. 2020. *Adding It Up: Investing in Sexual and Reproductive Health.* New York: Guttmacher Institute. https://www.guttmacher.org/report/adding-it-up-investing-in-sexual-reproductive-health-2019.

Sumpter, C., and B. Torondel. 2013. "A Systematic Review of the Health and Social Effects of Menstrual Hygiene Management." *PLoS One* 8 (4): e62004.

Sykes, A. G., J. Seyi-Olajide, E. A. Ameh, D. Ozgediz, A. Abbas, S. Abib, et al. 2022. "Estimates of Treatable Deaths within the First 20 Years of Life from Scaling Up Surgical Care at First-Level Hospitals in Low- and Middle-Income Countries." *World Journal of Surgery* 46 (9): 2114–22.

Sustainable Financing Initiative. 2022. "School Meals Programmes and the Education Crisis: A Financial Landscape Analysis." Education Commission, Washington, DC. https://educationcommission.org/wp-content/uploads/2022/10/School-Meals-Programmes-and-the-Education-Crisis-A-Financial-Landscape-Analysis.pdf.

Tam, E., E. C. Keats, F. Rind, J. K. Das, and Z. A. Bhutta. 2020. "Micronutrient Supplementation and Fortification Interventions on Health and Development Outcomes among Children Under-Five in Low- and Middle-Income Countries: A Systematic Review and Meta-Analysis." *Nutrient* 12 (2): 289.

Tzioumis, E., and L. S. Adair. 2014. "Childhood Dual Burden of Under- and Overnutrition in Low- and Middle-Income Countries: A Critical Review." *Food and Nutrition Bulletin* 35 (2): 230–43.

Tzioumis, E., M. C. Kay, M. E. Bentley, and L. S. Adair. 2016. "Prevalence and Trends in the Childhood Dual Burden of Malnutrition in Low- and Middle-Income Countries, 1990–2012." *Public Health Nutrition* 19 (8): 1375–88.

UN DESA (United Nations Department of Economic and Social Affairs, Population Division). 2015. *Population 2030: Demographic Challenges and Opportunities for Sustainable Development Planning.* New York: United Nations.

UNESCO (United Nations Educational, Scientific and Cultural Organization). 2023. *Ready to Learn and Thrive: School Health and Nutrition around the World.* Paris: UNESCO.

UNICEF (United Nations Children's Fund). 2011. *The State of the World's Children 2011: Adolescence, an Age of Opportunity.* New York: United Nations.

UNICEF (United Nations Children's Fund). 2021. *Counted, Included: Using Data to Shed Light on the Well-Being of Children with Disabilities.* New York: United Nations.

UNICEF (United Nations Children's Fund). 2021. *The State of the World's Children 2021: On My Mind—Promoting, Protecting and Caring for Children's Mental Health.* New York: United Nations.

van Eijk, A. M., M. Sivakami, M. B. Thakkar, A. Bauman, K. F. Laserson, S. Coates, et al. 2016. "Menstrual Hygiene Management among Adolescent Girls in India: A Systematic Review and Meta-analysis." *BMJ Open* 6 (3): e010290.

Warren, K., D. A. P. Bundy, R. Anderson, A. Davis, D. Henderson, and D. Jamison. 1993. "Helminth Infections." In *Disease Control Priorities in Developing Countries* (first edition), edited by D. T. Jamison, W. H. Mosley, A. R. Measham, and J. L. Bobadilla, 131–60. Oxford: Oxford University Press.

Watkins, D. A., D. T. Jamison, A. Mills, R. Atun, K. Danforth, A. Glassman, et al. 2018. "Universal Health Coverage and Essential Packages of Care." In *Disease Control Priorities* (third edition), Volume 9, *Disease Control Priorities: Improving Health and Reducing Poverty,* edited by D. T. Jamison, H. Gelband, S. Horton, P. Jha, R. Laxminarayan, C. Mock, and Rachel Nugent, 43–65. Washington, DC: World Bank.

WFP (World Food Programme). 2013. "Revised School Feeding Policy: Promoting Innovation to Achieve National Ownership." WFP, Rome.

WFP (World Food Programme). 2020. *State of School Feeding Worldwide 2020.* Rome: WFP.

WFP (World Food Programme). 2021. "Clean Cooking in Schools: A Lasting Shift to Clean Institutional Cooking." Climate & Disaster Risk Unit, WFP, Rome.

WFP (World Food Programme). 2023. *State of School Feeding Worldwide 2022.* Rome: WFP.

WHO (World Health Organization). 2014. *Global Status Report on Violence Prevention 2014.* Geneva: WHO.

WHO (World Health Organization). 2019. *Accelerated Action for the Health of Adolescents (AA-HA!): A Manual to Facilitate the Process of Developing National Adolescent Health Strategies and Plans.* Geneva: WHO.

WHO (World Health Organization). 2021a. *Ending the Neglect to Attain the Sustainable Development Goals: A Road Map for Neglected Tropical Diseases 2021–2030*. Geneva: WHO.

WHO (World Health Organization). 2021b. "Executive Summary. The Selection and Use of Essential Medicines 2021." Report of the 23rd WHO Expert Committee on the Selection and Use of Essential Medicines, virtual meeting, June 21–July 2, 2021, Geneva.

WHO (World Health Organization). 2022a. *WHO Guidelines for Malaria*. Geneva: WHO.

WHO (World Health Organization). 2022b. "Human Papillomavirus Vaccines: WHO Position Paper (2022 update)." *Weekly Epidemiological Record* 50 (97): 645–72.

WHO (World Health Organization) Regional Office for Europe. 2020. Spotlight on Adolescent Health and Well-Being. Findings from the 2017/2018 Health Behavior in School-Aged Children (HSBC) Survey in Europe and Central Asia." WHO, Geneva.

WHO (World Health Organization), UNAIDS (Joint United Nations Programme on HIV/AIDS), UNESCO (United Nations Educational, Scientific and Cultural Organization), UNFPA (United Nations Population Fund), UNICEF (United Nations Children's Fund), UN WOMEN (United Nations Entity for Gender Equality and the Empowerment of Women), the World Food Programme, and PMNCH (Partnership for Maternal, Newborn, and Child Health). 2023. *Global Accelerated Action for the Health of Adolescents (AA-HA!): Guidance to Support Country Implementation*, second edition. Geneva: World Health Organization.

WHO (World Health Organization) and UNESCO (United Nations Educational, Scientific and Cultural Organization). 2021a. *Making Every School a Health-Promoting School: Global Standards and Indicators*. Geneva: WHO.

WHO (World Health Organization) and UNESCO (United Nations Educational, Scientific and Cultural Organization). 2021b. *Making Every School a Health-Promoting School: Implementation Guidance*. Geneva: WHO.

WHO (World Health Organization) and UNESCO (United Nations Educational, Scientific and Cultural Organization). 2021c. *Making Every School a Health-Promoting School: Country Case Studies*. Geneva: WHO.

WHO (World Health Organization) and UNESCO (United Nations Educational, Scientific and Cultural Organization). 2021d. Global Standards for Health Promoting Schools and their Implementation Guidance. Geneva, Switzerland; 2021.

WHO (World Health Organization) and UNICEF (United Nations Children's Fund). 2018a. *WHO/UNICEF Guidance Note: Ensuring Sustained Protection Against Diphtheria: Replacing TT with Td Vaccine*. Geneva.

WHO (World Health Organization) and UNICEF (United Nations Children's Fund). 2018b. *Drinking Water, Sanitation and Hygiene in Schools: Global Baseline Report 2018*. New York.

World Bank. 1993. *World Development Report: Investing in Health*. Washington, DC: World Bank.

World Bank. 2013. *The What, Why, and How of the Systems Approach for Better Education Results (SABER)*. Washington, DC: World Bank.

World Bank. 2019. "Africa Human Capital Plan: Powering Africa's Potential through Its People." World Bank, Washington, DC.

World Bank, UNESCO (United Nations Educational, Scientific and Cultural Organization), and UNICEF (United Nations Children's Fund). 2021. *The State of the Global Education Crisis: A Path to Recovery*. Washington, DC, Paris, New York: World Bank, UNESCO, and UNICEF.

Wrottesley, S. V., E. Mates, E. Brennan, V. Bijalwan, R. Menezes, S. Ray, et al. 2023. "Nutritional Status of School-Age Children and Adolescents in Low- and Middle-Income Countries across Seven Global Regions: A Synthesis of Scoping Reviews." *Public Health Nutrition* 26 (1): 63–95.

Yap, A., A. Muzira, M. Cheung, J. Healy, N. Kakembo, P. Kisa, et al. 2018. "A Cost-Effectiveness Analysis of a Pediatric Operating Room in Uganda." *Surgery* 164 (5): 953–59.

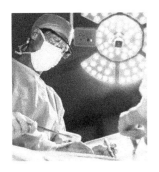

21

Implementation of *DCP3 Essential Surgery*: Cross-National Experiences

Peter Hangoma, Kristen Danforth, Lubna Samad, Peter Donkor, and Charles N. Mock

ABSTRACT

Most of the world's population, almost all in low- and middle-income countries (LMICs), lacks timely access to affordable surgical care. The first three editions of *Disease Control Priorities (DCP)* included surgery-relevant policy recommendations intended to address this gap, and the third edition *(DCP3)* devoted an entire volume to essential surgery. To better understand the extent to which recommendations from the *DCP* series informed national policy design and implementation, we conducted a two-step review, using a structured survey of DCP stakeholders complemented by an in-depth case study of the recent revision of the National Vision for Surgical Care 2020–2025 in Pakistan. Twenty individuals working across 25 countries responded to the survey and described the incorporation of *Essential Surgery* recommendations in national and global policy efforts. The most influential examples of uptake were of "wholesale" approaches to knowledge exchange, where *DCP3* informed academic or technical multicountry initiatives, which then filtered into national surgical, obstetric, and anesthesia plans, such as was seen in Ethiopia's Saving Lives through Safe Surgery initiative. In Pakistan, the package of 44 interventions included in *Essential Surgery* served as the starting point for surgical care included in the revised Essential Package of Health Services. However, the adaptation of *DCP3* for the Pakistan health system revealed several challenges, notably *DCP3*'s lack of policy implementation guidance, a mismatch between the *DCP3* conceptualization of health system platform levels and the reality in practice, and insufficient consideration of the distribution of specialty surgery providers across the platforms. Addressing these limitations in future iterations of *DCP* can improve the usefulness of *DCP* products to country-level policy makers and maximize the potential impact of recommendations.

INTRODUCTION

Surgical care is increasingly recognized as a vital component of overall health care. In the past, the broader fields of public health and global health neglected surgical care, considering it too expensive and complex. However, those viewpoints have been changing, with increasing recognition of the cost-effectiveness of surgery and its role in population health. Key milestones in that recognition include the Lancet Commission on Global Surgery (Meara et al. 2016) and the findings of the *Disease Control Priorities,* third edition (*DCP3*) volume on *Essential Surgery* (Debas et al. 2015). The Lancet Commission pointed out that conditions requiring surgical care as part of their management (for example, injuries and complications of pregnancy) accounted for 33 percent of all deaths worldwide. The commission also estimated that most (5 billion) of the world's population, almost all in low- and middle-income countries (LMICs), lacked timely access to affordable surgical care when they needed it. Even modest investments in surgical systems and improved access to emergency surgical care have the potential to translate into significant impacts in increased surgical procedures and health outcomes.

The *DCP3* volume *Essential Surgery* focused on components of surgical care that should be the highest priority to implement globally. They include surgical care that addresses health conditions that pose a large health burden and for which there are surgical procedures that are highly cost-effective and feasible to promote globally. *DCP3* undertook extensive economic analysis, showing that numerous surgical procedures are very cost-effective, with many costing US$10–US$100 per disability-adjusted life year averted—in the same cost-effectiveness range as immunizations, bed nets for prevention of malaria, antiretrovirals for HIV/AIDS, and other established interventions that have been the focus of major global implementation efforts.

In order to promote uptake of the most cost-effective aspects of surgical care, the 80 authors and editors of *DCP3 Essential Surgery* went on to define a set of 44 procedures (or sets of procedures) using the criteria of high disease burden, cost-effectiveness, and feasibility. Those procedures address conditions such as injuries, complications of pregnancy, surgical emergencies (for example, appendicitis), and several congenital anomalies (for example, cleft lip). *DCP3* estimated that increasing coverage of such procedures could avert 1.5 million deaths per year. The major conclusions and recommendations of *DCP3 Essential Surgery* were for more widespread access to that set of 44 procedures, with the goal of building capacity at first-level facilities to perform routine and less complex procedures safely, and to recognize and refer complex cases for tertiary care. To facilitate increased access, *DCP3 Essential Surgery* included recommendations on platforms and policies, including quality improvement programs, workforce innovations (such as task sharing), and use of specialized surgical platforms (such as mobile teams).

As with any set of health recommendations, implementation requires an active process. This chapter presents results of a structured review undertaken to better understand what has transpired with usage and implementation of the *DCP3 Essential Surgery* recommendations. The review sought to document examples of the usage and implementation of *DCP3 Essential Surgery* and related recommendations, as well as to understand how various pathways of impact compare to expected uptake of *DCP3* in policy (Bullock et al. 2021). Understanding what characteristics of *DCP3 Essential Surgery* have facilitated and hindered use should inform the creation of global recommendations that are more applicable to policy processes, especially in LMICs.

METHODS

To gain insight into the uptake of DCP publications on surgery programs and policies in LMICs, the review used a sequential, two-step approach, starting with a structured survey in REDCap. That survey was sent to 176 individuals who were authors of surgery-related chapters published in the first, second, and third editions of *Disease Control Priorities* (Debas et al. 2015; Jamison et al. 1993; Jamison et al. 2006) or selected experts on global surgery policy, primarily members of the Lancet Commission on Global Surgery (Meara et al. 2016). The survey included Likert and free-response questions on examples of DCP recommendations implemented in countries where the respondents have worked; whether, and how, respondents have used DCP recommendations in their own work; their evaluation of government commitment to increase surgery availability in the countries where they have worked; perceived challenges hindering the uptake of DCP recommendations; and their recommendations for addressing those challenges.

The second step involved an in-depth case study on the influence of DCP publications on essential surgery policy in Pakistan, using a combination of key informant interviews and desk review of policy agenda–setting documentation (for example, policy documents, statements of public officials, and national program data). Pakistan was selected as an illustrative example because of information collected through survey responses and the study team's prior knowledge of efforts to implement DCP recommendations. This chapter presents the case study to provide insight into the determinants of successful uptake of *DCP3* recommendations in national or subnational health programming and policy. For in-depth interviews, key informants with experience developing national surgery and health policy experts in Pakistan were approached. Interviews were conducted remotely via videoconferencing software (Zoom) between August and December 2021. The interviews also probed for qualitative data to understand features that detracted from *DCP3*'s utility as a policy guidance tool.

Analysis of quantitative survey data used basic descriptive statistics. Open-ended questions were summarized into common themes, such as *DCP3* influence and impact. Participant responses were triangulated with a review of published documents, when available. For the case study, a single data analyst coded interview data using a directed content analysis approach and integrated data from the desk review of documentation to confirm or disconfirm key themes from the interview findings. The study protocol was submitted to the University of Washington Institutional Review Board for determination and was considered exempt.

SURVEY RESULTS AND FINDINGS

Twenty individuals working across 25 countries responded to the survey. The primary outcome of interest was the uptake of DCP *Essential Surgery* recommendations. Slightly more people (11 versus 9) said they were not aware of examples of DCP recommendations having been used to inform health policy and planning.

The survey asked respondents to give details of the examples of DCP recommendations that they knew were used in health policies or planning of health services. Although the researchers envisioned that respondents would report uptake of DCP in both policies and practice, the cited examples provided by respondents suggest that use in influencing practice is uncommon. The survey asked about all three editions of DCP broadly, but examples exclusively focused on recommendations from *DCP3*'s *Essential Surgery* volume. At the country level, respondents noted the use of *Essential Surgery*'s recommendations in national surgical, obstetric, and anesthesia plans (NSOAPs) in Ethiopia, Malawi, and Rwanda. *DCP3* was a key contributor to the consolidation of surgery and anesthesia in the global health policy agenda in 2015 that in turn led to the creation of NSOAPs across LMICs (Truché et al. 2020).

The use of *Essential Surgery* recommendations in NSOAPs offers an informative case study of one channel of influence of DCP publications on national health policy. The NSOAPs result from the collaboration between ministries of health and the Program in Global Surgery and Social Change, an initiative based at Harvard University that focuses on strengthening surgical systems and improving surgery-specific leadership capacity in low-resource settings. In Ethiopia, that goal has manifested in the Saving Lives through Safe Surgery (SaLTS) initiative, which sits within the Directorate of Health Services Quality (Burssa et al. 2017; Iverson et al. 2020). The SaLTS Strategic Plan 2016–2020 makes multiple references to *DCP3 Essential Surgery* findings as justification for increased political commitment to surgical care. Further, the 44 essential surgical procedures recommended by *DCP3* are noted as the foundation for SaLTS to make available a package of essential surgical and anesthesia care, with a focus on strengthening delivery at the primary care level. That path of influence, most likely flowing from *DCP3* authors at US institutions through existing collaborations with national health leaders in a low-income country to inclusion in policy documentation, presents an example of the "wholesale" approach to knowledge exchange that global priority-setting publications such as *DCP3* are well positioned to leverage.

Respondents also mentioned *Essential Surgery* as a reference point for two global policy efforts. The volume informed the outline of minimum necessary services for primary health care delivery, funding, and management of the Primary Health Care Performance Initiative, a joint initiative of Ariadne Labs, the Bill & Melinda Gates Foundation, the United Nations Children's Fund, the World Bank, and the World Health Organization (Veillard et al. 2017). Additionally, Essential Surgery was influential in the Optimal Resources for Children's Surgery document developed by the Global Initiative for Children's Surgery and used in multiple countries (GICS 2019a). Specifically, the Optimal Resources for Children's Surgery recommendations adopted *DCP3*'s approach to capturing interventions by health system platform level, along with the platform definitions themselves (GICS 2019b).

On the use of *DCP Essential Surgery* recommendations in actual practice, respondents mentioned that the recommendations influenced the increased investments in burn care with improved referrals and reduced time to presentation in Malawi. Respondents also reported that *DCP3 Essential Surgery*'s recommendation on surgical task sharing was used in the implementation of training programs in hernia repair in Ghana. One respondent also noted that Ghana is embarking on a plan to construct new hospitals in all districts to improve access to health care, including surgery. Some respondents have also used the DCP recommendations to advocate for more availability of surgical services. Respondents indicated that, in India, the current estimates of population-based requirement of surgeries, their nature, and necessary government funding were based on DCP3 in conjunction with Global Burden of Disease 2017 estimates.

The survey also asked about locations or policy processes in which the respondents expected to see use of *DCP3 Essential Surgery* recommendations but did not see such use. Most of the respondents (14 out of 20) said there were no such places.

Country Commitments to Essential Surgery

The survey asked respondents if they have used *DCP3 Essential Surgery* recommendations in their own work. Over 70 percent of respondents reported using the recommendations. After asking respondents to identify up to three countries where they have worked, the survey then asked them to rate each country's commitment to increasing availability of essential surgery. Almost 40 percent of the ratings indicated low commitment that is increasing only slowly, 31 percent indicated moderate commitment, and 19 percent indicated high commitment (figure 21.1).

Figure 21.1 Survey Respondents' Ratings of Government Commitment to Increase Availability of Surgery in Countries Where They Have Worked

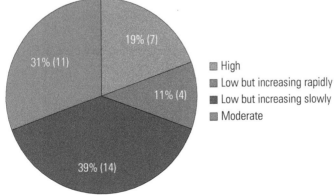

19% (7)

31% (11)

11% (4)

39% (14)

■ High
■ Low but increasing rapidly
■ Low but increasing slowly
■ Moderate

Source: Original figure for this publication.

The review also looked at ratings by region (Africa, Asia, and South America) and reasons given for the ratings, grouping the ratings into two categories for expository simplicity—low commitment and moderate or high commitment. Overall, Africa had a substantially high share of ratings classified as moderate or high commitment (70 percent) compared to Asia (25 percent) and South America (33 percent)—table 21.1. Respondents said they gave a rating of moderate to high commitment for Africa mainly because of strong commitment on the surgery policy front rather than on implementation. Across all regions, the cited reasons for providing low ratings include inadequate specialists and no appropriate training programs, inadequate infrastructure, limited efforts in providing services in rural/remote areas, and low prioritization and funding of health care with surgery viewed as too expensive (and not a disease).

Finally, the survey asked respondents to point out some of the challenges hindering adoption of *DCP3 Essential Surgery* recommendations in the countries where respondents have worked and what solutions they would propose. Table 21.2 shows their responses.

Table 21.1 Respondents' Evaluation of Country Commitment to Increasing Surgery Availability, Selected Regions

Region	Number of countries rated by authors	Share of ratings classified moderate to high commitment (versus low commitment)	Reasons
Africa	10	70%	**Moderate to high commitment:** 1. Surgery plans and guidelines developed, but with weak implementation or action 2. Presence of surgical societies dedicated to building capacity for essential surgery 3. One country highlighted as having implemented initiatives for surgery training and procurement of equipment. **Low commitment:** 1. Inadequate or absence of specialists with no commitment to training programs for important surgical specialties 2. Limited efforts in reaching remote or rural places where in some countries as much as 80% of the population resides 3. Low prioritization and limited funding 4. Limited investment in surgical infrastructure.

table continues next page

Region	Number of countries rated by authors	Share of ratings classified moderate to high commitment (versus low commitment)	Reasons
Asia	8	25%	**Moderate to high commitment:** 1. Substantial efforts in some countries to increase access to eye surgery. **Low commitment:** 1. Limited efforts in improving access to surgical and anesthesia capacity beyond big cities 2. Low prioritization with wide perception that surgery is expensive and is not a disease, like malaria, making advocacy difficult 3. Too much focus or private provision of health care and low prioritization of surgery in private provision 4. Limited investment in surgical infrastructure.
South America	6	33%	**Moderate to high commitment:** 1. In one country: implementation of surgical checklists, programs targeted at reaching out to rural areas, and restricting educational system to prioritize surgical capacity. **Low commitment:** 1. Systematic violence and weak social security systems that render health care low on the priority list 2. Limited efforts in expanding access to remote areas and reducing waiting times.

Source: Responses to open-ended survey questions sent to authors of previous *Disease Control Priorities* volumes.

Table 21.2 Challenges Hindering Adoption of DCP's *Essential Surgery* Recommendations and Proposed Solutions

Challenge	Proposed solution
Lack of political will, leadership, and governance	1. Systematically and proactively disseminate *DCP3 Essential Surgery* recommendations, leading to concrete action plans at the national level or a collective of institutions. 2. To change the perception of surgery as expensive, use simple infographics (rather than a bulky and hard-to-read *DCP4* full report) to promote the cost-effectiveness of surgery. 3. Hold dissemination workshops for stakeholders. 4. Align global surgery with public health and show the cost benefits of investments in surgery. 5. Disseminate case studies showing successful scaling capacity for essential surgery. 6. Present focused training topics on public health incorporating the importance of surgical care and anesthesia.

table continues next page

Table 21.2 Challenges Hindering Adoption of DCP Surgery Recommendations and Proposed Solutions (continued)

Challenge	Proposed solution
Lack of WHO and World Bank leadership	1. International institutions: establish funds, independent of national budgets, for supporting sustainable policies and implementation of DCP. 2. International donors: make a stronger commitment. 3. WHO: provide stronger recommendations. 4. Start by focusing on standardized metrics that countries are expected to collect and present, with action plans (and funding mechanisms) for how to close gaps in care noted when they identify issues.
Major funders not supporting efforts outlined in *DCP3*	None proposed
Poor dissemination to health authorities and lack of awareness	1. Partner with ministries of health and local academic bodies for dissemination. 2. More support to *DCP* authors as well as economists and surgeons for advocacy 3. Link with active researchers in Europe, the United States, and priority countries who are training economists and surgeons at the country level.
Financing	1. Make more specific recommendations for financing essential surgery. 2. Provide better guidance on how to spend funds most cost-effectively.
Human resources challenges	1. Expand the training of highly qualified surgical specialists and equip general doctors with surgical skills. 2. Upgrade health facilities for safe surgery. 3. Shift tasks.
Language too technical	1. Use more practical metrics than the DALY, which are easy to understand. 2. Bridge the clinical-policy divide by bringing clinicians together with policy makers in countries and regions. 3. Ensure that *DCP3* terms for elements of the health system directly correspond to those used by WHO (such as "district hospital" and "first-level hospital"). 4. Use more practical examples of implemented programs and their results rather than heavy use of modeling GBD data. 5. Make clearer connections with SDG targets, somehow including the voices/perspectives of patients and communities affected by surgical conditions. Do not rely overly on national surgical plans to wait for action. 6. Support in-country teams to advocate for policy change, helping them develop road maps and prioritize starting points among their many competing challenges. 7. Ensure better integration of anesthesia and nursing care and community health workers. 8. Work with policy makers to create concrete action plans. 9. Get political commitment from donor organizations and secure funding to implement policies and programs.
Limited involvement of professional surgical and anesthesia societies	None provided

table continues next page

Table 21.2 Challenges Hindering Adoption of DCP Surgery Recommendations and Proposed Solutions *(continued)*

Challenge	Proposed solution
Service delivery	1. Integrate surgical care more clearly with existing programs in NCDs (for example, oncology), trauma, emergency care, and infectious diseases.
Urgent problems such as COVID-19	1. Complete global COVID-19 vaccination.
DCP content	1. Provide more specific guidance on implementation and financial milestones.
	2. Start by focusing on standardized metrics that countries are expected to collect and present, with action plans (and funding mechanisms) for how to close gaps in care noted when they identify issues.

Source: Responses to open-ended survey questions sent to authors of previous *Disease Control Priorities* volumes.

Note: DALY = disability-adjusted life year; DCP = Disease Control Priorities; *DCP 1* = *Disease Control Priorities,* first edition; *DCP 2* = *Disease Control Priorities,* second edition; *DCP 3* = *Disease Control Priorities,* third edition; GBD = Global Burden of Disease; NCDs = noncommunicable diseases; SDG = Sustainable Development Goal; WHO = World Health Organization.

PAKISTAN: THE UNIVERSAL HEALTH COVERAGE, SURGERY, AND DCP AGENDAS CONVERGE

The experience of Pakistan provides an illuminating example of the convergence of timing in overcoming the challenges listed in the previous section to facilitate DCP's influence on a policy process. This case study of Pakistan is based on an integrated analysis of qualitative data, including interviews with key technical leaders in the policy development process, a review of policy documents, and results from the survey.

Toward a Unified National Approach to Surgery

Although many Pakistani surgical leaders have been working for decades to increase access to specific types of surgical care, the emergence of surgery in the national policy agenda and development of concrete strategy documents coincided with momentum provided by relevant global initiatives. Several key champions of the national surgical agenda in Pakistan participated in the Lancet Commission, as well as in DCP2 and DCP3 publications. Despite support for the value of those publications, interviewees remained skeptical of their potential applicability to Pakistan. As one individual noted, "a lot of the things that get trotted out for the LMIC world haven't been tried outside of Africa. There are certain generalizations that are possible in LMICs in an Africa context, but a lot of things mandated globally are not applicable to Pakistan at all."

Beginning in 2018, technical advisers and providers engaged with the Federal Ministry of National Health Services, Regulation and Coordination as well as with the provincial departments of health to bring up for debate Pakistan's National Vision for Surgical Care 2020–2025 (Fatima et al. 2020; MoNHSR&C 2021). That vision for surgical care, finalized in 2019 and launched in July 2021, acts as an addendum document to the National Health Vision 2025 (Fatima et al. 2020). Simultaneously, work had begun in parallel to revise the national essential package of health services (EPHS), also called the Universal Health Services Benefits Package. The DCP3 recommendations were distilled into a list of 218 interventions across six clusters; through a subsequent national consultative process, the 218 interventions were reviewed and adapted to Pakistan's health needs and priorities. The EPHS included 44 surgical interventions, which were then costed on the basis of technical requirements provided by surgical and anesthesia experts from Pakistan. For the first time, 19 surgical procedures were costed separately for adults and children (for example, neonatal colostomy versus adult colostomy and laparotomy in children versus in adults), establishing the difference in resources (surgical and anesthesia expertise, equipment, and neonatal care) required for newborns, infants, and children. Moreover, those surgical interventions form part of three clusters—health services (33); reproductive, maternal, newborn, and child health (6); and noncommunicable diseases and injury (5)—reemphasizing the fundamentally cross-cutting nature of surgical care. The EPHS revision process identified several concrete examples of areas needing further specification when applying the DCP recommendations to the context of Pakistan:

- While doing the costing workshop, contributors highlighted a real need to understand health system resource needs by age group (for example, a neonatal laparotomy cannot be done in a first-level hospital).
- Because not all district hospitals in Pakistan are the same, using a uniform label for "first level" as a synonymous category is insufficient for operationalizing intervention recommendations.
- All DCP recommended interventions need to be rationalized to the local context—for example, voluntary male medical circumcisions are not a priority in a Muslim majority country, so early infant circumcision at the primary level was included.

The adaptations speak to the value of DCP3 as a starting point but also to the need for an organized, resourced process for customizing DCP3 before it can effectively inform policy development.

Contextualizing Implementation

The implementation of EPHS in Pakistan has faced significant challenges because of a combination of factors, including political uncertainty, funding limitations, and delays due to the COVID-19 pandemic. Although the DCP3 recommendations provided the evidence that informed the development of the EPHS, the DCP3 volumes have no inherent structured policy guidelines. Importantly, however, *DCP3 Essential Surgery* was a key reference source for the Lancet Commission on Global Surgery, which in turn developed the NSOAP framework as a policy guide to strengthening surgical systems.

In the design phase of EPHS (and by extrapolation, the DCP3 recommendations), the following challenges became apparent:

- The first-level platform in *DCP3* does not correspond to a single level in Pakistan's health structure. A broad range of facilities exists between the primary and tertiary care levels—from Rural Health Centers to Tehsil Headquarter hospitals to District Headquarter hospitals. Even within the District Headquarter category, the service offering can range from outpatient clinics to comprehensive care that falls just short of the tertiary and teaching hospital capacity. Therefore, adapting the *DCP3* recommendations for platform of services does not easily translate into a practical service package.
- Recruitment and retention of qualified staff present a huge challenge, especially in rural facilities, with positions remaining chronically unfilled. Surgical care relies on a functioning ecosystem to deliver the end product—that is, a surgical procedure. The absence of any one essential component of the ecosystem leads to an inability to perform surgeries, with a resulting waste of resources. Moreover, the procedures recommended by *DCP3 for* the first-level platform can, in theory, be performed by a well-trained, generalist surgeon. In practice, because Pakistan does not have a training track for the "district" or "rural" surgeon, District Headquarter hospitals are staffed by specialists who are very difficult to recruit and retain. Moreover, the *DCP3*-recommended surgical procedures are performed by different specialist surgeons (for example OB/GYNs, orthopedic surgeons, and pediatric surgeons), bringing into serious question the cost-effectiveness of this model.
- Placing a surgical procedure in a particular level (primary, secondary, or tertiary care) detracts from the importance of training staff at all levels on the recognition and timely transfer or provision of care at the appropriate facility level. Informed and resource-appropriate bidirectional referral at all levels of the health care system is the key to effective surgical care provision. It is important to recognize that efficient referral does not just happen from the beginning: it requires investment in resources, systems to develop and sustain links, and level-appropriate sustained service components.

LIMITATIONS

The work presented in this chapter has several important limitations. First, as with most email-based surveys, the survey had a low response rate (11 percent). The chance of selection bias exists—that is, those who responded could have been more motivated or felt more strongly about issues. Responses showed varied perspectives, however, indicating a broad spectrum of views. Second, the findings could be skewed to the views of authors from specific regions. Although the survey did not collect specific demographic data, contact information provided by respondents indicates that they were more likely to be employed at US institutions (10 out of 20 respondents) and working in academic settings, regardless of country (11 out of 20); and only 6 out of 20 were from LMICs. Therefore, the data could be skewed toward activities and initiatives that have partnerships with those two organization types, and that thus may have more resources for implementation and evaluation. For the country case study, the researchers tried to address that risk in part by supplementing the survey data with qualitative data collected from individuals who participated in the policy development process. The findings should not be generalized, but instead viewed as likely transferable to areas with similar features. The findings should be understood as illustrative examples of the barriers and facilitators to uptake of DCP recommendations within a set of countries with a specific type of connection with the Essential Surgery volume—that is, a chapter author or volume editor with ongoing engagements there.

CONCLUSIONS

Efforts to trace the uptake of surgery-specific recommendations from DCP publications over time suggests that existing initiatives offer the most effective wholesale channel for DCP recommendations to influence policy that affects commitment to surgical care in LMICs. For example, the NSOAPs and the Primary Health Care Performance Initiative cited DCP documentation. Although limited, examples of direct use of DCP publications to inform global surgery at a national level do exist. When it was evident that such retail influence had occurred, its impact focused on guidelines informing provision of or access to specific surgical procedures (such as hernia repair) or subspecialties.

Pakistan presents a rich example of the ways countries can use *DCP3's* recommended essential package of surgical interventions broadly to facilitate the development of a wide-ranging national-level surgical policy. The timing of the country's push for a national surgery strategy—which occurred at the same time as the effort by key *DCP3* collaborators to facilitate a review of Pakistan's health benefits package—was instrumental in providing an avenue for realizing the impact of DCP. However, the Pakistan experience also reveals that the *DCP3* recommendations, although firmly grounded in evidence, have not translated into practical on-the-ground learnings in a real-world setting. It follows that *DCP3* recommendations revised using feedback from the field can take the impact of that body of work to the next level. Overall, future efforts to better promote uptake of the recommendations of *DCP3 Essential Surgery* could include development of more concrete policy recommendations, especially those focused on specific platforms of care delivery (such as first-level hospitals), and more specific recommendations for financing essential surgical care.

Although not broadly generalizable, the findings presented in this chapter suggest that country commitment to increasing availability of essential surgery remains low despite the compelling investment case presented in *DCP3 Essential Surgery*. Experts involved in programs to advance surgical care in LMICs point to the need to use language that policy makers can better understand and to partner with in-country organizations and champions in disseminating findings. Greater dissemination of the information in *DCP3 Essential Surgery* to several audiences (for example, policy makers, academics, and professional communities) is also needed. Development of advocacy tools, such as simple infographics, could help with that goal. Finally, as with the Pakistan case study, working with country governments during the development of concrete action plans, including supporting the identification of metrics to monitor policy implementation progress, presents an opportunity to directly link DCP recommendations to national needs.

REFERENCES

Bullock, H. L., J. N. Lavis, M. G. Wilson, G. Mulvale, and A. Miatello. 2021. "Understanding the Implementation of Evidence-Informed Policies and Practices from a Policy Perspective: A Critical Interpretive Synthesis." *Implementation Science* 16 (1): 18.

Burssa, D., A. Teshome, K. Iverson, O. Ahearn, T. Ashengo, D. Barash, E. Barringer, et al. 2017. "Safe Surgery for All: Early Lessons from Implementing a National Government-Driven Surgical Plan in Ethiopia." *World Journal of Surgery* 41 (12): 3038–45.

Debas, H. T., P. Donkor, A. Gawande, D. T. Jamison, M. E. Kruk, and C. N. Mock. 2015. *Disease Control Priorities*, (third edition), Volume 1, *Essential Surgery*. Washington, DC: World Bank.

Fatima, I., H. Shoman, A. W. Peters, L. Samad, and S. Nishtar. 2020. "Pakistan's National Surgical, Obstetric, and Anesthesia Plan: An Adapted Model for a Devolved Federal-Provincial Health System." *Canadian Journal of Anesthesia* 67 (9): 1212–16.

GICS (Global Initiative for Children's Surgery). 2019a. "Optimal Resources for Children's Surgical Care: Executive Summary." *World Journal of Surgery* 43 (4): 978–80.

GICS (Global Initiative for Children's Surgery). 2019b. "Optimal Resources for Children's Surgical Care: Guidelines for Different Levels of Care." GICS. https://www .globalchildrenssurgery.org/wp-content/uploads/2019/03/OReCS-Supplement-1.pdf.

Harris, P. A., R. Taylor, R. Thielke, J. Payne, .N Gonzalez, and J. G. Conde. 2009. "Research Electronic Data Capture (REDCap): A Metadata-Driven Methodology and Workflow Process for Providing Translational Research Informatics Support." *Journal of Biomedical Informatics* 42 (2): 377–81.

Harris, P. A., R. Taylor, B. L. Minor, V. Elliott, M. Fernandez, L. O'Neal, L. McLeod, et al. 2019. "The REDCap Consortium: Building an International Community of Software Partners." *Journal of Biomedical Informatics* 95. https://doi.org/10.1016/j.jbi.2019.103208.

Iverson, K. R., O. Ahearn, I. Citron, K. Garringer, S. Mukhodpadhyay, A. Teshome, A. Bekele, et al. 2020. "Development of a Surgical Assessment Tool for National Policy Monitoring & Evaluation in Ethiopia: A Quality Improvement Study." *International Journal of Surgery* 80 (August): 231–40.

Jamison, D. T., J. G. Breman, A. R. Measham, G. Alleyne, M. Claeson, D. B. Evans, P. Jha, et al. 2006. *Disease Control Priorities in Developing Countries* (second edition), Washington, DC: World Bank.

Jamison, D. T., W. H. Mosley, A. R. Measham, and J. L. Bobadilla. 1993. *Disease Control Priorities in Developing Countries*. New York: Oxford University Press; Washington, DC: World Bank.

Meara, J. G., A. J. M. Leather, L. Hagander, B. C. Alkire, N. Alonso, E. A. Ameh, S. W. Bickler, et al. 2016. "Global Surgery 2030: Evidence and Solutions for Achieving Health, Welfare, and Economic Development." *International Journal of Obstetric Anesthesia* 25: 75-78.

MoNHSR&C (Pakistan, Ministry of National Health Services Regulations and Coordination). 2021. *National Vision for Surgical Care 2020–2025 Launch Report*. Islamabad: Government of Pakistan.

Truché, P., H. Shoman, C. L. Reddy, D. T. Jumbam, J. Ashby, A. Mazhiqi, T. Wurdeman, et al. 2020. "Globalization of National Surgical, Obstetric and Anesthesia Plans: The Critical Link between Health Policy and Action in Global Surgery." *Globalization and Health* 16 (1): 1.

Veillard, J., K. Cowling, A. Bitton, H. Ratcliffe, M. Kimball, S. Barkley, L. Mercereau, et al. 2017. "Better Measurement for Performance Improvement in Low- and Middle-Income Countries: The Primary Health Care Performance Initiative (PHCPI) Experience of Conceptual Framework Development and Indicator Selection." *Milbank Quarterly* 95 (4): 836–83.

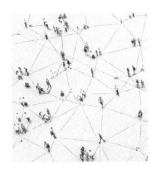

22

Lessons Learned from the Use of Disease Control Priorities Recommendations to Address Noncommunicable Diseases in Low- and Middle-Income Countries

David A. Watkins, Neil Gupta, Ana O. Mocumbi, and Cherian Varghese

ABSTRACT

Noncommunicable diseases (NCDs) are a rapidly growing challenge worldwide, and priority setting is essential for making progress on NCDs in limited-resource settings. This chapter reviews the evolution of NCDs within the Disease Control Priorities (DCP) project over the years. It then presents two recent case studies where DCP recommendations were used in priority-setting processes. The chapter concludes with suggestions for expanding and improving the analyses and recommendations that will come from the fourth edition of DCP and related projects.

INTRODUCTION

The term "noncommunicable diseases" (NCDs) largely comes from the nosology of global health measurement, starting with the 1990 Global Burden of Disease study that accompanied the first edition of the *Disease Control Priorities* (DCP) series and the 1993 *World Development Report* (Jamison et al. 1993; World Bank 1993). Practically, NCDs capture every health condition that is not part of the "unfinished agenda" of communicable, maternal, perinatal, and nutritional diseases and cannot be classified as an injury. Although NCDs account for most premature deaths in low- and middle-income countries (LMICs), actions at the global and national levels to implement NCD interventions and packages have encountered numerous political, financial, and logistical challenges (Nishtar et al. 2018).

In the 2000s, efforts to raise awareness on NCDs focused on a subset of four groups of NCDs (cardiovascular diseases, cancers, chronic respiratory diseases, and diabetes) that were emerging in LMICs as a by-product of economic development and increased exposure to a small set of common risk factors (tobacco use, harmful use of alcohol, unhealthy diets, and insufficient physical activity). Those NCDs had the additional characteristics of chronicity and complexity of disease management. That conceptualization culminated in the "4 × 4" framing of the NCD problem reflected in the first United Nations high-level meeting on NCDs in 2011 (Schwartz, Shaffer, and Bukhman 2021) and persists to this day in the form of Sustainable Development Goal (SDG) target 3.4.[1] In 2021, the World Health Organization (WHO) developed a road map for countries to get back on track for SDG target 3.4, with a renewed focus on high-priority interventions (WHO 2021). The United Nations community plans to meet again in 2025 to review progress on that target and the NCD agenda, and to begin looking beyond 2030 and the SDGs (NCD Countdown 2030 Collaborators 2022). The COVID-19 pandemic, and its impact on health care systems and on progress on NCDs, will inevitably serve as the backdrop for that assessment.

Still, the 4 × 4 framing—four major diseases and four major risk factors—can be critiqued as an oversimplification that fails to address important NCDs in very resource-constrained environments (Schwartz, Shaffer, and Bukhman 2021). In 2015, the Lancet Commission on Noncommunicable Diseases and Injuries in the Poorest Billion (hereafter, "Lancet NCDI Poverty Commission") was launched as an attempt to broaden the NCD agenda beyond the top four diseases to endemic conditions like sickle cell anemia and rheumatic fever, and to link NCDs to injuries because they have similar implications for health care systems and have been neglected in the global health agenda (Bukhman et al. 2020). The Lancet NCDI Poverty Commission launched a series of national commissions to provide context for the global report and begin to take action to implement interventions (box 22.1).

This chapter reviews the contribution of the DCP enterprise to the global NCD agenda over the past 30 years, especially the influence of DCP recommendations for priority interventions. It presents two case studies on the use of DCP evidence in practice: (1) the Lancet NCDI Poverty Commission and (2) the NCD Countdown 2030 Collaborators and related efforts on WHO's road map for NCDs in the post-COVID-19 era. The chapter aims to critically review the strengths and limitations of existing recommendations, particularly from DCP3, to inform work on NCDs in subsequent volumes in this series.

Box 22.1

National- and State-Level NCDI Poverty Commissions

The Lancet Commission on Noncommunicable Diseases and Injuries in the Poorest Billion (the "Lancet NCDI Poverty Commission") developed a two-step analytic framework to support national and subnational NCDI poverty commissions in defining local NCDI epidemiology, determining an expanded set of priority NCDI conditions, and recommending cost-effective, equitable health sector interventions (Bukhman et al. 2020). National NCDI poverty commissions were established in 22 countries with country-level commissions and one state-level commission in India that have more than 25 percent prevalence of extreme poverty in at least one subnational region (determined by a modified multidimensional poverty index). The commissions were established from 2016 to 2022 following application and approval by respective ministry of health officials in collaboration with in-country implementers.[a]

As of October 2024, 17 commissions had completed the NCDI priority-setting exercise using recommendations from the third edition of *Disease Control Priorities*, and 21 have published reports (Gupta et al. 2021). The first six published reports had an average of 25 prioritized noncommunicable disease (NCD) and injury conditions based on prevalence, severity, disability, and equity metrics. All commissions selected the following 15 conditions: asthma, breast cancer, cervical cancer, diabetes mellitus (types 1 and 2), epilepsy, hypertensive heart disease, intracerebral hemorrhage, ischemic heart disease, ischemic stroke, major depressive disorder, motor vehicle road injuries, rheumatic heart disease, sickle cell disorders, and subarachnoid hemorrhage. On average, the commissions prioritized 35 health sector interventions on the basis of cost-effectiveness, financial risk protection, and equity-enhancing characteristics. The prioritized interventions were estimated to cost an additional US$4.7 to US$14.0 per capita, or approximately 9.7 percent to 36.0 percent of current total health expenditure (0.6 percent to 4.0 percent of current gross domestic product), depending on the country.

Participants have reported positive outcomes of the commissions in informing national planning and implementation of NCD and injury interventions, improving governance and coordination for those conditions, and advocating for an expanded NCD agenda. In Ethiopia, Kenya, and Nepal, commission recommendations were incorporated into the development of national universal health coverage policies and benefits packages and formed the basis for primary research in the delivery of integrated NCDI interventions from the third edition of *Disease Control Priorities* (Memirie et al. 2022; Mwangi et al. 2021). In Liberia and Malawi, commission findings formed the basis for a National Operational Plan for addressing severe NCDs, and 13 commissions have overseen the implementation of the integrated package of health services for severe NCDs at the primary referral hospital level ("PEN-Plus"), endorsed by the World Health Organization Africa Region (Boudreaux et al. 2022).

In 2020, the commissions formed the NCDI Poverty Network, hosted by co-secretariats at the Center for Integration Science at Brigham & Women's Hospital and the Universidade Eduardo Mondlane (Bukhman et al. 2021). That network, governed by a steering committee of 10 commission leaders, provides an active platform for collective policy, research, and advocacy to improve health sector interventions and financing for NCDIs in low- and lower-middle-income countries within national and regional commitments for universal health coverage.

a. For a full list of countries and partners, refer to the NCDI Poverty Network home page, www.ncdipoverty.org.

THE EVOLUTION OF NCD RECOMMENDATIONS OVER DCP1–DCP3

Broadly speaking, the DCP enterprise has been integral to the NCD agenda and to recent efforts to accelerate progress. The 1990 Global Burden of Disease study, the first *Disease Control Priorities (DCP1)* volume, and the 1993 *World Development Report* (all produced around the same time) were the first international publications to emphasize the growing burden of NCDs in LMICs and their relationship, at the population level, to trends in risk factors like tobacco use (Bobadilla et al. 1993). In fact, although the development community at the time focused almost exclusively on eradicating communicable childhood diseases, 9 out of 25 of DCP1's disease-specific chapters addressed NCDs or injuries. Table 22.1 presents a summary of NCD interventions recommended in DCP1.

Table 22.1 Recommended NCD interventions in DCP1

Disease group	Specific interventions
Cancers	• Screening (Pap smear) and treatment of cervical cancer • Screening (clinical exam) and treatment of breast cancer • Treatment of early-stage oral and rectal cancers • Palliative care and pain relief for all cancer cases • Smoking cessation classes • Tobacco taxes
Cardiovascular diseases	• Screening and counseling regarding individual risk, plus medical management of hypertension and hypercholesterolemia • Medical management of stable angina • Low-cost management of unstable angina and acute myocardial infarction at district hospitals • Secondary prevention medications post myocardial infarction or stroke • Secondary prevention of rheumatic heart disease • Where resources allow, angioplasty or bypass graft surgery • Where resources allow, surgery for rheumatic heart disease
Chronic respiratory diseases	• Treatment of exacerbations including mechanical ventilation, steroids, and fluids • Tobacco control measures (refer to "cancers" in the first row)
Diabetes	• Health education regarding diet and exercise to prevent diabetes • Screening of high-risk groups (pregnant, obese) and treatment of diabetes (both type 1 and type 2)
Mental disorders	• Antipsychotic therapy for schizophrenia • Lithium therapy for bipolar disorder
Other NCDs	• Cataract repair • Plaque and calculus removal, fissure sealants, and topical fluoride • Extraction of teeth with advanced caries

Source: Jamison et al. 1993.

Note: DCP1 = *Disease Control Priorities*, first edition; NCD = noncommunicable disease.

NCDs also featured prominently in DCP2 (Jamison et al. 2006), with updates to the cost-effectiveness estimates provided in DCP1. Still, DCP2 had very similar main messages around value for money and featured many of the interventions in table 22.1 in its chapters. Cross-fertilization of DCP2 with the WHO Choosing Interventions that are Cost-Effective (WHO-CHOICE) project also shaped a package of "Best Buy" interventions that accompanied WHO's Global Action Plan on NCDs (WHO 2013).[2] One important distinction between the DCP2 approach and WHO's Best Buys was a greater focus on clinical interventions in DCP2, a distinction that persisted through DCP3 (Jamison et al. 2018).

The initiation of DCP3 (2010–17) provided an opportunity to do a more in-depth treatment on specific NCDs (defined broadly) and intervention areas. Three entire volumes (3, 4, and 5) and substantial portions of other volumes (1, 7, 8, and 9) were devoted to NCD topics; out of 21 intervention packages, 6 focused exclusively on NCDs, with another 4 in the "health services cluster" (surgery, rehabilitation, palliative care, and pathology) having major implications for NCDs. DCP3 volumes included systematic reviews of cost and cost-effectiveness analyses that informed the essential intervention packages. Online annex 22A UR (https://dcp4.w.uib.no/volumes/volume-1-country-led-priority-setting-for-health) provides a list of the interventions found throughout DCP3 that addressed NCDs.

Generally speaking, DCP recommendations and WHO recommendations for NCDs have had a high degree of concordance over the years. Both sets of recommendations have placed a strong emphasis on cross-cutting preventive interventions like tobacco control and on clinical interventions to address cardiovascular disease, for which cost-effectiveness evidence is easiest to find. DCP has tended to go further on clinical care (for example, recommending pharmacological treatment of chronic and acute heart failure in DCP3) whereas WHO has tended to emphasize promotion and behavior change interventions (for example, mass media campaigns on physical activity and diet). However, many of the apparent differences appear at the surface level and relate to differences in naming and aggregation of activities and technologies into unique interventions rather than reflecting substantive differences.

Although DCP3 was not resourced to do original cost and cost-effectiveness analyses, two working papers for volume 9 included estimates of the overall cost and mortality impact of the interventions included in the volumes. Across all low- and lower-middle-income countries, the packages of NCD interventions will cost an estimated US$140 billion annually by 2030 but would prevent about 2.6 million premature deaths annually (that is, about US$54,000 per death averted).

Cost-effectiveness is not the only relevant criterion for priority setting for universal health coverage (UHC). Health systems also seek to improve the distribution of health in the population (that is, equity) and, through public financing of health services, to provide financial protection from the risks of seeking health care (WHO 2014). DCP3 included new attempts to consider equity and financial protection alongside cost-effectiveness in a new methodological approach called "extended cost-effectiveness analysis" (Watkins, Nugent, and Verguet 2017). Five country-level extended cost-effectiveness analyses were done on NCD interventions in DCP3. Despite the data challenges inherent in conducting them, those studies have come to be seen as helpful additions to the cost-effectiveness literature, with 60 publications indexed in PubMed as of June 26, 2024.

One concrete example of the usefulness of extended cost-effectiveness analysis, a study of the equity impact of tobacco taxes in China, provides compelling evidence to counter the tobacco industry's long-standing argument that taxes are regressive (Verguet, Gauvreau, et al. 2015). Another study shows that NCD interventions were relatively more favorable in financial protection terms than in cost-effectiveness terms. It follows that a UHC benefits package that seeks both to improve health and provide financial protection would invest relatively more in NCD interventions than a package focused solely on health gains (Verguet, Olson, et al. 2015).

USE IN THE LANCET NCDI POVERTY COMMISSION

During 2016–17, substantial cross-fertilization occurred between the DCP3 enterprise and the Lancet NCDI Poverty Commission. DCP3 collaborators developed a priority-setting framework for NCDI national commissions that balanced disease burden data, cost-effectiveness, equity, and financial protection. The collaborators provided draft lists of interventions and packages, with semiquantitative assessments of cost-effectiveness, equity, and financial protection as well as cost estimates. Those data were prepared as a series of Excel spreadsheets used in commission priority-setting exercises (refer to online annex 22B for a sample spreadsheet from the Uganda commission, https://dcp4.w.uib.no/volumes/volume-1-country-led-priority-setting-for-health/). Additionally, the official report of the global commission, published in 2020, features updates to the DCP3 estimates of intervention cost and impact mentioned previously (Bukhman et al. 2020).

The global and national commissions also influenced the direction of DCP3, especially the synthesis chapters in volume 9. Commissioners pointed out some areas that DCP3 initially missed, such as congenital and genetic disorders, which prompted new evidence reviews and revision of chapter content (Watkins et al. 2017). They also served as an informal network for validating quantitative estimates (for example, intervention costs) and the final lists of interventions.

The general feedback from commissioners was that DCP3 provided a useful starting point and a structured process for deliberating on NCD priorities. Messages regarding priority interventions contained in the commission reports were frequently used for advocacy within countries and especially to ministries of health (Gupta et al. 2021). Strong collaborations between the NCDI poverty network and the DCP team also unlocked new resources from the Norwegian Agency for Development Cooperation to work on priority setting and capacity building in several countries and with the Africa Centres for Disease Control and Prevention.

The commissions did, however, identify several challenges and limitations. First, some disease areas were not well represented by DCP3 evidence because of the structure of the volumes. For example, DCP3 did not deal comprehensively with management of digestive disorders. Some relevant interventions were interspersed throughout the volumes—such as surgery for perforated ulcers in volume 1, childhood hepatitis B immunization in volume 2, and care for alcohol and opioid use disorders in volume 4—but basic clinical questions (such as medical management of decompensated cirrhosis) were not addressed at all.

Second, and related, the DCP3 packages were largely constructed around cost-effectiveness studies, which did not always account for the continuum of care for certain conditions. For example, the congenital and genetic disorders package contained an intervention around sickle cell disease screening and infection prophylaxis in under-five children, based on evidence for the cost-effectiveness of the approach in highly endemic settings (Kuznik et al. 2016). At the time of DCP3 writing, however, later-life management of sickle cell anemia had not been addressed in any economic evaluations in low- or middle-income countries, so potentially beneficial interventions (for example, hydroxyurea or basic management of acute crises) were not even assessed. A more systematic approach to sickle cell disease interventions—including original cost-effectiveness analyses for areas with evidence gaps—and with a life course perspective could address those limitations.

Third, despite the helpfulness of the spreadsheets of intervention lists and properties in facilitating dialogue, commissioners found them cumbersome and not very user-friendly. Relatedly, because of data gaps, many interventions did not have an assessment of equity or financial risk protection properties, making it difficult to systematically weigh the pros and cons of alternative intervention options.

Additionally, commissioners found that the definition of an "intervention" was inconsistent in terms of aggregation. On one end of the spectrum was "aspirin for suspected cases of acute coronary syndrome," a clear statement on use of a specific medicine for a specific indication. On the other end of the spectrum was a "basic package of palliative care," a recommendation based on aggregating numerous medications and tasks for various serious diseases into one intervention. Surgical procedures emerged as another challenging area, with some commissioners expecting detailed information on the cost-effectiveness of specific procedures and others advancing the idea of an integrated approach to surgery (for example, "basic district hospital services that can be performed by a nonspecialist physician or clinical officer").

From an analytic standpoint, one of the biggest challenges—and not unique to DCP—was identifying data on the current (or baseline) coverage level of various interventions. An intervention's baseline coverage, and the target coverage level that policy makers set, is a major driver of incremental costs and benefits, yet very few indicators for NCD service coverage are available. Hypertension is a notable exception, with numerous population-based surveys (STEPwise Approach to NCD Risk Factor Surveillance, sometimes Demographic and Health Surveys, and so on) capturing hypertension awareness, treatment, and control (NCD Risk Factor Collaboration 2021). Future efforts to measure NCD service coverage and quality need to address that critical evidence gap.

Finally, and also not unique to DCP3, the commissions reported challenges incorporating their work into routine ministry of health policy processes. Feedback from policy makers indicated a desire to conduct sector-wide priority setting, for example, through national strategic plans and health benefits package revisions rather than siloed priority setting just for NCDs. At the same time, DCP3 recommendations were very useful for advocacy efforts, including the global surgery movement (refer to chapter 21, this volume). There are several plausible ways to balance disease-specific content and cross-cutting/synthetic approaches, and forthcoming volumes of *Disease Control Priorities,* fourth edition (*DCP4*), will need to consider the range of readership and structure their content accordingly.

CONTRIBUTION OF DCP IN UPDATING WHO'S GLOBAL AND REGIONAL NCD ACTION PLANS

The NCD Countdown 2030 was launched in 2018 as a collaboration between *The Lancet*, WHO, the NCD Alliance, and Imperial College London to track progress on reducing NCD mortality to achieve SDG 3.4 (NCD Countdown Collaborators 2018). In 2019, the Countdown collaborators approached Bergen Center for Ethics and Priority Setting collaborators (and DCP3 alumni) to prepare a paper on NCD intervention priorities for the SDG period (NCD Countdown 2030 Collaborators 2022). The onset of the COVID-19 pandemic led to a reframing of the paper to focus on how countries could get back on track to achieving SDG 3.4 in the face of pandemic-related disruptions to health systems.

The foundation of that paper was a list of 15 clinical interventions (for example, treatment of hypertension and hypercholesterolemia to prevent cardiovascular disease) and six intersectoral policies (for example, tobacco excise taxes) taken from the DCP3 essential packages related to NCDs. Importantly, the interventions represented a subset of the scores of interventions for NCDs in DCP3. The paper focused on interventions that (1) addressed the four most common NCDs among adults and (2) could substantially reduce mortality by 2030. The analysis did not include numerous high-value NCD interventions that did not meet those criteria (for example, HPV immunization, treatment of childhood cancers, palliative care, and rehabilitation).

The paper's authors estimated that, under realistic implementation conditions, scaling up that package of interventions across 123 LMICs could allow 55 percent of countries to achieve SDG target 3.4, preventing 39 million deaths between 2023 and 2030 at a cost of about US$140 billion (or about US$2.6 per person per year) (NCD Countdown 2030 Collaborators 2022). If innovations in delivery science occur to allow NCD interventions to be scaled up as fast as HIV treatment and childhood immunization programs have been, then about 85 percent of countries could achieve the target. Intersectoral policies to reduce behavioral risk factors would be responsible for about two-thirds of the package's health gains and would reduce the need for more costly clinical services.

Around the same time that the Countdown paper was being prepared and under peer review, WHO initiated an effort to update its Global Action Plan for NCDs and provide a road map for countries to get back on track for SDG target 3.4 (WHO 2021). During much of 2021, the WHO NCDs department collaborated closely with the Bergen Center team and representatives from other Countdown partners. The Countdown report, published in *The Lancet* in March 2022, helped inform WHO's overall strategy and especially the road map document. Part of the context for the Countdown report was the observation that the pandemic disproportionately affected persons living with NCDs, who had higher rates of severe disease and case fatality. The Countdown report emphasized the links between NCDs, pandemic preparedness, and health security, and the need for advocacy efforts to acknowledge those links (NCD Countdown 2030 Collaborators 2022). Framing NCD prevention and management as a health systems resilience issue might also be helpful in the argument for additional investment.

After launch of the Countdown report, WHO commissioned a team from the University of Washington to develop two web-based tools to help countries implement the recommendations from the report. The first simulation tool provided estimates of intervention impact in 123 LMICs, under different implementation scenarios (Pickersgill et al. 2022).[3] The second impact simulation tool, commissioned by the WHO South-East Asia Regional Office, was tailored to the 11 countries in the region and incorporated estimates of intervention cost and cost-effectiveness.[4] The second tool was a key component of the WHO Regional Office's implementation road map for NCDs in South-East Asia, endorsed at the Regional Committee Meeting in 2022 in Paro, Bhutan (WHO 2022). The road map sought to help countries assess their status, sustain their good work, prioritize interventions, accelerate the most effective and feasible approaches, and promote accountability (figure 22.1). During late 2022 and early 2023, WHO disseminated its tool for South-East Asia to its country offices and to ministries of health in the region, which used the tool for national strategic planning on NCDs (figure 22.2).

Figure 22.1 Scope of the NCD Road Map Developed by WHO for Countries in Its South-East Asia Region

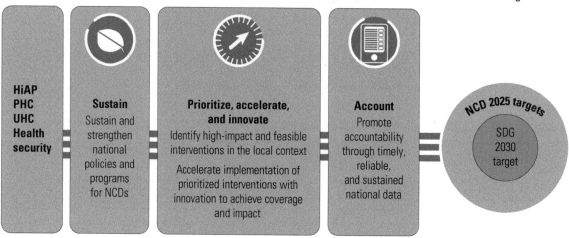

| HiAP PHC UHC Health security | **Sustain** Sustain and strengthen national policies and programs for NCDs | **Prioritize, accelerate, and innovate** Identify high-impact and feasible interventions in the local context

 Accelerate implementation of prioritized interventions with innovation to achieve coverage and impact | **Account** Promote accountability through timely, reliable, and sustained national data | **NCD 2025 targets** SDG 2030 target |

Source: Adapted from the World Health Organization Regional Office for South-East Asia, "WHO South-East Asia Regional NCD Roadmap," https://apps.searo.who.int/whoroad/.

Note: The World Health Organization's South-East Asia Region consists of the following countries: Bangladesh, Bhutan, Democratic People's Republic of Korea, India, Indonesia, Maldives, Myanmar, Nepal, Sri Lanka, Thailand, and Timor-Leste. HiAP = Health in All Policies; NCD = noncommunicable disease; PHC = primary health care; SDG = Sustainable Development Goal; UHC = universal health coverage.

The tools developed for WHO generally received very positive feedback, though some stakeholders raised concerns about the alignment of the tools with WHO recommendations, including those from the latest Global Action Plan, updated the Best Buy recommendations. Others noted the potential for confusion at the country level about how to use the tools relative to the Spectrum toolkit, including the OneHealth Tool[5] and WHO-CHOICE generalized cost-effectiveness analysis. Most relevant, however, was that countries could use the tool to do their own exercises and arrive at context-specific priorities. Global tools, lists, and instruments can guide this process.

The analyses and tools developed for the NCD road map had an immediate impact by enabling scale-up of cardiovascular disease interventions through the SEAHEARTS program, an adaptation of the WHO HEARTS program for countries in WHO's South-East Asia region (Joshi et al. 2024). The SEAHEARTS initiative represents the world's largest expansion of NCDs in primary health care and includes a target of 100 million people with hypertension and diabetes on treatment by 2025. India has set its own target of 75 million by 2025 and had reached 30 million as of June 2024. Experience with WHO's South-East Asia modeling tool demonstrates that, in the right political and policy context, DCP evidence can have a rapid and major impact.

Figure 22.2 Screenshots from the NCD Prioritization Tool Developed for WHO Using DCP3 Evidence

a. Introduction

b. Dashboard of health outcomes, India

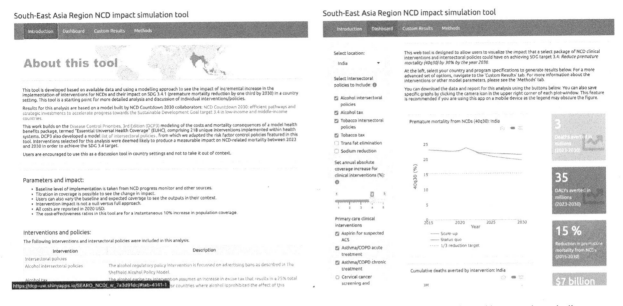

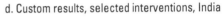

c. Cost-effectiveness and impacts of selected interventions, India

d. Custom results, selected interventions, India

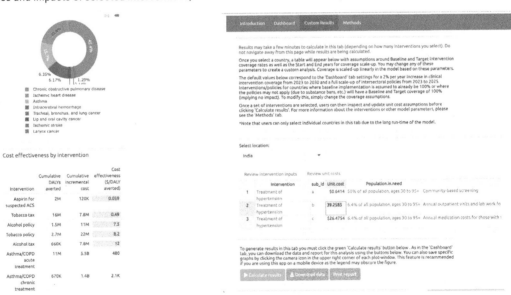

Source: World Health Organization, South-East Asia Region NCD Impact Simulation Tool, https://apps.searo.who.int/whoroad/south-east-asia-region-ncd-impact-simulation-tool.

Note: Panel a shows the landing page for the simulation tool. Panel b shows the tool's dashboard, with India selected as the location and a given mix of interventions. Panel c, also for India, shows the cost-effectiveness of selected interventions and their impact on cause-specific deaths. Panel d shows the tool's ability to dynamically incorporate, for example, different hypertension treatment costs for India. WHO's South-East Asia Region consists of the following countries: Bangladesh, Bhutan, Democratic People's Republic of Korea, India, Indonesia, Maldives, Myanmar, Nepal, Sri Lanka, Thailand, and Timor-Leste. DCP3 = *Disease Control Priorities*, third edition; NCD = noncommunicable disease; WHO = World Health Organization.

RECOMMENDATIONS FOR FUTURE DCP4 VOLUMES

Close collaboration with the NCDI Poverty Commission and WHO has provided the DCP/Bergen Center team with important opportunities for learning, with the following implications for the subsequent volumes of DCP4, even beyond NCDs.

First, efforts need to be made to ensure that DCP4's treatment of various health topics is as comprehensive as possible, indicating the need for a more systematic approach to identifying and appraising interventions. The WHO's UHC Compendium is intended to be a comprehensive repository of health interventions across the continuum of care for most diseases of public health relevance.[6] DCP4 analysts should consider engaging more broadly with disease experts in areas underrepresented in DCP3 (for example, hepatology and otolaryngology) to ensure that no important topics are neglected, and they should consider aligning their work with the structure of the UHC Compendium to ensure appraisal of a full range of interventions for each health issue. When available, resources should go toward original cost-effectiveness analysis of the interventions in different settings to allow for a more evenhanded treatment. At the same time, comprehensive lists of interventions might be overwhelming, with costs that are off-putting to financing and planning stakeholders. An alternative approach could be to create several "tiers" of investment that account for both differential cost-effectiveness and the interdependencies of interventions (for example, a set of interventions that can be efficiently delivered by the same cadre). Those tiers could be tied to different levels of incremental and total resources and different contexts—for example, what sorts of interventions are realistic to consider in a low-income country with US$5 per capita versus in a low-income country with US$10 per capita versus in a lower-middle-income country with US$20 per capita.

Second, it will be important to review the content of health benefits packages in a range of countries to help DCP contributors and analysts better understand what constitutes an "intervention" from a policy standpoint. Although something like a tobacco tax could reasonably be considered a standalone intervention, most interventions require the co-implementation of multiple clinical services and technologies, and cost-effectiveness evidence needs to adapt to that reality. For example, in the context of diabetes care, it is incoherent to assess the cost-effectiveness of glycemic control separately from the cost-effectiveness of blood pressure and lipid management in diabetes, because the drugs are co-deployed and form a coherent "package" of care for persons with diabetes. At the same time, health technology assessment (for example, for new, costly, branded diabetes drugs) clearly has a somewhat separate role from the more fundamental question of what constitutes the health system building blocks for a national NCD program in a low-income setting.

Third, and related to the issue of intervention aggregation, is the presentation of results for aggregations of countries. DCP4 analytics could be done at the country level but then flexibly grouped for presentation purposes into country typologies with relevance for specific policy questions and to avoid the politically fraught issue of publishing country-level data without sufficient local engagement and review. For example, analysis of the cost-effectiveness of direct-acting antivirals for hepatitis C could take place by level of endemicity (such as high, medium, and low seroprevalence) rather than by World Bank income group or WHO region. Other cross-cutting groupings that might be useful include the small island developing states and fragile and conflict zones.

Fourth, the scientific and technical community is clearly moving more into the digital and online space with each passing year. Printed books and Excel spreadsheets have extremely limited use in the setting of rapid growth in research and evidence in LMICs. The DCP4 team should consider alternative ways of disseminating findings, potentially by focusing on producing continuously updated online content and open-access online analytical tools that can incorporate local data. The experience with WHO's South-East Asia prioritization tool provides a case in point: the tool has undergone several revisions since 2022 as new data have emerged and the modeling has improved.

Finally, DCP4 collaborators need to take countries along on the process and create champions within countries. DCP4 development itself should provide an opportunity for learning within national ministries of health. Ultimately, DCP4 could benefit from a "co-production" model whereby a network of academics and technical experts in selected ministries from around the world collaborates to continuously improve the outputs of the DCP enterprise. Because many of the specific actions on NCDs take place outside the health sector, it will also be important to engage other stakeholders within government (for example, legislatures that draft laws and appropriate funds to health and finance ministries that implement health taxes) as well as nongovernment stakeholders (for example, civil society organizations, persons with lived experience, and other advocates). Fostering durable multisectoral coalitions can help ensure that political commitment to NCDs translates into financial commitment, implementation, and impact.

NOTES

1. United Nations, "Goal 3: Ensure healthy lives and promote well-being for all at all ages," http://www.un.org/sustainabledevelopment/health/.
2. For more on WHO-CHOICE, refer to the WHO-CHOICE web page, https://www.who.int/news-room/questions-and-answers/item/who-choice-frequently-asked-questions.
3. For more on the tool, visit "Simulation tool for countries to assess the impact of interventions on the SDG target for NCDs," https://dcp-uw.shinyapps.io/NCDC/.
4. WHO, South-East Asia Region NCD impact simulation tool, https://dcp-uw.shinyapps.io/SEARO_NCD/. WHO's South-East Asia Region consists of the following countries: Bangladesh, Bhutan, Democratic People's Republic of Korea, India, Indonesia, Maldives, Myanmar, Nepal, Sri Lanka, Thailand, and Timor-Leste.
5. WHO, OneHealth Tool, https://www.who.int/tools/onehealth.
6. WHO, UHC Compendium, https://www.who.int/universal-health-coverage/compendium.

REFERENCES

Bobadilla, J. L., J. Frenk, R. Lozano, T. Frejka, and C. Stern. 1993. "The Epidemiologic Transition and Health Priorities." In *Disease Control Priorities in Developing Countries*, edited by D. T. Jamison, W. H. Mosley, A. Measham, and J. L. Bobadilla. New York: Oxford University Press.

Boudreaux, C., P. Barango, A. Adler, P. Kabore, A. McLaughlin, M. O. S. Mohamed, P. H. Park, et al. 2022. "Addressing Severe Chronic NCDs across Africa: Measuring Demand for the Package of Essential Non-communicable Disease Interventions-Plus (PEN-Plus)." *Health Policy and Planning* 37 (4): 452–60. https://doi.org/10.1093/heapol/czab142.

Bukhman, G., A. O. Mocumbi, R. Atun, A. E. Becker, Z. Bhutta, A. Binagwaho, C. Clinton, et al. 2020. "The Lancet NCDI Poverty Commission: Bridging a Gap in Universal Health Coverage for the Poorest Billion." *The Lancet* 396 (10256): 991–1044. https://doi.org/10.1016/S0140-6736(20)31907-3.

Bukhman, G., A. O. Mocumbi, N. Gupta, M. Amuyunzu-Nyamongo, M. Echodu, A. Gomanju, Y. Jain, et al. 2021. "From a Lancet Commission to the NCDI Poverty Network: Reaching the Poorest Billion through Integration Science." *The Lancet* 398 (10318): 2217–20. https://doi.org/10.1016/S0140-6736(21)02321-7.

Gupta, N., A. Mocumbi, S. H. Arwal, Y. Jain, A. M. Haileamlak, S. T. Memirie, N. C. Larco, et al. 2021. "Prioritizing Health-Sector Interventions for Noncommunicable Diseases and Injuries in Low- and Lower-Middle Income Countries: National NCDI Poverty Commissions." *Global Health: Science and Practice* 9 (3): 626–39. https://doi.org/10.9745/GHSP-D-21-00035.

Jamison, D. T., J. G. Breman, A. R. Measham, G. Alleyne, M. Claeson, D. B. Evans, P. Jha, et al. 2006. *Disease Control Priorities in Developing Countries* (second edition). Washington, DC: World Bank.

Jamison, Dean T., Hellen Gelband, Susan Horton, Prabhat Jha, Ramanan Laxminarayan, and Charles N. Mock, eds. 2018. *Disease Control Priorities,* (third edition), Volume 9, *Disease Control Priorities: Improving Health and Reducing Poverty*. Washington, DC: World Bank. https://doi.org/10.1596/978-1-4648-0527-1.

Jamison, D. T., W. H. Mosley, A. R. Measham, and J. L. Bobadilla, eds. 1993. *Disease Control Priorities in Developing Countries*. New York: Oxford University Press. https://documents.worldbank.org/en/publication/documents-reports/documentdetail/705591468320064221/disease-control-priorities-in-developing-countries.

Joshi, P., M. R. Amin, F. A. Dorin, L. Dzed, P. Lethro, S. Swarnkar, Y. Setoya, et al. 2024. "The Dhaka Call to Action to Accelerate the Control of Cardiovascular Diseases in South-East Asia." *Nature Medicine* 30, 19–20. https://doi.org/10.1038/s41591-023-02678-w.

Kuznik, A., A. G. Habib, D. Munube, and M. Lamorde. 2016. "Newborn Screening and Prophylactic Interventions for Sickle Cell Disease in 47 Countries in Sub-Saharan Africa: A Cost-Effectiveness Analysis." *BMC Health Services Research* 16: 304. https://doi.org/10.1186/s12913-016-1572-6.

Memirie, S. T., W. W. Dagnaw, M. K. Habtemariam, A. Bekele, D. Yadeta, A. Bekele, W. Bekele, et al. 2022. "Addressing the Impact of Noncommunicable Diseases and Injuries (NCDIs) in Ethiopia: Findings and Recommendations from the Ethiopia NCDI Commission." *Ethiopian Journal of Health Science* 32 (1): 161–80. https://doi.org/10.4314/ejhs.v32i1.18.

Mwangi, K., G. Gathecha, M. Nyamongo, S. Kimaiyo, J. Kamano, F. Bukachi, F. Odhiambo, et al. 2021. "Reframing Non-communicable Diseases and Injuries for Equity in the Era of Universal Health Coverage: Findings and Recommendations from the Kenya NCDI Poverty Commission." *Annals of Global Health* 87 (1): 3. https://doi.org/10.5334/aogh.3085.

NCD Countdown 2030 Collaborators. 2022. "NCD Countdown 2030: Efficient Pathways and Strategic Investments to Accelerate Progress towards the Sustainable Development Goal Target 3.4 in Low-Income and Middle-Income Countries." *The Lancet* 399 (10331): 1266–78. https://doi.org/10.1016/S0140-6736(21)02347-3.

NCD Countdown Collaborators. 2018. "NCD Countdown 2030: Worldwide Trends in Non-communicable Disease Mortality and Progress towards Sustainable Development Goal Target 3.4." *The Lancet* 392 (10152): 1072–88. https://doi.org/10.1016/S0140 -6736(18)31992-5.

NCD Risk Factor Collaboration. 2021. "Worldwide Trends in Hypertension Prevalence and Progress in Treatment and Control from 1990 to 2019: A Pooled Analysis of 1201 Population-Representative Studies with 104 Million Participants." *The Lancet* 398 (10304): 957–80. https://doi.org/10.1016/S0140-6736(21)01330-1.

Nishtar, S., S. Niinisto, M. Sirisena, T. Vazquez, V. Skvortsova, A. Rubinstein, F. G. Mogae, et al. 2018. "Time to Deliver: Report of the WHO Independent High-Level Commission on NCDs." *The Lancet* 392 (10143): 245–52. https://doi.org/10.1016/S0140-6736(18)31258-3.

Pickersgill, S. J., D. A. Watkins, B. Mikkelsen, and C. Varghese. 2022. "A Tool to Identify NCD Interventions to Achieve the SDG Target." *The Lancet Global Health* 10 (7): e949–50. https://doi.org/10.1016/S2214-109X(22)00124-3.

Schwartz, L. N., J. D. Shaffer, and G. Bukhman. 2021. "The Origins of the 4 x 4 Framework for Noncommunicable Disease at the World Health Organization." *SSM–Population Health* 13: 100731. https://doi.org/10.1016/j.ssmph.2021.100731.

Verguet, S., C. L. Gauvreau, S. Mishra, M. MacLennan, S. M. Murphy, E. D. Brouwer, R. A. Nugent, et al. 2015. "The Consequences of Tobacco Tax on Household Health and Finances in Rich and Poor Smokers in China: An Extended Cost-Effectiveness Analysis." *The Lancet Global Health* 3 (4): e206–16. https://doi.org/10.1016/S2214-109X(15)70095-1.

Verguet, S., Z. D. Olson, J. B. Babigumira, D. Desalegn, K. A. Johansson, M. E. Kruk, C. E. Levin, et al. 2015. "Health Gains and Financial Risk Protection Afforded by Public Financing of Selected Interventions in Ethiopia: An Extended Cost-Effectiveness Analysis." *The Lancet Global Health* 3 (5): e288–96.

Watkins, D. A., D. T. Jamison, T. Mills, T. Atun, K. Danforth, A. Glassman, S. Horton, et al. 2017. "Universal Health Coverage and Essential Packages of Care." In *Disease Control Priorities* (third edition), Volume 9: *Disease Control Priorities: Improving Health and Reducing Poverty*, edited by D. T. Jamison, H. Gelband, S. Horton, P. Jha, R. Laxminarayan, C. N. Mock, and R. Nugent. Washington, DC: World Bank.

Watkins, D., R. Nugent, and S. Verguet. 2017. "Extended Cost-Effectiveness Analyses of Cardiovascular Risk Factor Reduction Policies." In *Disease Control Priorities* (third edition), Volume 9, *Disease Control Priorities: Improving Health and Reducing Poverty*, edited by D. T. Jamison, H. Gelband, S. Horton, P. Jha, R. Laxminarayan, C. N. Mock, and R. Nugent. Washington, DC: World Bank.

WHO (World Health Organization). 2013. *Global Action Plan for the Prevention and Control of Noncommunicable Diseases 2013–2020*. Geneva: WHO.

WHO (World Health Organization). 2014. *Making Fair Choices on the Path to Universal Health Coverage. Final Report of the WHO Consultative Group on Equity and Universal Health Coverage*. Geneva: World Health Organization.

WHO (World Health Organization). 2021. *Mid-point Evaluation of the Implementation of the WHO Global Action Plan for the Prevention and Control of Noncommunicable Diseases 2013–2020*. A74/10 Add.1. Geneva: WHO.

WHO (World Health Organization). 2022. *Implementation Roadmap for Accelerating the Prevention and Control of Noncommunicable Diseases in South-East Asia 2022–2030*. New Delhi: WHO, Regional Office for South-East Asia.

World Bank. 1993. *World Development Report 1993: Investing in Health*. New York: Oxford University Press. https://openknowledge.worldbank.org/handle/10986/5976.

Acknowledgments

Disease Control Priorities, fourth edition (*DCP4*), draws on the global health knowledge of institutions and experts from around the world, including volume editors, chapter authors, peer reviewers, and research and staff assistants. The finalization of this first volume would not have been possible without the intellectual vision, enduring support, and invaluable contributions of these individuals.

We owe gratitude to the financial sponsors of this effort. We are indebted to the Bill & Melinda Gates Foundation for supporting and funding the DCP Country Translation and DCP-Ethiopia projects that have informed many of the chapters in this volume and helped us stake out the direction for future work in DCP4. We acknowledge the Research Council of Norway that—through its Centre of Excellence grant to the Bergen Center for Ethics and Priority Setting (BCEPS) at the University of Bergen—has enabled us to set up and develop a core analytics team for evidence collection, mathematical modeling, and economic evaluations. A special thank you to the Norwegian Development Cooperation Agency (Norad) and the Trond Mohn Foundation, which have co-funded much of the ongoing country engagement work, including local capacity strengthening and master's and PhD training in health economics, ethics, and priority setting.

We are grateful to the University of Bergen, the Department of Global Public Health and Primary Care, and BCEPS for supporting the training of numerous students and creating a home base for the DCP4 Secretariat, a base that provides intellectual collaboration, logistical coordination, and administrative and social support. We thank those who worked behind the scenes within the department to ensure this work ran smoothly, including Wafa Aftab, Austen Davis, Øystein Ariansen Haaland, Kjell Arne Johanson, Solomon Memirie, Omar Mwalim, Jan-Magnus Økland, Bjarne Robberstad, Guri Rørtveit, Ingvild Sandøy, Sid Sharma (based in Perth, Western Australia), Maria Sollohub, Mieraf Tadesse, and Jana Wilbricht.

Journal editors have been important in encouraging greater diversity in global health publications, and we especially thank the editors of *BMJ Global Health* and the *International Journal of Health Policy Management* for publishing special supplements covering all aspects of the DCP country translation work.

The DCP country work has benefited immensely from the collaboration with the country offices of the World Health Organization (refer to the list of contributors), as well as at World Health Organization headquarters in Geneva. We especially thank Melanie Bertram, Alarcos Cieza, Tessa Tan-Torres Edejer, Bente Michelsen, Andrew Mirelman, Teri Reynolds, Karin Stenberg, Soumya Swaminathan, and Anna Vassall.

The World Bank provided exceptional guidance and support throughout the planning phase, the review process, and the demanding production and design process. Within the World Bank, we especially want to thank Jung-Hwan Choi, Magnus Lindelow, Martin Mpungu Lutalo, Juan Pablo Uribe, Monique Vledder, and Feng Zhao who served as champions of *DCP4*; and we thank the numerous expert reviewers of all chapters (refer to the list of reviewers). Mary Fisk oversaw the editing and publication of the series with diligence and expertise, and we are pleased to have had designer Debra Naylor who developed the beautiful and crisp design for this volume and the series as a whole. Additionally, we thank Jewel McFadden, acquisitions editor in the World Bank's formal publishing unit, for providing professional counsel on contracts, communications, and marketing strategies.

Volume Editors

Ala Alwan

Ala Alwan is Regional Director Emeritus, World Health Organization (WHO). He was Professor of Global Health and Principal Investigator of the Disease Control Priorities Country Translation Project at London School of Hygiene & Tropical Medicine; Affiliate Professor, Global Health, University of Washington; and Honorary Professor at Imperial College London and University of Oxford. At WHO, Dr. Alwan was Assistant Director-General for Noncommunicable Diseases (NCDs) and Mental Health, Representative of the WHO Director-General for Emergencies and Health Action in Crises, and Regional Director for the WHO Eastern Mediterranean Region. Dr. Alwan coordinated the development of the Global Strategy for the Prevention and Control of NCDs and led the work of WHO and the United Nations (UN) in preparing for the first UN General Assembly High-Level Meeting on NCDs, which resulted in the adoption of the UN Political Declaration on NCDs in September 2011. In Iraq, he was Professor of Medicine and Dean of Faculty of Medicine, Minister of Health and Minister of Education (2003–05), and again Minister of Health and Environment (2018–19).

Mizan Kiros Mirutse

Mizan Kiros Mirutse is a global health expert, holding a PhD in global health from the University of Bergen, Norway, and currently a postdoctoral researcher at Bergen Centre for Ethics and Priority Setting. With over 12 years of professional experience in the Ethiopian health sector, Dr. Mizan has held pivotal roles, including Director for Resource Mobilization, Director General of the Ethiopia Health Insurance Agency, Senior Health Financing Advisor to the Minister of Health, and National COVID-19 Response Coordinator. His leadership has been instrumental in shaping health financing reforms, improving access to health insurance, and coordinating the national response to the COVID-19 pandemic.

Dr. Mizan is engaged in international health policy and financing platforms, such as the Joint Learning Network for Universal Health Coverage and the International Society for Priorities in Health, and serves as a Senior Contributor to the Global Burden of Disease study.

Pakwanja Desiree Twea

Pakwanja Desiree Twea is an economist with the Ministry of Health in Malawi and a PhD candidate at the Bergen Centre for Ethics and Priority Setting in Health at the University of Bergen, Norway. Her professional expertise includes policy development and analysis, strategic planning, and project management. Pakwanja's research centers on evidence generation, priority setting, and policy analysis, currently focusing on the economic analysis of orthopedic care in specialist hospitals in Malawi and other low-income settings. Her academic pursuits and professional interests converge on bridging the gap between evidence and policy across the health sector.

Ole F. Norheim

Ole F. Norheim is a physician and Mary B. Saltonstall Professor of Ethics and Population Health at the Department of Global Health and Population, Harvard T. H. Chan School of Public Health. He co-founded the Bergen Centre for Ethics and Priority Setting in Health at the University of Bergen, Norway, and is an Adjunct Researcher at the center.

Norheim's research interests include theories of distributive justice, inequality in health, priority setting in health systems, and how to achieve universal health coverage in low- and middle-income countries. He is the Lead Series Editor of *Disease Control Priorities* (fourth edition) and a member of the Lancet Commission on Investing in Health and the Lancet Commission on Sustainable Healthcare. Norheim is an elected member of the Norwegian Academy of Science and Letters.

He has served as Head of the Norwegian Biotechnology Advisory Board (2019–23), as Chair of the World Health Organization's Consultative Group on Equity and Universal Health Coverage (2012–14), and on the third Norwegian National Committee on Priority Setting in Health Care (2013–14).

Series Editors

Ole F. Norheim

Refer to the list of volume editors.

David A. Watkins

David A. Watkins is an associate professor in the Division of General Internal Medicine and in the Department of Global Health at the University of Washington. He currently leads the University of Washington site for the Disease Control Priorities Project and is affiliated with the Implementation Science Program in the Department of Global Health. Additionally, he is the Co-Director of the Learning for Action in Policy Implementation and Health Systems Initiative. He studies health system reform and policy challenges, with a particular emphasis on universal health coverage and the growing burden of noncommunicable diseases in low-income countries. His team works in three thematic areas: (1) population and economic modeling to support policy analysis, (2) integrated health care delivery, and (3) use of evidence in policy formulation. In addition to his scholarly work, Dr. Watkins teaches on global noncommunicable diseases and quantitative research methods and practices as a hospitalist at Harborview Medical Center.

Kalipso Chalkidou

Kalipso Chalkidou is the Director of the Department of Health Financing and Economics at the World Health Organization headquarters. Before that she founded and ran the Department of Health Finance at the Global Fund to Fight AIDS, Tuberculosis and Malaria. She is a Visiting Professor of Global Health at the School of Public Health, Imperial College London. Before moving to Geneva she was Director of Global Health Policy and a Senior Fellow at the Center for Global Development.

Her past work has concentrated on helping governments build technical and institutional capacity for using evidence to inform health policy as they move toward universal health coverage. She is interested in how local information, local expertise, and local institutions can drive scientific and legitimate health care resource allocation decisions. She has been involved in the Chinese rural health reforms and in national health reform projects in Colombia, Ghana, India, South Africa, Türkiye, and the Middle East, working with the Inter-American Development Bank; Pan American Health Organization; UK Foreign, Commonwealth & Development Office; and World Bank as well as national governments.

Victoria Y. Fan

Victoria Y. Fan is a senior economist in health financing at the World Bank. She previously served at the Center for Global Development over 2011–14 and 2022–24. From 2014 to 2024, she was on the faculty at the University of Hawaii, including tenured associate professor and interim director of the Center on Aging. At the university, she founded the Pacific Health Analytics Collaborative, a lab with more than 120 employees and an annual operating budget of $10 million, which conducted policy research on social determinants of health and mental health. During the COVID-19 pandemic, she established and chaired the Hawaii Pandemic Applied Modeling workgroup advising state leaders while serving as executive director of Hawaii CARES, the state's integrated call center and managed care network for mental health and substance use. She has more than 200 publications, including 70 in peer-reviewed journals. She holds a doctorate in health systems from Harvard and a bachelor's in mechanical engineering from the Massachusetts Institute of Technology. She was born and raised in Hawaii.

Muhammad Ali Pate

Muhammad Ali Pate serves as the coordinating Minister of Health and Social Welfare, Federal Republic of Nigeria. He formerly served as the Global Director, Health, Nutrition and Population Global Practice at the World Bank and was Julio Frenk Professor of the Practice of Public Health Leadership in the Department of Global Health and Population at the Harvard T. H. Chan School of Public Health.

Dr. Pate is an MD trained in both internal medicine and infectious diseases, with an MBA from Duke University. Previously, he studied at the University College London. He also holds a master's in health system management from the London School of Hygiene & Tropical Medicine.

Dean T. Jamison

Dean T. Jamison is professor emeritus of health economics at the University of California, San Francisco. He has worked at the World Bank as manager of both its education policy division and of its health, nutrition, and population division. His subsequent career was in academia including eight years as Director of UCLA's Center for Pacific Rim Studies. At the World Bank he initiated the *Disease Control Priorities* series. Jamison studied at Stanford University and then at Harvard University, where he received his PhD in economics under Kenneth Arrow. He is a member of the Academy of Medicine of the US National Academies of Science, Engineering, and Medicine.

Contributors

Mohsen Aarabi

- Department of Family Medicine, School of Medicine, Mazandaran University of Medical Sciences, Tehran, Islamic Republic of Iran

Tayseer Abdelgader

- National Consultant, Sudan

Seye Abimbola

- School of Public Health, Faculty of Medicine and Health, University of Sydney, Sydney, Australia
- Editor in Chief of *BMJ Global Health*

Ibrahim Abubakar

- University College London, London, United Kingdom

Wafa Aftab

- Bergen Centre for Ethics and Priority Setting in Health, Department of Global Public Health and Primary Care, University of Bergen, Bergen, Norway
- Department of Community Health Sciences, Aga Khan University, Pakistan

Ahsan Ahmad

- Center for Global Public Health, Pakistan
- Affiliate, Institute of Global Public Health, University of Manitoba, Canada

Robert Akparibo

- University of Sheffield, Sheffield, United Kingdom

Ala Alwan

- DCP3 Country Translation Project, London School of Hygiene & Tropical Medicine, London, United Kingdom
- World Health Organization, Geneva, Switzerland

Amir Aman

- Former Minister of Health, Ethiopia
- Former Country Operation Lead at the Global Financing Facility, World Bank

Emmanuel Ameh

- National Hospital, Abuja, Nigeria

Blake Angell

- Centre for Health Systems Science, The George Institute for Global Health, University of New South Wales, Sydney, Australia

Noam Angrist

- Oxford University, Oxford, United Kingdom
- Youth Impact, Gaborone, Botswana

Fatma Bakar

- Ministry of Health, Zanzibar

Rob Baltussen

- IQ Health, Radboud University Medical Center, Nijmegen, The Netherlands

Louise Banham

- Foreign, Commonwealth & Development Office, United Kingdom

Mariana Barraza-Lloréns

- Founding Partner, Blutitude, Mexico
- Formerly Policy Advisor, Ministry of Health, Mexico

Mark Bassett

- Bassett Consulting Services
- Formerly IFHP Health Insurance Fellow, World Bank

Biniam Bedasso

- Center for Global Development, London, United Kingdom

Melanie Y. Bertram

- Department of Health Systems Governance and Financing, World Health Organization, Geneva, Switzerland
- Department of Delivery for Impact, World Health Organization, Geneva, Switzerland

Zulfiqar A. Bhutta

- Aga Khan University, Karachi, Pakistan
- Centre for Global Child Health, Hospital for Sick Children, Toronto, Canada

Karl Blanchet

- Geneva Centre of Humanitarian Studies, Faculty of Medicine, University of Geneva, Geneva, Switzerland

Mary Brennan

- University of Edinburgh, Edinburgh, United Kingdom

Donald A. P. Bundy

- Research Consortium for School Health and Nutrition, London School of Hygiene & Tropical Medicine, London, United Kingdom

Carmen Burbano

- World Food Programme, Rome, Italy

Manuel Carballo

- International Centre for Migration, Health and Development, Geneva, Switzerland

Sudha Chandrashekar

- Formerly Health Policy and Hospital Management, National Health Authority, India

Collins Chansa

- Health, Nutrition and Population Global Practice, World Bank

Sheena Chhabra

- Health, Nutrition, and Population in South Asia Region, World Bank, New Delhi, India

Tim Colbourn

- Institute for Global Health, Faculty of Population Health Sciences, University College London, London, United Kingdom

Faihaa Dafalla

- Federal Ministry of Health, Sudan

Kristen Danforth

- Department of Global Health, University of Washington, Seattle, Washington, United States

Margaret Anne Defeyter

- Northumbria University, Newcastle, United Kingdom

Peter Donkor

- Department of Surgery, Kwame Nkrumah University of Science and Technology, Kumasi, Ghana

Lesley Drake

- Partnership for Child Development, Imperial College London, London, United Kingdom

Christina Economos

- Tufts University, Boston, Massachusetts, United States

Getachew Teshome Eregata

- Federal Ministry of Health of Ethiopia, Addis Ababa, Ethiopia
- Bergen Centre for Ethics and Priority Setting in Health, Department of Global Public Health and Primary Care, University of Bergen, Bergen, Norway

Wael Fakiahmed

- National Health Insurance Fund, Sudan

Farhad Farewar

- Formerly with the Ministry of Health, Afghanistan

Ferozuddin Feroz

- Ministry of Public Health, Kabul, Afghanistan

John Fogarty

- World Health Organization, Geneva, Switzerland

Basant Garg

- National Health Authority, India
- Ayushman Bharat Digital Health Mission, India

Sylvestre Gaudin

- Department of Economics, Oberlin College, Oberlin, Ohio, United States

Pratibha Gautam

- Harvard T. H. Chan School of Public Health, Boston, Massachusetts, United States

Lia Tadesse Gebremedhin

- Former Minister of Health, Ethiopia
- Harvard Ministerial Leadership Program, Harvard T. H. Chan School of Public Health, Boston, Massachusetts, United States

Zelalem Adugna Geletu

- Office of the Minister, Ministry of Health of Ethiopia, Addis Ababa, Ethiopia
- HANZ Consulting, Addis Ababa, Ethiopia

Ugo Gentilini

- Social Protection and Labor in the Middle East and North Africa Unit, World Bank Group, Washington, DC, United States

Boitshepo Giyose

- AUDA-NEPAD, Johannesburg, South Africa

Eduardo González-Pier

- Palladium, Global Fellow, Wilson Center, Washington, DC, United States
- Formerly Deputy Minister of Health, Mexico

Andre Griekspoor

- World Health Organization, Geneva, Switzerland

Ina Gudumac

- Country Translation Project, London School of Hygiene & Tropical Medicine, London, United Kingdom

Neil Gupta

- Center for Integration Science, Division of Global Health Equity, Brigham and Women's Hospital, Boston, Massachusetts, United States
- Program in Global NCDs and Social Change, Department of Global Health and Social Medicine, Harvard Medical School, Boston, Massachusetts, United States

Javier Guzman

- Global Health Policy Program and Senior Policy Fellow, Center for Global Development, Washington, DC, United States

Hassan Haghparast-Bidgoli

- Centre for Global Health Economics, University College London, London, United Kingdom

Alemayehu Hailu

- Federal Ministry of Health of Ethiopia, Addis Ababa, Ethiopia
- Bergen Centre for Ethics and Priority Setting in Health, Department of Global Public Health and Primary Care, University of Bergen, Bergen, Norway
- Department of Global Health and Population, Harvard T. H. Chan School of Public Health, Boston, Massachusetts, United States
- Section for Global Health and Rehabilitation, Western Norway University of Applied Sciences, Bergen, Norway

Abdul-latif Haji

- Ministry of Health, Zanzibar

Peter Hangoma

- Bergen Centre for Ethics and Priority Setting in Health, Department of Global Public Health and Primary Care, University of Bergen, Bergen, Norway

Maryam Huda

- Health Policy & Management Unit, Department of Community Health Sciences Medical College, Aga Khan University, Karachi, Pakistan

Abdullahi A. Ismail

- Ministry of Health and Human Services, Federal Government of Somalia, Mogadishu, Somalia

Mohamed Jama

- Ministry of Health and Human Services, Federal Government of Somalia, Mogadishu, Somalia

Dean T. Jamison

- University of California San Francisco, San Francisco, California, United States

Guru Rajesh Jammy

- Health, Nutrition, and Population in South Asia Region, World Bank, New Delhi, India

Ahmad Jan

- Formerly with the Ministry of Health, Afghanistan

Gerard J. Abou Jaoude

- Centre for Global Health Economics, University College London, London, United Kingdom

Abdulmajid Jecha

- Office of Chief Government Statistician, Zanzibar

Kjell Arne Johansson

- Bergen Centre for Ethics and Priority Setting in Health, Department of Global Public Health and Primary Care, University of Bergen, Bergen, Norway

Matthew Jowett

- Department of Financing and Economics, World Health Organization, Geneva, Switzerland

Ritsuko Kakuma

- London School of Hygiene & Tropical Medicine, London, United Kingdom

Muhammad Khalid

- Health Planning Systems Strengthening and Information Analysis Unit, Ministry of National Health Services, Regulations and Coordination, Pakistan

Haji Khamis

- Ministry of Health, Zanzibar

Hannah Kuper

- London School of Hygiene & Tropical Medicine, London, United Kingdom

Marina Madeo

- World Health Organization, Somalia

Reza Majdzadeh

- School of Health and Social Care, University of Essex, Colchester, United Kingdom

Wahid Majrooh

- Former Minister of Public Health, Afghanistan
- Afghanistan Center for Health and Peace, Geneva, Switzerland

Sk Md Mamunur Rahman Malik

- World Health Organization, Eastern Mediterranean Regional Office

Jacqueline Mallender

- Economics By Design, London, United Kingdom

Gerald Manthalu

- Malawi Ministry of Health and Population, Lilongwe, Malawi

Awad Mataria

- Universal Health Coverage and Health Systems, World Health Organization Regional Office for the Eastern Mediterranean, Cairo, Arab Republic of Egypt

Arianna Rubin Means

- Department of Global Health, University of Washington, Seattle, Washington, United States

Solomon Tessema Memirie

- Addis Centre for Ethics and Priority Setting in Health, Addis Ababa University, Addis Ababa, Ethiopia
- Department of Paediatrics and Child Health, College of Health Sciences, Addis Ababa University, Addis Ababa, Ethiopia

Peiman Milani

- Rockefeller Foundation, Nairobi, Kenya

Ingrid Miljeteig

- Bergen Centre for Ethics and Priority Setting in Health, Department of Global Public Health and Primary Care, University of Bergen, Bergen, Norway

Shafiq Mirzazada

- Geneva Centre of Humanitarian Studies, Faculty of Medicine, University of Geneva, Geneva, Switzerland

Charles N. Mock

- Department of Surgery, University of Washington, Seattle, Washington, United States

Ana O. Mocumbi

- Faculty of Medicine, Eduardo Mondlane University, Maputo, Mozambique
- Instituto Nacional de Saúde, Ministério da Saúde, Maputo, Mozambique

Dhameera Mohammed

- Ministry of Health, Zanzibar

Nur A. Mohamud

- Ministry of Health and Human Services, Federal Government of Somalia, Mogadishu, Somalia

Sakshi Mohan

- Centre for Health Economics, University of York, York, United Kingdom

Mohammed Musa

- World Health Organization Country Office, Sudan

Omar Mussa

- President's Office, Labour, Economic Affairs and Investment, Zanzibar

Mohammed Mustafa

- Formerly Director General of Health Planning and Development, Sudan

Omar Mwalim

- Ministry of Health, Zanzibar
- Bergen Centre for Ethics and Priority Setting in Health, Department of Global Public Health and Primary Care, University of Bergen, Bergen, Norway

Safi Najibullah

- World Health Organization, Kabul, Afghanistan

Bill Newbrander

- Management Sciences for Health, Cambridge, Massachusetts, United States

Dominic Nkhoma

- Health Economics and Policy Unit, Kamuzu University of Health Sciences, Lilongwe, Malawi

Justice Nonvignon

- School of Public Health, University of Ghana, Legon, Ghana

Ole F. Norheim

- Department of Global Health and Population, Harvard T. H. Chan School of Public Health, Boston, Massachusetts, United States
- Bergen Centre for Ethics and Priority Setting in Health, Department of Global Public Health and Primary Care, University of Bergen, Bergen, Norway

Fawziya A. Nur

- Ministry of Health and Human Services, Federal Government of Somalia, Mogadishu, Somalia

Ibrahim M. Nur

- Ministry of Health and Human Services, Federal Government of Somalia, Mogadishu, Somalia

Alireza Olyaeemanesh

- National Institute of Health Research and Health Equity Research Center, Tehran University of Medical Sciences, Tehran, Islamic Republic of Iran

Obinna Onwujekwe

- Health Policy Research Group, University of Nigeria Enugu Campus, Enugu, Nigeria

Doruk Ozgediz

- University of California San Francisco, San Francisco, California, United States

Shankar Prinja

- Department of Community Medicine & School of Public Health Post Graduate Institute of Medical Education and Research Chandigarh, India

A. Venkat Raman

- Faculty of Management Studies, University of Delhi, Delhi, India

Wajeeha Raza

- Centre for Health Economics, University of York, York, United Kingdom

Paul Revill

- Centre for Health Economics, University of York, York, United Kingdom

Teri Reynolds

- Department of Integrated Health Services, World Health Organization, Geneva, Switzerland

David A. Ross

- Institute for Life Course Health Research, Stellenbosch University, South Africa
- Consultant to the Child Health Initiative of the FIA Foundation

Shwetlena Sabarwal

- Education in the Middle East and North Africa Unit, World Bank Group, Washington, DC, United States

Sayed Ataullah Saeedzai

- Formerly with the Ministry of Health, Afghanistan

Hamidreza Safikhani

- Board Member of the Iranian Health Economics Association, Islamic Republic of Iran

Sanaa Said

- Bergen Centre for Ethics and Priority Setting in Health, Department of Global Public Health and Primary Care, University of Bergen, Bergen, Norway
- State University of Zanzibar, Zanzibar

Haniye Sadat Sajadi

- Knowledge Utilization Research Center and University Research and Development Center, Tehran University of Medical Sciences, Tehran, Islamic Republic of Iran

Ahmad Salehi

- Formerly with the Ministry of Health, Afghanistan

Lubna Samad

- Global Surgery Program, IRD Global, Pakistan

Susan Sawyer

- University of Melbourne, Melbourne, Australia
- Murdoch Children's Research Institute, Melbourne, Australia
- Centre for Adolescent Health, Royal Children's Hospital, Melbourne, Australia

Linda Schultz

- Research Consortium for School Health and Nutrition, London School of Hygiene & Tropical Medicine, London, United Kingdom

Jaime Sepúlveda

- Institute for Global Health Sciences, University of California San Francisco, San Francisco, California, United States

Justina Seyi-Olajide

- Lagos University Teaching Hospital, Lagos, Nigeria

Sameen Siddiqi

- Department of Community Health Sciences, Aga Khan University, Karachi, Pakistan

Neha Singh

- London School of Hygiene & Tropical Medicine, London, United Kingdom

Samrat Singh

- Imperial College London, London, United Kingdom

Jolene Skordis

- Centre for Global Health Economics, University College London, London, United Kingdom

Agnès Soucat

- Health and Social Protection, Agence Française de Développement

Karin Stenberg

- Department of Health Financing and Economics, World Health Organization, Geneva, Switzerland
- Swiss Tropical and Public Health Institute, Allschwil, Switzerland
- University of Basel, Basel, Switzerland

Subira Suleiman

- Ministry of Health, Zanzibar

Mieraf Taddesse

- Division of Health Economics and Financing, Africa Centres for Disease Control and Prevention, African Union Commission, Addis Ababa, Ethiopia

Ajay Tandon

- Health, Nutrition, and Population in South Asia Region, World Bank, New Delhi, India

Neil Thalagala

- Ministry of Health, Colombo, Sri Lanka

Pakwanja Desiree Twea

- Bergen Centre for Ethics and Priority Setting in Health, Department of Global Public Health and Primary Care, University of Bergen, Bergen, Norway
- Department of Planning and Policy Development, Ministry of Health, Lilongwe, Malawi

Cherian Varghese

- Prasanna School of Public Health, Manipal University, Manipal, Karnataka, India

Marcela Brun Vergara

- Independent Researcher/Consultant

Wubaye Walelgne

- Federal Ministry of Health of Ethiopia, Addis Ababa, Ethiopia

David A. Watkins

- Division of General Internal Medicine, Department of Medicine, University of Washington, Seattle, Washington, United States
- Department of Global Health, University of Washington, Seattle, Washington, United States

Kevin Watkins

- London School of Economics, London, United Kingdom

Helen Weiss

- London School of Hygiene & Tropical Medicine, London, United Kingdom

Thomas Wilkinson

- Health Economics Lead for iDSI in Sub-Saharan Africa

Samia Yahia

- Department of Health Economics, Federal Ministry of Health, Sudan

Amanuel Yigezu

- Federal Ministry of Health of Ethiopia, Addis Ababa, Ethiopia

Raza Zaidi

- Health Planning, System Strengthening and Information Analysis Unit, Evidence for Health, Pakistan
- Ministry of National Health Services, Regulations and Coordination, Islamabad, Pakistan

Collins Owen Francisco Zamawe

- Health, Nutrition and Population Global Practice, World Bank

Reviewers

Wafa Aftab

- Bergen Centre for Ethics and Priority Setting in Health, Department of Global Public Health and Primary Care, University of Bergen, Bergen, Norway

Ala Alwan

- DCP3 Country Translation Project, London School of Hygiene & Tropical Medicine, London, United Kingdom
- World Health Organization, Geneva, Switzerland

Aneesa Arur

- Human Development in Africa Unit, World Bank, Dar Es Salaam, Tanzania

Maria Eugenia Bonilla-Chacin

- Human Development in Latin America and the Caribbean Unit, World Bank, Bogotá, Colombia

Mickey Chopra

- Health, Nutrition, and Global Engagement Unit, World Bank, Washington, DC, United States

Agnes Couffinhal

- Health, Nutrition, and Population Global Engagement, World Bank, Washington, DC, United States

Zelalem Yilma Debebe

- Health, Nutrition, and Population in East Asia and Pacific Unit, World Bank, Jakarta, Indonesia

Laura Di Giorgio

- Health, Nutrition, and Population in Latin America and the Caribbean Unit, World Bank, Samana, Dominican Republic

Patrick Eozenou

- Health, Nutrition, and Population Global Engagement, World Bank, Washington, DC, United States

Getachew Teshome Eregata

- Federal Ministry of Health of Ethiopia, Addis Ababa, Ethiopia

Sayed Ghulam

- Senior Health Specialist, World Bank, Kinshasa, Democratic Republic of Congo

Tseganeh Amsalu Guracha

- Health, Nutrition, and Population in Africa Unit, World Bank, Addis Ababa, Ethiopia

Reem Hafez

- Health, Nutrition, and Population in the Middle East and North Africa Unit World Bank, Washington, DC, United States

Alemayehu Hailu

- Federal Ministry of Health of Ethiopia, Addis Ababa, Ethiopia
- Bergen Centre for Ethics and Priority Setting in Health, Department of Global Public Health and Primary Care, University of Bergen, Bergen, Norway
- Department of Global Health and Population, Harvard T. H. Chan School of Public Health, Boston, Massachusetts, United States

Ali Hamandi

- Health, Nutrition, and Population in Europe and Central Asia Unit, World Bank, Vienna, Austria

Mohini Kak

- Health, Nutrition, and Population in Europe and Central Asia Unit, World Bank, Vienna, Austria

Roberto Lunes

- World Bank, Washington, DC, United States

Reza Majdzadeh

- School of Health and Social Care, University of Essex, Colchester, United Kingdom

Mizan Kiros Mirutse

- Federal Ministry of Health of Ethiopia, Addis Ababa, Ethiopia
- Bergen Centre for Ethics and Priority Setting in Health, Department of Global Public Health and Primary Care, University of Bergen, Bergen, Norway

Somil Nagpal

- Health, Nutrition, and Population in East Asia and Pacific Unit, World Bank, Jakarta, Indonesia

Son Nam Nguyen

- Health, Nutrition, and Population in the Middle East and North Africa Unit, World Bank, Washington, DC, United States

Ole F. Norheim

- Department of Global Health and Population, Harvard T. H. Chan School of Public Health, Boston, Massachusetts, United States
- Bergen Centre for Ethics and Priority Setting in Health, Department of Global Public Health and Primary Care, University of Bergen, Bergen, Norway

Naoko Ohno

- Health, Nutrition, and Population in East Asia and Pacific Unit, World Bank, Washington, DC, United States

Olumide Olaolu Okunola

- Health Nutrition, and Population in Africa Unit, World Bank, Abuja, Nigeria

Bernard O. Olayo

- Health in Africa Unit, World Bank, Nairobi, Kenya

Karima Saleh

- Health, Nutrition and Population in Africa Unit, World Bank, Washington, DC, United States

Pia Helene Schneider

- Health, Nutrition, and Population in Africa Unit, World Bank, Washington, DC, United States

Karin Stenberg

- Department of Health Financing and Economics, World Health Organization, Geneva, Switzerland
- Swiss Tropical and Public Health Institute, Allschwil, Switzerland
- University of Basel, Basel, Switzerland

Chiho Suzuki

- Health, Nutrition, and Population in East Asia and Pacific Unit, World Bank, Phnom Penh, Cambodia

Pakwanja Desiree Twea

- Bergen Centre for Ethics and Priority Setting in Health, Department of Global Public Health and Primary Care, University of Bergen, Bergen, Norway
- Department of Planning and Policy Development, Ministry of Health, Lilongwe, Malawi

Jeremy Henri Maurice Veillard

- Health, Nutrition, and Population in Latin America and the Caribbean Unit, World Bank, Bogotá, Colombia

Stéphane Verguet

- Harvard T. H. Chan School of Public Health, Boston, Massachusetts, United States

Huihui Wang

- Health, Nutrition, and Global Engagement Unit, World Bank, Washington, DC, United States

David A. Watkins

- Division of General Internal Medicine, Department of Medicine, University of Washington, Seattle, Washington, United States
- Department of Global Health, University of Washington, Seattle, Washington, United States

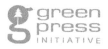